STUDY GUIDE TO PSYCHIATRY

A Companion to *The American Psychiatric Association Publishing Textbook of Psychiatry*, Seventh Edition

STUDY GUIDE TO PSYCHIATRY

A Companion to
The American Psychiatric Association Publishing Textbook of Psychiatry, Seventh Edition

Edited by

Philip R. Muskin, M.D., M.A.
Anna L. Dickerman, M.D.
Claire C. Holderness, M.D.
Vivian P. Liu, M.D.

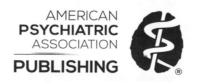

AMERICAN
PSYCHIATRIC
ASSOCIATION
PUBLISHING

Contents

Part II: Answer Guide

Contributors

Volume Editors

Philip R. Muskin, M.D., M.A.
Dr. Muskin is Professor of Psychiatry and Senior Consultant in Consultation-Liaison Psychiatry in the Department of Psychiatry at Columbia University Irving Medical Center in New York, New York.

Anna L. Dickerman, M.D.
Dr. Dickerman is Associate Professor of Clinical Psychiatry and Chief of Consultation-Liaison Psychiatry at Weill Cornell Medical College/New York-Presbyterian Hospital in New York, New York.

Claire C. Holderness, M.D.
Dr. Holderness is Associate Clinical Professor in the Department of Psychiatry at Columbia University Vagelos College of Physicians and Surgeons in New York, New York.

Vivian P. Liu, M.D.
Dr. Liu was a PGY1 Resident in Psychiatry at Mt. Sinai Beth Israel Hospital in New York, New York, at the time of her work on this Study Guide.

Resident and Faculty Teams

Baylor Scott & White Medical Center / Texas A&M University

Residents
Hongjing Cao, M.D., M.P.H.   Shadi Lavasani, M.D.
Brian Vu Clinton, M.D.   Daniel Robert Lavin, D.O.

Faculty Mentors
Faculty Leader: James A. Bourgeois, O.D., M.D.
Virginia Maxanne Flores, M.D.   Kael Anton Kuster, M.D.
Paul Brently Hicks, M.D., Ph.D.   Chinonyerem Okwara, M.D.

New York State Psychiatric Institute / Columbia University Irving Medical Center

Residents

Simon Dosovitz, M.D.

Sophia Ebel, M.D.

Ian Hsu, M.D.

Samuel Kolander, M.D.

Taber Lightbourne, M.D., M.H.S.

Ruth McCann, M.D.

Rita Elena Morales, M.D.

Emily Nash, M.D.

Meredith Senter, M.D.

Daniel Shalev, M.D.

Aaron Slan, M.D.

Samantha Slomiak, M.D.

Jennifer Sotsky, M.D., M.S.

Joseph Villarin, M.D., Ph.D.

Niesha Voigt, M.D.

Lisa Wang, M.D.

Faculty Mentors

Faculty Leader: Claire C. Holderness, M.D.

Mary E. Bongiovi, M.D. Ph.D.

Stephanie G. Cheung, M.D.

Elizabeth Leimbach, M.D.

Alison Lenet, M.D.

Jon Levenson, M.D.

Philip R. Muskin, M.D., M.A.

Akhil Shenoy, M.D.

Oliver M. Stroeh, M.D.

Stanford University, Department of Psychiatry and Behavioral Sciences

Residents

Neal Dilip Amin, M.D., Ph.D.

Giovanni Dandekar, M.D.

Charles Fagundes, M.D.

Karen Li, M.D.

Csilla Lippert, M.D., Ph.D.

Dexter Louie, M.D.

Alissa M. Rogol, M.D., J.D.

Jonathan Updike, M.D., M.P.H.

Jackie Wang, M.D.

Dina Wang-Kraus, M.D.

Faculty Mentors

Faculty Leader: Sallie G. De Golia, M.D., M.P.H.

Laura Dunn, M.D.

George M. Freeman Jr., M.D., Ph.D.

Aazaz Haq, M.D.

Margaret May, M.D.

Michael Ostacher, M.D., M.P.H., M.M.Sc.

Kristin S. Raj, M.D.

Katherine Sanborn, M.D.

Katherine E. Williams, M.D.

Tufts University Medical Center

Residents

Daniel Augustadt, M.D.

Amy Blood, M.D.

Lisa Bosco, M.B., B.Ch., BAO

Joshua D. Brown, M.D.

Colleen Curtin, M.D.

Erin Dunn, M.D.

Krista Ferretti, M.D.

Michael Heneghan, M.D.

Sandra Lucio, D.O.

Hareesh Pillai, M.D.

Thomas Scary, M.D.

Sina Shah, M.D.

Whitney Snyders, M.D.

Faculty Mentors

Faculty Leader: Paul Summergrad, M.D.

Manuel Pacheco, M.D.

John Sargent, M.D.

Karen L. Saroca, M.D.

Neha Sharma, D.O.

Edward Silberman, M.D.

Weill-Cornell Medical Center

Residents

Abigail Benudis, M.D.

Ariel Claman, M.D.

Ariella Dagi, M.D.

Heather Kawalick, M.D.

Paul McCormick Jr., M.D.

Benjamin Scherban, M.D.

Faculty Mentors

Faculty Leader: Anna L. Dickerman, M.D.

Benjamin D. Brody, M.D.

Elaina DellaCava, M.D.

Diana Feldman, M.D.

Liliya Gershengoren, M.D.

Joseph F. Murray, M.D.

Anna Salajegheh, M.D.

Jessica Simberlund, M.D.

Jess Zonana, M.D.

Disclosure of Interests

The volume editors have indicated that they have no financial interests or other affiliations that represent a competing interest with their contributions to this book.

Preface

The *Study Guide to Psychiatry* is a companion to, but not a replacement for reading, *The American Psychiatric Association Publishing Textbook of Psychiatry*, Seventh Edition. This self-examination guide has special meaning to the contributors, mentors, and editors, as it was written during an extraordinary time in the world, and especially in the United States. Many of the physicians involved in the project were redeployed to care for critically ill patients with coronavirus disease 2019 (COVID-19). Nevertheless, they persevered to carefully read the *Textbook* in order to create this self-examination guide. All of the contributors were psychiatric residents or fellows at the time of writing the questions. This is a unique book, as it was written entirely by residents who were mentored by faculty at each institution. We hope that using this guide will prepare readers to educate themselves in the assessment and treatment of patients with psychiatric disorders.

This study guide is organized around the chapters in the *Textbook*. As you work through the self-examination questions, let them guide you to focus on the chapter content in the *Textbook* as a path to your self-education. Some questions will seem obvious or easy, whereas others will be quite difficult. In the 400-plus questions included in this study guide, we have endeavored to use the style of question writing found in certification examinations; however, this is not a board preparation book. For each question or vignette, we provide explanations for both the correct and the incorrect options.

The contributors have graciously agreed that the proceeds from this study guide will be donated to charitable foundations dedicated to mental health.

Philip R. Muskin, M.D., M.A.
Anna L. Dickerman, M.D.
Claire C. Holderness, M.D.
Vivian P. Liu, M.D.

PART I

Questions

CHAPTER 1

The Psychiatric Interview and Mental Status Examination

1.1   Which of the following statements could most appropriately be used as the chief complaint?

    A. The patient was brought to the hospital by Emergency Medical Services after being found lying on the street surrounded by bottles.
    B. "My brother seems more depressed and isolative recently."
    C. Depression and suicide attempt.
    D. "I'm not answering any of your questions."

1.2   When considering the biopsychosocial model, which of the following would be the most pertinent *social* contributor to a patient's clinical picture?

    A. Ego defenses.
    B. Comorbid medical diagnoses.
    C. Race.
    D. Medication adherence.

1.3   Which of the following interviewer techniques or practices may be potentially *unhelpful* in the assessment of an agitated ("revved-up") patient?

    A. Remain near the doorway during the interview.
    B. Use open-ended questions.
    C. Ensure that staff members and security guards are available during the interview.
    D. Use a clear, gentle, and pleasantly firm tone of voice with the patient.

1.4   During an emergency room psychiatric evaluation, which of the following represents the most important concern?

A. Accurate diagnosis.
B. Treatment strategy.
C. Safety assessment.
D. Patient disposition.

1.5   A patient knowingly neglects to mention his recent escalating cocaine use when discussing his depression related to his wife leaving him. Which of the following terms best describes what causes the patient to leave out this information?

A. Conscious resistance.
B. Malingering.
C. Repression.
D. Factitious disorder.

1.6   Which of the following sample patient descriptions best fulfills the requirements for the *general appearance and behavior* component of the mental status examination (MSE)?

A. "Middle-aged man, appearing older than stated age, poor hygiene, numerous tattoos across his arms, uncooperative with interview."
B. "Elderly woman wearing hospital gown, disheveled, alert but psychomotor agitated and with loosening of associations."
C. "Young woman, unusually dressed, poor grooming, eye contact intense, psychomotor retarded, responding to internal stimuli."
D. "Adolescent boy, appearing younger than stated age, cooperative with interview, euthymic mood and congruent affect."

1.7   Which of the following components of therapeutic interviewing is most helpful in encouraging patients to speak freely, particularly regarding potentially embarrassing or illegal activities?

A. Attentive listening.
B. Therapeutic alliance.
C. Confidentiality.
D. Therapeutic neutrality.

C H A P T E R 2

DSM-5 as a Framework for Psychiatric Diagnosis

2.1   What U.S. organization currently oversees the process of making country-specific changes in the International Classification of Diseases (ICD)?

      A. The World Health Organization.
      B. The National Center for Health Statistics.
      C. The American Psychiatric Association.
      D. The U.S. Census Bureau.

2.2   Which of the following statements correctly describes how the DSM-5 Task Force attempted to address the imprecision in DSM-IV and earlier editions regarding the definition of *mental disorder*?

      A. In DSM-5, the terms *distress* and *impairment* were eliminated from the definition of *mental disorder*.
      B. In DSM-5, the definition of *mental disorder* specified a threshold for diagnosis.
      C. DSM-5 introduced a new effort to apply dimensional measures to determine clinical significance.
      D. DSM-5 no longer provides a definition for *mental disorder*.

2.3   In what year was the first DSM published?

      A. 1917.
      B. 1949.
      C. 1952.
      D. 1968.

2.4   What were the initial goals of the DSM?

A. To be used in judicial proceedings and social welfare systems.
B. To provide extensive information beyond the criteria in an effort to help clinicians understand the disorder.
C. To provide a framework to record nondiagnostic data about a patient's condition and use five "axes" of diagnostic formulation.
D. To serve as a diagnostic manual and a guide to statistical reporting.

2.5   What problems did DSM-5 Work Group members identify as they reviewed DSM-IV criteria?

A. Underutilization of the "not otherwise specified" (NOS) category.
B. Inappropriate characterization of distinct disorders as different presentations of a single disorder.
C. High rates of reported comorbidity.
D. Excessive coverage of clinical conditions so that no new disorders could be added.

2.6   What change was made to substance use disorders in DSM-5?

A. Collapse of abuse and dependence categories.
B. Use of a categorical approach to grade severity.
C. Restriction of clinical assessment scope to a single diagnostic category.
D. Removal of withdrawal as a substance use disorder category.

2.7   Which of the following was added in DSM-5 as an independent diagnosis?

A. Grief reaction.
B. Binge-eating disorder.
C. Asperger's disorder.
D. Somatoform disorder.

2.8   How is the *reliability* of a given diagnosis defined?

A. Accuracy of the criteria in making a diagnosis.
B. Demonstration of a clear etiology and pathogenic mechanism.
C. Agreement between raters that a disorder is or is not present.
D. Percentage of total variance specifically from the signal.

2.9   Which of the following diagnoses is addressed most differently between DSM-5 and ICD-11?

A. Binge-eating disorder.
B. Personality disorder.
C. Autism spectrum disorder.
D. Schizoaffective disorder.

2.10 Which of the following options best describes the Research Domain Criteria (RDoC) approach to investigating mental disorders?

   A. A "bottom-up" strategy to examine basic cognitive, psychological, social, or biological processes and then determine how any dysfunctions in them are expressed clinically.
   B. A "top-down" approach that uses the prespecified disorder in a classification like DSM or ICD as the starting point for an investigation.
   C. A diagnostic system meant to help develop a precision medicine approach to mental disorders.
   D. A simplified organizational framework for the definition of mental disorders that reduces time and funding needs.

CHAPTER 3

Normal Child and Adolescent Development

3.1 How does family systems theory define the term *attractor states*?

A. Attractor states provide coherence and social meaning to the individual narrative.
B. Attractor states are phases that are recognizable but infinitely variable and often unevenly achieved in any individual child at any given moment.
C. Attractor states arise from the interaction between emerging ego capacities, the interpersonal world, unconscious fantasy, and the pull toward the next level of mental organization.
D. Attractor states form the basis of the autobiographical narrative that is part of everyone's mental life, whether conscious or unconscious.

3.2 A father with a 6-month-old baby makes a sad face when his infant son cries, and accurately identifies a dirty diaper. He stays calm but responds immediately and alleviates the baby's distress. The father also shows excitement when the baby is enjoying a new toy, and the two share a big laugh together. This reciprocal relationship between father and baby is most likely to help the infant achieve which of the following tasks?

A. Moving toward psychological differentiation and individuation from parents.
B. Develop foundation for identity consolidation.
C. Achieve an objective and separate sense of self, with rudimentary grasp of gender distinctions.
D. Manifest beginning self-regulatory capacities as representations of shifting psychosomatic states.

3.3 A 13-year-old boy has noticed his body starting to change. As he looks in the mirror, he thinks about whether his classmates in his all-male school will make comments. He contemplates what it would be like to go to a coed school after his parents have "the talk" with him. He knows it is time to ask for a later curfew and decides to communicate this to his parents. What underlying factor is propelling this boy's current developmental process?

A. Ego capacities.

B. Physical maturation.

C. Environmental effects.

D. A false sense of identity.

3.4   A new mother with postpartum depression is experiencing sleep deprivation and is feeling completely overwhelmed. When she hears her baby crying, she huddles in bed, covering her ears, and is unable to respond appropriately to the infant's distress. Which of the following infant developmental tasks would likely be most affected as a result of this mother's depression?

A. Self-regulation.

B. Joint attention.

C. Rapprochement.

D. Object constancy.

3.5   As a 4-year-old boy, Mike got into trouble with his parents and preschool teacher for pulling wings off insects and plucking hairs off cats. What process best explains his becoming a veterinarian as an adult?

A. Internal conflict.

B. Rapprochement crisis.

C. Object constancy.

D. Oedipal complex.

3.6   A 5-year-old boy places potatoes inside a cookie jar and says, "Mom is going to be tricked because she will think there are cookies in there." Which of the following developmental concepts is illustrated by this child's actions?

A. Theory of mind.

B. Superego precursors.

C. Formal operations.

D. Hatching.

3.7   Which of the following stages of normal development is best characterized by an inward drive toward independence along with a newfound sense of vulnerability?

A. Infancy.

B. Toddlerhood.

C. Oedipal phase.

D. Emerging adulthood.

3.8   Which of the following tasks is associated with toddlerhood?

A. Establishment of peer relationships and pursuit of group activities.

B. Acquisition of basic concepts of the world through sensorimotor practice.

C. Use of sublimation to deal with feelings and impulses.

D. Begin the process of socialization via the establishment of superego precursors.

3.9 A 4-year-old girl picks up a tennis ball and "hops" it along the surface of a table while saying, "This is Mister Kangaroo, we are going to find all of the other kangaroos!" Which of the following developmental tasks is this child's behavior illustrating?

A. Fantasy play.

B. Rudimentary understanding of gender distinctions.

C. Formal operations and abstract thinking.

D. Hatching.

3.10 Which of the following terms is used to describe the coalescence of a child's sexual and aggressive drives with feelings of jealousy and rivalry?

A. Internal conflict.

B. Object constancy.

C. Sublimation.

D. Oedipal complex.

3.11 In normal childhood development, *preadolescence* is most strongly associated with which of the following tasks?

A. Entering the cognitive period of preoperational thinking.

B. Entering the cognitive period of concrete operations.

C. Entering the cognitive period of formal operations.

D. Entering the cognitive phase of acquiring an understanding of triadic relationships.

3.12 Robin, as an irrepressible 7-year-old, loved to spend her evenings talking with her father about her day, but as she grew older, she became less inclined to engage in these conversations. She would often call from school asking if she could sleep over at a friend's house or "hang out" at the mall. She would frequently shut the door to her room to call classmates, often spending her evenings on the phone. Which of the following developmental tasks of preadolescence is illustrated in Robin's changing behavior?

A. Turning away from parental intimacy and toward peer socialization.

B. Integration of the sexual self and romantic longings into the self-representation.

C. Adjustment to the subjective experience of bodily changes.

D. Development of the capacity to love.

3.13   At age 11, Katie had a crush on a popular boy named Austin. She liked his "skater boy" clothing and style. At age 16, in her photography class, Katie was paired with a 17-year-old senior named Patrick. They had never interacted much before, but after an hour it was clear that while they were both very different, they recognized and appreciated each other's quirks. They soon became inseparable. Their common interests in books, music, and photography connected them deeply. The differences in Katie's romantic interests demonstrate which developmental change in adolescence?

   A. Solidifying of the gender identity.
   B. The "midadolescence shift" toward romance.
   C. Demonstrating the ability to commit to and depend on a significant other outside of familial relations.
   D. Completing identity exploration to achieve a role in contemporary society.

3.14   Gideon started college as a freshman and moved into a 1-bedroom apartment with a junior named Gus. He idealized Gus's charm, intelligence, and ability to easily navigate a world that to Gideon was still overwhelming and novel. He emulated Gus's mannerisms and aspired to be as successful as Gus. The influence of Gus in Gideon's life at this developmental stage illustrates_____, which largely occurs in_____?

   A. The revision of the superego; late adolescence.
   B. Gender identity; late adolescence.
   C. Rejection of infantile ties; middle adolescence.
   D. Risky behaviors; early to middle adolescence.

3.15   Jared, a 26-year-old man, had a strife-filled relationship with his father and mother while growing up. As a young adult first starting out, he had minimal communication with them; however, after working at a steady job for a few years, he felt more open to reengaging with his parents. To his surprise, he and his parents were able to successfully interact, both feeling more equipped to navigate the complexity of the past, and remaining respectful of each other's boundaries. Which of the following tasks of emerging adulthood (ages 22 or 23 years through 30 years) does Jared's newfound ability to interact with his parents illustrate?

   A. Renegotiating family relationships toward equality.
   B. Achieving formal operations.
   C. Integrating sexuality.
   D. Transformation of self-representation.

CHAPTER 4

Assessment of Suicide Risk

4.1 A psychiatry resident is evaluating a patient who was brought to the hospital after she told a coworker that she was hearing voices and having suicidal thoughts. The resident begins the interview by asking questions about the patient's thoughts. He observes that the patient is responding in short phrases and is not answering his questions about hallucinations and suicidal ideation. Which of the following actions would be the best initial approach for the resident to take?

A. Ask if the patient has access to a firearm.
B. Address the patient's fear of answering questions as understandable and offer basic information about suicidal thoughts.
C. Ask the patient if she had taken objective or preparatory steps to act on her suicidal thoughts.
D. Consider that the patient may be experiencing perceptual disturbances and ask about auditory hallucinations.

4.2 A patient is experiencing increasing severity of suicidal thoughts. He states that he is going through a divorce and has been struggling to find a job. He admits to feeling like he has no future. Which of the following, if communicated by the patient, would indicate a higher risk of suicide?

A. He reports having increased thoughts about what death is like.
B. He reports that he has been seeing a supportive therapist weekly over the past 4 months.
C. He discloses that he has been feeling consistently hopeless for the past 3 weeks.
D. He states that he has been having a difficult time talking to his children.

4.3 A 28-year-old woman with major depressive disorder was brought to the hospital after taking 24 pills of her duloxetine 90 mg/day prescription. She was found by her sister, who called the ambulance. Which of the following factors, if disclosed by or discovered about this patient, would place her at highest risk of suicide?

A. She has a coping card in her bag.
B. She was discharged from inpatient hospitalization 3 weeks ago.
C. She confides that her sister is her own main reason for living.
D. She reports having thoughts that life is not worth living for many years.

4.4   A 54-year-old woman who was referred to your outpatient clinic for depression reports that she has been experiencing low mood, anhedonia, and insomnia for the past 6 weeks. She becomes tearful, stating that she has been feeling worthless and that "life has been tough to tolerate lately." What approach should you take when raising the issue of this patient's suicidal thoughts?

   A. Approach questioning of the patient more broadly rather than focusing solely on the suicidal thoughts.
   B. Refrain from asking directly about suicidal thoughts, because direct questioning increases the risk of the patient committing suicide.
   C. Ask detailed and explicit questions about the patient's suicidal thoughts.
   D. Avoid addressing any ambivalence expressed by the patient regarding suicide.

4.5   A 60-year-old woman discloses that she has been depressed for the past 6 months, ever since her husband died. She reports staying in bed most days and having little motivation to do the things she used to enjoy. She also describes having thoughts about wishing she were dead and about what her family would do if she died. Which of the following statements best characterizes this patient's thoughts?

   A. The patient is having active suicidal thoughts.
   B. The patient's thoughts are focused on self-harm.
   C. The patient's thoughts express an intention to end her own life.
   D. The patient's thoughts represent morbid rumination.

4.6   While exploring a patient's history, you learn that she has made suicide attempts in the past. You attempt to learn the details and the overall pattern of the patient's behavior. Which of the following features of the patient's past suicide attempts would provide the most useful information about her current risk?

   A. The patient's emotional response to each previous attempt.
   B. The method most often used in past attempts.
   C. The overall presence of chronic suicidality.
   D. The first attempt and the most serious of past attempts.

4.7   You are interviewing a 45-year-old man with a history of major depressive disorder (diagnosed when he was in his twenties). He reports that he had done well for almost a decade without being in treatment; however, over the past 4 weeks, his depressive symptoms have returned and have been progressing. He discloses that at times he has been having thoughts of wanting to end his life. Which of the following domains would be most important for you to inquire about during the interview with this patient?

   A. Family history of completed suicide.
   B. Previous history of morbid rumination.
   C. History of scratching his thigh when feeling overwhelmed.
   D. Access to bottles of medications.

4.8   You are assessing a 16-year-old Native American girl who was sent in from her school after a teacher noticed multiple scratch marks on her arms. The patient discloses that she has been struggling in school, and her grades have dropped. Her father has been traveling more for work, and she reports that her father's absence has been hard on her mother and siblings. The girl is close to her mother, and they both are active in their local church. She reports depressed mood, insomnia, and a 5-pound weight loss. When asked about suicidal thoughts, the patient becomes quiet. Which of the following factors in this patient's profile may place her at greater risk of suicide?

A. The patient is a Native American teenager.
B. The patient is female.
C. The patient has a close relationship with her mother.
D. The patient is active in her local church.

4.9   Before a clinician begins a patient evaluation, it can be helpful to communicate the purpose of the interview to the patient. Which of the following best expresses the goal of the initial interview of a patient with new suicidal thoughts?

A. To obtain a thorough report regarding the events leading up to the patient's presentation.
B. To develop a deep understanding of the patient's psychiatric history.
C. To help the patient recover a sense of personal agency, safety, and hope.
D. To point out the patient's unrealistic thinking about suicide.

CHAPTER 5

Laboratory Testing and Neuroimaging Studies in Psychiatry

5.1   A 51-year-old patient with a prior history of alcohol use disorder is brought to the emergency room for evaluation for danger to self and is being considered for psychiatric admission. The complete blood count (CBC) and comprehensive metabolic panel (CMP) were unremarkable, the chest X ray was normal, and the blood alcohol level (BAL) was 0.03%. Which of the following statements accurately describes the clinical utility of an electrocardiogram (ECG) for medical clearance prior to psychiatric admission of this patient?

A. ECG screening for prolonged QT interval is cost-effective in reducing the risk of sudden cardiac death in patients admitted to psychiatric hospitals.
B. This patient's BAL is low and does not indicate increased risk of an acute cardiac event.
C. Because this patient is younger than 60 years, he is at low risk of a cardiac event and does not need an ECG.
D. A normal chest X ray is an appropriate substitute for an ECG.

5.2   A multiple sleep latency test (MSLT) demonstrated that a patient's average time to sleep onset was 12 minutes, and three sleep-onset rapid eye movement (REM) periods were observed. The baseline electrocardiogram (EEG) was within normal limits. Which of the following disorders can be diagnosed on the basis of these findings?

A. Narcolepsy without cataplexy.
B. Hypersomnolence.
C. Delirium.
D. Subacute sclerosing panencephalitis.

5.3   Which of the following imaging modalities detects cerebrospinal fluid (CSF) with high-intensity (white) signal?

A. Computed tomography.
B. Proton density–weighted magnetic resonance imaging.
C. T1-weighted magnetic resonance imaging.
D. T2-weighted magnetic resonance imaging.

5.4   Which of the following imaging modalities would be most effective for detecting damage to the structural integrity of white matter tracts?

A. Magnetic resonance spectroscopy (MRS).
B. Magnetoencephalography.
C. Diffusion tensor imaging (DTI).
D. Functional magnetic resonance imaging (fMRI).

5.5   A 44-year-old woman with a history of alcohol use disorder presents to the emergency room. She has a blood alcohol level (BAL) that is below the threshold of detection. A laboratory test of which of the following would provide the most reliable indicator of recent alcohol consumption in this patient?

A. Aspartate transaminase.
B. Gamma-glutamyltransferase.
C. Alkaline phosphatase.
D. Alcohol breath analysis.

5.6   Which of the following is a commonly observed laboratory abnormality in patients with alcohol use disorder?

A. Low magnesium.
B. Elevated phosphate.
C. Low mean corpuscular volume.
D. Low serum total homocysteine.

5.7   Which of the following statements about single photon emission computed tomography (SPECT) is *true*?

A. SPECT measures cerebral glucose metabolism.
B. SPECT is typically more expensive than positron emission tomography (PET).
C. SPECT uses a radiotracer that is attached to a drug.
D. SPECT provides higher structural anatomic visualization than magnetic resonance imaging (MRI).

5.8   A patient has abnormal liver function test findings on a comprehensive metabolic panel (CMP) after initiation of chlorpromazine. Which of the following, if elevated to more than three times the upper limit of normal, would point to a cholestatic drug reaction?

A. Aspartate transaminase (AST).
B. Alanine aminotransferase (ALT).
C. Alkaline phosphatase.
D. Bilirubin.

5.9   A patient with low thyroid-stimulating hormone (TSH) and normal free thyroxine (T_4) is most likely to have which of the following conditions?

A. Hypothyroidism.
B. Subclinical hypothyroidism.
C. Hyperthyroidism.
D. Subclinical hyperthyroidism.

5.10   Which of the following findings on an electroencephalogram (EEG) would be most consistent with delirium?

A. Alpha power highest over occipital areas.
B. Generalized slow-wave activity.
C. Reactivity to eye opening and closure.
D. Periodic complexes consisting of 2–4 high-amplitude delta waves repeated every 5–7 seconds.

CHAPTER 6

The Social Determinants of Mental Health

6.1   As described by scholars of public health and global health, what are *social determinants of mental health*?

    A. Aspects of daily socialization with friends, family, and coworkers that affect an individual's mental health.

    B. The impact of religious and cultural traditions on how mental health symptoms are expressed within a given society.

    C. Environmental, societal, and economic conditions that affect mental health outcomes at a population level.

    D. Legal, psychiatric, and medical consensus definitions of psychiatric disorders, used mainly by social service entities.

6.2   As used in public health and public policy contexts, what does the term *health inequities* mean?

    A. Disparities in health that result from unjust and avoidable social and economic policies.

    B. Marked interpersonal variations in health that result entirely from genetic risk factors.

    C. Observed health differences between segments of the population, which have many causes.

    D. Discrepancies in how behavioral health care and medical care are covered by insurance.

6.3   You are working as an embedded psychiatrist in a primary care clinic. You are asked to evaluate an 18-year-old who recently immigrated from Ecuador who was referred to you by her primary care physician for a major depressive episode. This patient was born biologically male and currently identifies as female. She is living with family members who are critical of her gender identity and presentation. While at her workplace, she has experienced derogatory comments regarding her gender identity and immigration status. Which of the following adverse social determinants of health would be of greatest relevance to you, the psychiatrist, in considering the best approach to caring for this patient?

A. Hormonal treatment should be encouraged for this patient, because untreated gender dysphoria increases the likelihood that the patient's depressive symptoms will worsen.
B. Psychiatric care is stigmatized in immigrant communities; thus, it would most likely be preferable for this patient's depression to be treated by her primary care physician.
C. Depressive symptoms arising in the context of psychosocial stressors are likely to self-resolve and do not require medication.
D. Experiences of discrimination are associated with adverse mental health symptoms, placing this patient at increased risk for depression.

6.4   You are a community psychiatrist who receives a referral of an 18-year-old woman who is aging out of a local child psychiatry clinic, where she is being treated for persistent depressive disorder (dysthymia). The evaluation provided by the clinic comments that this patient is at increased risk for poor mental health outcomes based on her multiple "adverse childhood experiences." You recognize *adverse childhood experiences* as a term from the public psychiatry literature. To what does this term refer?

A. Childhood experiences of interpersonal abuse or neglect.
B. Childhood experiences of displacement or forced migration.
C. Childhood experiences of school-based bullying or exclusion.
D. Childhood experiences of being adopted or in foster care.

6.5   You recently started working at a community psychiatry clinic. You are wondering what approach to use for patients who are affected by adverse determinants of mental health. What would a public psychiatry expert most likely recommend that you do?

A. Avoid asking new patients about childhood abuse or neglect, as such questions may trigger traumatic memories.
B. Educate patients that concerns about employment would be best shared with a social worker.
C. Screen patients routinely for food insecurity, and provide them with lists of local resources.
D. Encourage patients who are victims of discrimination to find a provider with a similar background.

CHAPTER 7

Ethical Considerations in Psychiatry

7.1   A 45-year-old woman with a history of schizophrenia and end-stage renal disease on hemodialysis is admitted to the hospital for acute psychotic decompensation. She is disheveled, and her thinking is disorganized. She denies suicidal/homicidal ideation. She is alert and can tell you why she gets hemodialysis, although in very simple, concrete terms. She scores 20/30 on the Montreal Cognitive Assessment. Since her admission, she has been adamantly and consistently refusing hemodialysis, because she believes that the admitting medical team is trying to "poison the blood" with the dialysis machine. She cannot tell you the medical consequences of refusing this treatment. What are the conflicting ethical considerations in this situation?

   A. Clinical indications and patient preferences.
   B. Clinical indications and patient quality of life.
   C. Contextual influences and patient preferences.
   D. Patient quality of life and contextual influences.

7.2   A 65-year-old woman with Stage IV breast cancer with metastasis to the brain has decided she does not want to pursue chemotherapy. She is cachectic appearing and reports to be in a lot of pain. She can tell you details of her diagnosis, which treatment is recommended and why. She demonstrates an understanding of the consequences of refusing treatment, which could include death. On examination, she is alert throughout and able to attend to the interview. She has mild cognitive impairment on formal testing, with a Montreal Cognitive Assessment score of 22/30. She denies suicidal ideation but she expresses pessimism that treatment would help to improve her quality of life or extend her survival. A psychiatrist has been asked to perform a decisional capacity evaluation to determine this patient's capacity to refuse proposed treatment. The psychiatrist happens to be a friend of the patient's intimate partner. Which essential ethical skills must the psychiatrist make particular use of when evaluating this patient?

A. The ability to identify ethical dilemmas, to understand how one's personal biases may affect one's care of patients, and to know one's own scope of clinical competence and be willing to work within those boundaries.
B. The ability to identify ethical dilemmas, to anticipate ethically high-risk situations, and to understand how one's personal biases may affect one's care of patients.
C. The ability to identify ethical dilemmas and to know one's own scope of clinical competence and be willing to work within those boundaries.
D. The ability to understand how one's personal biases may affect one's care of patients, to anticipate ethically high-risk situations, and to seek information and consultation and make use of advice received when faced with difficult situations.

7.3   A psychiatrist working in a private practice of three psychiatrists notices that her colleague has not shown up to work twice this week and also noticed that he was stumbling toward his car after work one day. She is unaware of any adverse patient outcomes based on these observed behaviors. What is the appropriate action to be taken by the psychiatrist?

A. Respect her colleague's confidentiality and keep this information private.
B. Do nothing until she has enough information to make a definitive judgment about whether or not the colleague is practicing competently.
C. Wait until her colleague confides in her that he has a substance use disorder.
D. Report her colleague to the appropriate professional bodies.

7.4   A patient with bipolar disorder is admitted to the hospital due to shortness of breath and found to have an acute coronary syndrome requiring cardiac catheterization. On exam, he is intermittently hypotensive and somnolent. He is not able to tell you why he is in the hospital. His Montreal Cognitive Assessment score is 8/30. When informed of his medical diagnosis and the proposed treatment, the patient decides he does not want a cardiac catheterization. You are asked to assess the patient's decisional capacity to refuse the procedure. A judgment of decisional capacity is based primarily on which of the following?

A. The judgment depends on whether the procedure is deemed high risk or low risk.
B. The judgment depends on the psychiatric diagnosis of the patient.
C. The judgment is based on an assessment of the adequacy of the patient's understanding, appreciation, reasoning, and indication of a choice regarding the proposed intervention.
D. The judgment is determined on the basis of whether the patient has a severe mental illness such as schizophrenia.

7.5   A third-year medical student often works long hours and spends his weekends studying for exams. Despite this busy schedule, he enjoys spending his free time volunteering at a child advocacy center, where he helps to organize fundraising events and cook meals for families. Which of the following ethical principles is this man practicing by his participation in such volunteer activity?

   A. Fidelity.
   B. Autonomy.
   C. Integrity.
   D. Beneficence.

7.6   A 65-year-old man with diabetes mellitus type 2, chronic obstructive pulmonary disease (COPD), congestive heart failure (CHF), and schizophrenia is admitted to the medical floor for cellulitis. His COPD and CHF are end stage, with an estimated 6-month survival. He is not actively psychotic and does not need medication adjustments. His Montreal Cognitive Assessment score is 27/30. In the discussion of code status, his understanding of his systemic illnesses and prognosis is adequate, and after the discussion, he chooses to be listed as DNR/DNI (Do Not Resuscitate/Do Not Intubate). Which of the following statements most accurately describes the ethical basis of the informed consent process for a decisionally intact patient to exercise his/her autonomy regarding a code status decision?

   A. Given that the patient has schizophrenia, the philosophical basis for informed consent resides in what the clinician thinks would be the best treatment decision for the patient.
   B. Promoting autonomy alone creates an environment for true informed consent that enhances a patient's meaningful decision making.
   C. The clinician must also appraise whether the patient has the opportunity to make a choice consistent with the preferences of his or her family and friends.
   D. Informed consent is the process by which individuals make free, knowledgeable decisions about whether to accept a proposed plan for assessment and/ or treatment.

7.7   Which of the following statements regarding decisional capacity and competency is *true*?

   A. Legal jurisdictions have differing standards for establishing decisional capacity.
   B. *Decisional capacity* refers to a determination made by a clinical professional, and *competency* is a legal determination.
   C. *Competency* refers to a determination made by a clinical professional, and *decisional capacity* in a particular life domain is a legal determination.
   D. A decisional capacity assessment must be performed by a psychiatrist.

7.8   Dr. Jones is a first-year resident, working more than 80 hours per week and sleeping, at most, 5 hours each night. She is not involved in health-promoting recreation or exercise and is often isolated from family and friends. She has finished a particularly long day of work and is exhausted. She is sitting down to chart and notices after reviewing her patient list that she ordered laboratory work on the wrong patient, a medical error. Other than increasing the likelihood of medical error, which of the following is an additional negative consequence of diminished physician well-being?

A. Substance use.
B. Delivering high-quality care.
C. Improved health and service outcomes.
D. Increased empathy and engagement.

C H A P T E R   8

Legal Considerations in Psychiatry

8.1   Which of the following legal terms refers to the concept of "guilty mind"?

    A. *Actus reus.*
    B. *Mens rea.*
    C. *Voir dire.*
    D. *Pro se.*

8.2   Which of the following legal rulings has served as the basis for many state sanity statutes, by which a legal defendant may claim that he did not know right from wrong because of a mental illness?

    A. *Tarasoff.*
    B. *M'Naghten.*
    C. *Cruzan.*
    D. *Jaffee.*

8.3   Three weeks after being discharged from an inpatient psychiatric unit, a 40-year-old female patient commits suicide. Dr. Jones had treated the patient during a 10-day voluntary hospitalization for a major depressive episode. The patient came to the hospital on her own to seek help and had specifically asked Dr. Jones not to tell her family members about her diagnosis and hospitalization. In the days prior to discharge, Dr. Jones completed a competent suicide risk assessment. The patient adamantly denied any thoughts of self-harm, including intent or plan to commit suicide. Which of the following elements must the patient's family prove by a preponderance of the evidence to win a malpractice claim against Dr. Jones?

    A. Dr. Jones should have been able to predict that a patient suffering from a major depressive episode would have attempted suicide after leaving the hospital.
    B. The patient's suicide occurred as a direct result of Dr. Jones's actions during the patient's treatment.

C. In letting the patient leave the hospital without completing a "no-harm con-tract," Dr. Jones violated his duty of care.

D. The patient's family suffered psychic harm damages as a result of the patient's death.

8.4 Which of the following is an accurate characterization of patient confidentiality under the Health Insurance Portability and Accountability Act of 1996 (HIPAA)?

A. Before HIPAA was implemented, there were no guidelines governing the scope of patient confidentiality with regard to the therapist–patient relation-ship.

B. Following HIPAA's implementation, psychotherapy notes cannot be released without explicit authorization from the patient even if they are stored with the remainder of a patient's medical records.

C. Under HIPAA, a patient's psychiatric symptoms, treatment plan, and progno-sis cannot be released without explicit authorization from the patient.

D. HIPAA prohibits insurers from making treatment and/or payment for a pa-tient's psychiatric condition contingent on whether psychotherapy notes are disclosed.

8.5 Which of the following statements about determinations of competence is *true*?

A. A determination of competence or incompetence must be made by a judge sit-ting in a court of law.

B. Although determination of competence can be made by any physician, psy-chiatrists may be more capable of conducting competence evaluations in clin-ical contexts.

C. A determination of competence has no impact on whether a person can pro-vide informed consent for treatment.

D. A determination of competence is based solely on a patient's underlying cog-nitive abilities.

8.6 In which of the following situations would it be considered risky for a physician to proceed with treatment before obtaining informed consent?

A. A patient requires emergent treatment to save her life but is unconscious and therefore unable to communicate with the treatment provider.

B. A patient who is able to make his own medical decisions knowingly waives the right to informed consent, preferring to defer to his physician's judgment.

C. A psychiatrist believes that her patient may become so ill or emotionally dis-traught by the disclosure of certain information that it would complicate or hinder treatment.

D. A patient has been deemed unable to make his own medical decisions but has a readily available legal guardian who can provide informed consent on his behalf.

8.7 A 55-year-old financial executive with a diagnosis of bipolar I disorder is scheduled to be discharged from an inpatient psychiatric unit where he has been treated with lithium and olanzapine for an acute manic episode. He plans to return to the home which he owns and where he lives with his wife and two young children. Two years ago, after being discharged from the psychiatric hospital under similar circumstances, the patient threw a glass vase at the wall while intoxicated. Six months ago, the patient's wife bought him a vintage baseball bat that he proudly displays in the living room. In the violence risk assessment conducted by the psychiatrist, which of the following features in this patient's profile would likely represent the most serious risk factor for violence?

A. The patient's planned return to live with his wife and two young children.
B. The patient's history of relapsing to alcohol use when he returns to the outpatient setting.
C. The patient's recent acquisition of a baseball bat that is readily accessible.
D. The fact that the patient is undergoing treatment with multiple psychiatric medications.

8.8 Which of the following populations is protected in all 50 states by statutes mandating that psychiatrists report suspected maltreatment?

A. Children who might be experiencing abuse.
B. Patients who have been medically or psychiatrically hospitalized within the last year.
C. Physically disabled adults.
D. Middle-aged adult patients living alone.

8.9 A psychiatrist is subpoenaed to testify as a fact witness in his patient's civil case after the patient is suspended from her teaching position following accusations of sexual misconduct with a student. The psychiatrist has been treating the patient with both psychotherapy and medication management for the past 10 years. During this time, the patient has revealed her sexual fantasies involving her male students, but has consistently insisted that she would never act upon them. Which of the following would be considered an appropriate action by the psychiatrist in this case?

A. Providing expert witness testimony in addition to serving as a fact witness on the patient's behalf.
B. Thoroughly reviewing the subpoena with a psychiatric colleague before deciding whether to respond.
C. Altering the patient's psychotherapy records to remove information told to him in confidence that he fears might prove damaging to the patient's husband and minor children if publicly revealed.
D. Explaining to the patient that patient–psychiatrist privilege does not extend to all psychotherapeutic communications and that the scope of confidentiality will be determined by the court.

CHAPTER 9

Neurodevelopmental Disorders

9.1   The mother of a 10-year-old boy reports that for the past 9 months, she has noticed her son making pouting movements with his mouth every day. He also frequently clears his throat and shrugs his shoulders. The boy's teachers have commented that they have noticed similar behavior. What is the most appropriate diagnosis for this child?

    A. Tourette's disorder.
    B. Persistent tic disorder.
    C. Provisional tic disorder.
    D. Unspecified tic disorder.

9.2   A child whose development tracked closely with that of her peers during early childhood, but then diverged in later childhood, would best be described as having which kind of developmental trajectory?

    A. Typical.
    B. Regressing.
    C. Remitting.
    D. Persisting–delayed.

9.3   Which of the following findings on evaluation would satisfy Criterion B for the DSM-5 diagnosis of intellectual disability?

    A. Onset of difficulties during adolescent period.
    B. Intelligence testing scores more than 2 standard deviations below average.
    C. Impaired adaptive functioning in everyday life across multiple domains.
    D. Deficits in intellectual functions on clinical assessment.

9.4   A persistent deficit in articulation of spoken language should prompt consideration of which of the following disorders?

A. Speech sound disorder.
B. Language disorder.
C. Childhood-onset fluency disorder.
D. Social communication disorder.

9.5   Which of the following is considered a first-line treatment for attention-deficit/hyperactivity disorder (ADHD)?

A. Bupropion.
B. Tricyclic agents.
C. Alpha-agonists.
D. Atomoxetine.

9.6   Behaviors such as excessive motor activity or restlessness in inappropriate contexts, fidgeting, and talkativeness are examples of which of the following?

A. Inattention.
B. Hyperactivity.
C. Impulsivity.
D. Stereotypies.

9.7   Which of the following disorders is defined by difficulties in the acquisition or application of specific core academic skills?

A. Language disorder.
B. Intellectual disability.
C. Attention deficit/hyperactivity disorder.
D. Specific learning disorder.

9.8   A young child has deficits in social–emotional reciprocity and in nonverbal communicative behaviors used for social interaction, stereotyped motor movements, and highly restricted interest of abnormal intensity. What additional deficit must be present to meet criteria for a DSM-5 diagnosis of autism spectrum disorder (ASD)?

A. Ritualized patterns of verbal or nonverbal behavior.
B. Unusual interest in sensory aspects of the environment.
C. Deficits in developing, maintaining, and understanding relationships.
D. Inaccuracy of performance of gross and/or fine motor skills.

9.9   Which of the following interventions is widely used and effective for treating the core symptoms of autism spectrum disorder (ASD)?

A. Habit reversal training.
B. Early Intensive Behavioral Intervention.
C. Organizational skills planning.
D. Motor skills intervention.

9.10   Which of the following disorders is characterized by involuntary, coordinated, repetitive, seemingly driven but apparently purposeless motor behaviors?

A. Stereotypic movement disorder.
B. Developmental coordination disorder.
C. Autism spectrum disorder.
D. Unspecified tic disorder.

9.11   Which of the following features would preclude a diagnosis of social communication disorder?

A. Onset of symptoms at an early age.
B. Difficulty observing rules of typical conversation.
C. Difficulty understanding implicit meanings.
D. Presence of repetitive behaviors.

9.12   A 13-year-old boy is referred by a school nurse to a local clinic for evaluation of school difficulties due to forgetting to complete school assignments and poor exam scores. The boy's mother recalls that her son was slow to begin speaking as a toddler and used to throw tantrums when she dropped him off at daycare. Given this patient's history, which of the following characteristics, if found to be present, would be consistent with a diagnosis of intellectual disability?

A. He requires frequent reminders to wear a coat and closed-toed shoes when it is snowing outside.
B. His memory deficits appeared after a concussion at age 12 years.
C. He has an IQ one standard deviation below the expected population mean.
D. He has difficulty completing assignments when at school but is able to complete homework assignments at home without assistance.

9.13   Which of the following statements correctly describes a way in which autism spectrum disorder (ASD) differs from social (pragmatic) communication disorder (SPCD)?

A. Deficits in nonverbal communication are found in SPCD but not in ASD.
B. Restrictive and repetitive behaviors are found in ASD but not in SPCD.
C. Onset of symptoms occurs at an early age in ASD but not in SPCD.
D. Evidence-based treatments are available for SPCD but not for ASD.

9.14   A 40-year-old man is transferred to your care with a diagnosis of schizoid personality disorder. As a child, the patient was moved to multiple different schools due to behavioral dysregulation and was brought to the emergency room numerous times due to head banging. The patient is socially isolated due to difficulty engaging in conversation. Which of the following additional characteristics, if discovered about this patient, would lead you to suspect autism spectrum disorder (ASD) as the correct diagnosis rather than schizoid personality disorder?

A. He is uninterested in socializing.
B. He has a counting compulsion, which he finds distressing.
C. He exhibits stereotypic movements.
D. He has no activities that he enjoys.

9.15   A 35-year-old man comes to your office because he is concerned that he might have attention-deficit/hyperactivity disorder (ADHD). Which of the following details, if present or discovered about this patient, would strongly support an ADHD diagnosis?

A. He reports having experienced an improved ability to concentrate after taking his friend's ADHD medication.
B. He reports that he is more restless as an adult than he was as a child.
C. He is able to provide a history of symptoms from when he was less than 12 years old.
D. He is male.

9.16   A 14-year-old girl is brought to your office by her mother because of worsening social isolation at school. The girl's teacher reports that she frequently appears to be daydreaming during class. The teacher also reports that the girl is always having to borrow her classmates' books because she forgets to bring her own. The patient was recently seen by a neurologist to evaluate the possibility of absence seizures, and her electroencephalogram was normal. In conjunction with the patient's history, which of the following features would lead you to suspect attention-deficit/hyperactivity disorder (ADHD) as the primary diagnosis?

A. The onset of the patient's problem was 1 year ago.
B. The patient is having symptoms only at school.
C. The patient is female.
D. The patient has trouble completing tasks at home as well as at school.

9.17   A 15-year-old girl with a provisional diagnosis of tic disorder presents for evaluation. She has been experiencing symptoms of finger flexing and nose twitching. These symptoms have been bothersome, leading to difficulty completing tasks at school. Workup for underlying medical causes of the patient's symptoms has been negative. Which of the following characteristics would lead you to suspect that Tourette's disorder is the correct diagnosis?

A. The patient's symptoms have been present for the past 6 months.
B. The patient also has a phonic tic (throat clearing).

C. The patient is female.

D. The patient's symptoms have been worsening since the start of adolescence.

9.18 Which of the following statements about stereotypic movement disorder (SMD) is *true*?

A. It is idiopathic by definition.

B. It is associated with higher cognitive functioning.

C. It typically involves movements such as eye blinking or mouth pouting.

D. There are multiple evidence-based therapies for its treatment.

9.19 A 9-year old boy presents to your clinic for evaluation of speech. He frequently repeats sounds and syllables when he speaks. His mother notes that the symptoms are worse in certain situations, and he tends to say he is sick on days when he has to present a project in front of the class. The boy's symptoms have responded well to therapy by a speech and language pathologist. On the basis of this presentation, you suspect that the patient has childhood-onset fluency disorder. Which of the following statements about this disorder is *true*?

A. Childhood-onset fluency disorder cannot co-occur with other language-based disorders.

B. Childhood-onset fluency disorder symptoms are more severe in a relaxed and familiar setting.

C. Childhood-onset fluency disorder symptoms usually start after age 10.

D. Childhood-onset fluency disorder specifically affects the rate and continuity of speech production.

9.20 Which of the following disorders is defined by deficits in the articulation or phonology of spoken language such as difficulty using phonemes to produce intelligible speech?

A. Speech sound disorder.

B. Social (pragmatic) communication disorder.

C. Childhood-onset fluency disorder.

D. Language disorder.

CHAPTER 10

Schizophrenia Spectrum and Other Psychotic Disorders

10.1 *Posturing* is classified as what type of psychotic symptom?

A. Positive.
B. Negative.
C. Disorganization.
D. Cognitive impairment.

10.2 A patient's psychosis was well controlled on clozapine 300 mg/day when he was discharged. from the hospital. Two weeks later, he experiences a reemergence of psychotic symptoms, although his dosage has not changed and he has been observed taking his medication daily. Which of the following is the most likely reason for this symptom reemergence?

A. The patient began drinking copious amounts of grapefruit juice after leaving the hospital.
B. The patient began smoking heavily after leaving the hospital.
C. The patient began taking cimetidine for gastritis after leaving the hospital.
D. The patient began taking diltiazem for atrial fibrillation after leaving the hospital.

10.3 Which of the following is *not* a standard part of the workup for first-episode psychosis?

A. Thyroid-stimulating hormone (TSH).
B. HIV and syphilis testing.
C. Computed tomography (CT) scan of the head.
D. Urine toxicology.

10.4   Temporal lobe seizures are often associated with which of the following types of psychotic symptoms?

A. Visual hallucinations.
B. Olfactory hallucinations.
C. Bizarre behavior.
D. Echolalia.

10.5   A patient presents with subacute-onset psychotic symptoms, changes in behavior, seizures, and memory loss. Which of the following is the most likely cause of these symptoms?

A. Mitochondrial disease.
B. HIV-associated central nervous system (CNS) infection.
C. Cocaine intoxication.
D. Limbic encephalitis.

10.6   Which of the following stages of schizophrenia is associated with the highest risk of suicide as well as neuroimaging evidence of cortical thinning?

A. Premorbid stage.
B. Prodromal stage.
C. Progressive stage.
D. Chronic–residual stage.

10.7   A patient develops a temperature of 102°F, rigidity, confusion, and hypotension after a rapid increase in his fluphenazine dosage. Which of the following is the most likely diagnosis?

A. Serotonin syndrome.
B. Neuroleptic malignant syndrome.
C. Drug reaction with eosinophilia and systemic symptoms.
D. Central nervous system (CNS) infection.

10.8   There are low levels of this neurotransmitter in patients with schizophrenia in comparison with healthy control subjects. Moreover, psychotic symptoms result from administration of agents that are antagonists for the receptors that mediate this neurotransmitter. Based on these findings, which of the following neurotransmitters *not targeted by current medications* has been hypothesized to play an important role in schizophrenia?

A. Glutamate.
B. Dopamine.
C. Serotonin.
D. GABA.

CHAPTER 11

Bipolar and Related Disorders

11.1 A 35-year-old woman with a history of bipolar disorder is brought to the emergency department by her husband for suicidal ideation. He reports that his wife abruptly quit her job as a computer programmer 10 days ago to start working on a book about climate change. He notes that this behavior is very atypical for her, and she has been staying up day and night filling notebooks with senseless writing. She apparently never gets tired. Over the past week, she has been increasingly irritable and moody, cries frequently, and has been talking about death. On interview, the patient states that she needs to be discharged immediately so that she can get back to writing an "extremely important" book about the global climate crisis. She reports strong feelings of guilt regarding her own role in the "destruction of the environment." The mental status exam is notable for rapid and pressured speech, "depressed" mood, labile affect, tangential thought processes, and suicidal ideation. Which of the following diagnoses best describes this patient's current mood episode?

A. Manic episode with anxious distress.
B. Hypomanic episode with mixed features.
C. Major depressive episode with mixed features.
D. Manic episode with mixed features.

11.2 Which of the following statements accurately describes how suicide rates among patients with bipolar disorder differ from rates in the general population?

A. Compared with individuals in the general population, patients with bipolar disorder have increased rates of both attempted and completed suicide.
B. Compared with individuals in the general population, patients with bipolar disorder have increased rates of attempted suicide but not of completed suicide.
C. Compared with individuals in the general population, patients with bipolar disorder have increased rates of completed suicide but not of attempted suicide.
D. The rates of attempted and completed suicide among patients with bipolar disorder are about the same as those in the general population.

11.3 You are treating a 25-year-old man with bipolar I disorder who was admitted 5 days ago to an inpatient psychiatric unit for treatment of acute mania with mixed features. On admission, he received a loading dose of divalproex 20 mg/ kg and was started on divalproex 750 mg/day, which 2 days ago was increased to 1,000 mg/day. The patient continues to be euphoric with an irritable edge, is intrusive, and is sleeping only 3 hours a night. You order a 12-hour serum divalproex trough level and find it to be 75 µg/mL. Which of the following would be the most appropriate next step in managing this patient's mood stabilizer?

A. Decrease divalproex to 750 mg/day.
B. Increase divalproex to 1,250 mg/day.
C. Switch to lithium 300 mg bid.
D. Switch to lamotrigine 25 mg bid daily.

11.4 A 38-year-old woman with a history of bipolar I disorder presents to her outpatient psychiatrist reporting 3 weeks of a symptom constellation consistent with an episode of acute bipolar depression. What U.S. Food and Drug Administration (FDA)–approved medications are currently available to treat this patient?

A. Olanzapine-fluoxetine (combination), sertraline, and quetiapine.
B. Olanzapine-fluoxetine (combination), quetiapine, and lurasidone.
C. Lithium, lurasidone, and quetiapine.
D. Divalproex, lurasidone, and quetiapine.

11.5 The patient described in question 11.4 is started on quetiapine, and the dosage is increased to 300 mg/day (taken nightly). She continues on this medication for 4 weeks and experiences improvement in her sleep quality, but her low mood, poor concentration, poor appetite, decreased interest, and feelings of guilt persist. She denies any concurrent manic symptoms and does not have a history of rapid cycling. She reports that a number of years ago, her depression was effectively treated with escitalopram, and she asks her psychiatrist whether it might be possible/appropriate for her to receive this medication again. How should the psychiatrist respond?

A. "No, patients with a diagnosis of bipolar I disorder should never be treated with antidepressants because of the risk of inducing mania."
B. "No, patients with a diagnosis of bipolar I disorder should never be treated with antidepressants because they are ineffective."
C. "Yes, we can taper off and discontinue the quetiapine, and then start escitalopram."
D. "Yes, you could start taking escitalopram in addition to quetiapine."

11.6 A 31-year-old man is admitted to an inpatient unit for treatment of acute mania. His psychiatrist is pondering whether to initiate treatment with lithium or divalproex. Which of the following features, if present in the patient's current presentation or history, might support use of divalproex rather than lithium?

A. A history of rapid cycling (i.e., four or more mood episodes within 1 year).

B. A family history of bipolar disorder in the patient's mother, who has been stable on lithium for many years.

C. A current presentation consistent with euphoric mania.

D. No prior history of manic episodes.

11.7   Which of the following statements regarding the use of psychotherapy in treatment of patients with bipolar disorder is *true*?

A. Psychotherapy is most effective in treatment of acute manic episodes.

B. Psychotherapy is most effective in treatment of acute depressive episodes.

C. Psychotherapy has demonstrated benefit in preventing mood episode recurrence in euthymic patients.

D. Psychotherapy alone (without medications) is the first-line treatment for patients with bipolar disorder.

11.8   A 46-year-old man with a history of hypertension and bipolar I disorder is brought to the emergency department by his wife because he has been acting sleepy and "confused" for the last few hours. She explains that both of them have recently had a stomach virus, with several days of vomiting and diarrhea. She is now recovered, but her husband continues to have vomiting and diarrhea. This morning, she was concerned that he seemed to be sleepier than usual and forgot where to get a water glass in their kitchen. On exam, the patient is lethargic, is not fully oriented, and shows a coarse tremor and an ataxic gait. He does not have any rigidity or myoclonus. Among medications routinely prescribed for maintenance treatment of bipolar disorder, which of the following would be most likely to account for the patient's presentation?

A. Lamotrigine.

B. Olanzapine.

C. Lithium.

D. Divalproex.

11.9   An 18-year-old woman presents to the emergency room because of suicidal ideation. She reports a month of low mood, anhedonia, poor sleep, daytime fatigue, and feelings of worthlessness in addition to the recent onset of suicidal thoughts. She has not previously experienced a depressive episode. Which of the following aspects of this patient's presentation might lead the evaluating psychiatrist to consider bipolar disorder (in addition to unipolar depression) in the differential diagnosis?

A. Presence of suicidal ideation.

B. The patient's age.

C. Presence of insomnia.

D. The patient's gender.

11.10 A 31-year-old man with a history of bipolar disorder consults his psychiatrist about changing his maintenance medication regimen. He is tired of taking pills every day and asks if he could be treated with a long-acting injectable medication. Which of the following medications is U.S. Food and Drug Administration (FDA) approved for the maintenance treatment of bipolar disorder and is available in a long-acting injectable formulation?

A. Ziprasidone.
B. Haloperidol.
C. Fluphenazine.
D. Aripiprazole.

CHAPTER 12

Depressive Disorders

12.1 An 8-year-old boy is brought to clinic by his parents, who report that for the past year, their son has had severe behavioral outbursts, including punching and kicking his parents. He appears very irritable throughout the day, and his parents state that over the past year, he has screamed and lashed out multiple times each week, including at home, school, and soccer practice. His parents say he is almost never calm and happy. Which of the following interventions should be considered for this child?

A. Sertraline.
B. Lithium.
C. Insight-oriented psychotherapy.
D. Play therapy.

12.2 Which of the following is a key feature of disruptive mood dysregulation disorder (DMDD) that can help distinguish it from other disorders that also cause behavioral problems?

A. Boredom and poor concentration.
B. Chronic irritability punctuated by periodic outbursts.
C. Periods of irritability combined with increased energy.
D. Normal mood punctuated by periodic outbursts.

12.3 A 66-year-old man presents to your clinic at the urging of his wife, for "not being himself" for the past 6 months. He complains of poor sleep, poor appetite, slowed movements, and low energy; however, he denies depressed mood, saying he feels "fine." Which of the following additional symptoms would be required to meet criteria for a diagnosis of major depressive disorder (MDD)?

A. Anhedonia.
B. Insomnia.
C. Change in weight.
D. Feelings of worthlessness.

12.4   Which of the following symptoms, if present only during a major depressive episode, would *not* be suggestive of a separate diagnosis?

A. Bizarre delusions.
B. Weight loss.
C. Hypersomnia.
D. Panic attacks.

12.5   A 45-year-old man with major depressive disorder presents to your clinic 1 week after starting an antidepressant. The patient had an abusive childhood and is recently divorced. He reports that work colleagues have commented that he "seems more motivated," but he still feels depressed and anxious and continues to experience some suicidal thoughts and feelings of despondency. Which of the following features in this patient's history portends a good initial response to antidepressant medication?

A. Stressor immediately prior to current episode.
B. The patient's adverse childhood experiences.
C. Prominent anxious features.
D. Increased motivation and energy.

12.6   A 76-year-old man with major depressive disorder (MDD) and chronic kidney disease returns to clinic for follow-up. He started escitalopram 8 weeks ago at 20 mg/day, with a dosage increase to 30 mg/day 4 weeks ago. He reports mild improvement, and his Patient Health Questionnaire–9 score has improved by 50%. He has experienced mild side effects, which he states are tolerable, but he does not want to increase the dosage. What is the next best step in management?

A. Augment with lithium.
B. Augment with aripiprazole.
C. Switch to another selective serotonin reuptake inhibitor.
D. Recommend electroconvulsive therapy (ECT).

12.7   A 62-year-old woman with a history of major depressive disorder (MDD) is brought in by her son for evaluation and treatment. She reports having depression off and on for many years, dating back to her adolescence. She is reluctant to start treatment due to a dislike of doctors. Which of the following elements in this patient's profile and history most strongly suggest that she will experience more severe recurrences in the future?

A. She is an older adult.
B. She is female.
C. She had previous untreated episodes of depression.
D. She was brought to treatment by her son.

12.8 Which of the following is a major clinical feature that differentiates persistent depressive disorder (dysthymia) from major depressive disorder (MDD)?

A. Concomitant presence of anxious features.
B. Lack of changes in appetite and sleep.
C. Chronic subthreshold low mood.
D. Greater response to psychotherapy.

12.9 A 37-year-old woman with a history of premenstrual dysphoric disorder (PMDD) presents to your clinic for treatment. You initiate treatment with a selective serotonin reuptake inhibitor (SSRI) and she quickly reports a benefit; however, she complains of sexual dysfunction and asks for some way to reduce this side effect. Which of the following is the best strategy to do so while maintaining a good therapeutic effect?

A. Continue the SSRI unchanged.
B. Increase her caffeine intake.
C. Take the SSRI only in the days prior to the onset of menses.
D. Decrease physical activity.

12.10 A 45-year-old man with a long history of alcohol use disorder presents to your clinic. He states that he has been sober for the past 6 months. He remains very depressed and despondent, and his wife confirms his history. Which of the following is the most likely diagnosis?

A. Alcohol withdrawal syndrome.
B. Demoralization.
C. Substance/medication-induced depressive disorder (SMIDD).
D. Major depressive disorder (MDD).

CHAPTER 13

Anxiety Disorders

13.1 Which of the following factors increases the likelihood of having an anxiety disorder?

A. Male sex.
B. Married marital status.
C. White race.
D. High socioeconomic status.

13.2 Which of the following anxiety disorders carries the highest lifetime prevalence in the United States?

A. Specific phobia.
B. Panic disorder.
C. Generalized anxiety disorder.
D. Agoraphobia.

13.3 What is the most likely comorbid diagnosis in patients with generalized anxiety disorder?

A. Major depressive disorder.
B. Another anxiety disorder.
C. Alcohol use disorder.
D. Borderline personality disorder.

13.4 A 30-year-old woman comes to your office for evaluation. She reports several visits to the emergency room in the past 2 months for evaluation of new-onset episodes of paroxysmal chest pain and shortness of breath, often accompanied by diaphoresis and intense fears of dying. Despite negative findings from a thorough medical workup, the patient remains convinced she has a heart condition that will kill her and spends a significant amount of time worrying that her symptoms will return. She has been avoiding strenuous physical activity, although she is still unsure about what triggered her previous episodes. What is the most likely diagnosis for this patient?

A. Panic disorder.
B. Generalized anxiety disorder.
C. Illness anxiety disorder.
D. Specific phobia.

13.5   A patient comes to the emergency room reporting symptoms consistent with a panic attack. Which of the following, if found in the patient's medical history, would most likely be the direct cause of the patient's panic attacks?

A. Mitral valve prolapse.
B. Sleep apnea.
C. Asthma.
D. Hyperthyroidism.

13.6   The medical history and emergency department workup of the patient described in question 13.5 reveal no significant abnormalities, and he appears calmer after administration of oral lorazepam 1 mg. However, the patient continues to appear distressed and tearful. When you evaluate him, he tells you "This is the third time this month that I've come to the emergency room and they can't find anything wrong with me and tell me that it's all in my head. I'm going to walk out of here still feeling terrible." What is the next best course of action to take?

A. Offer another dose of lorazepam 0.5 mg.
B. Provide reassurance and empathic listening.
C. Refer the patient for Holter monitor and cardiac consultation.
D. Ask about symptoms of depression and suicidal ideation.

13.7   A 55-year-old man comes to your office for an evaluation. He describes an intense fear of traveling on the subway since he had a panic attack 10 years ago on a very crowded car. Now he refuses to travel on the subway and avoids many social situations with friends because of similar fears of "being trapped somewhere." What is the most likely diagnosis for this patient?

A. Social anxiety disorder.
B. Posttraumatic stress disorder.
C. Agoraphobia.
D. Specific phobia.

13.8   A 40-year-old man with a history of a specific phobia of needles comes to your office seeking treatment. He is due for routine but required blood work in 6 weeks, and he describes significant anticipatory anxiety surrounding the appointment. Which of the following pharmacological options would be most appropriate for this patient?

A. Escitalopram.
B. Lorazepam.
C. Duloxetine.
D. Buspirone.

13.9   A 7-year-old boy is brought to your office for an evaluation prompted by recent disruptive behavior in school. His teachers report frequent tantrums and yelling, daily stomachaches with trips to the nurse's office, and excessive crying that interferes with his ability to focus in class. In your office, he continually fidgets with his mother's skirt, does not direct his attention toward you, and cries when his mother steps out of the office. What is the most likely diagnosis for this patient?

A. Panic disorder.
B. Social anxiety disorder.
C. Generalized anxiety disorder.
D. Separation anxiety disorder.

13.10   A 25-year-old graduate student who is in ongoing psychotherapy with a clinical social worker is referred to you by his therapist for a pharmacological consultation. He gives a history of severe anxiety that is interfering with his ability to complete his thesis. On questioning, the young man admits to using alcohol to help control his symptoms, stating that drinking 3–4 beers is the only thing that reduces his anxiety. He is ambivalent about decreasing his current intake of alcohol because he experiences overwhelming anxiety when he does not drink. His symptoms are consistent with severe generalized anxiety, and he informs you that he was diagnosed with generalized anxiety disorder as a teenager. Which of the following medications would you recommend at this time?

A. Naltrexone.
B. Gabapentin.
C. Sertraline.
D. Lorazepam.

CHAPTER 14

Obsessive-Compulsive and Related Disorders

14.1   Which of the following psychiatric disorders has the highest rate of comorbidity with obsessive-compulsive disorder (OCD) and should be screened for when making that diagnosis?

    A. Autism spectrum disorder.
    B. Tourette's disorder.
    C. Major depressive disorder.
    D. Stereotypic movement disorder.

14.2   A 23-year-old patient with obsessive-compulsive disorder (OCD) has tried sertraline, fluoxetine, and fluvoxamine at full therapeutic dosages for 2 months each without improvement. Which of the following pharmacological augmentation strategies would be the most appropriate in this situation?

    A. Continue fluvoxamine and add bupropion.
    B. Continue fluvoxamine and add aripiprazole.
    C. Continue fluvoxamine and add imipramine.
    D. Discontinue fluvoxamine and start citalopram.

14.3   A 42-year-old divorced woman (BMI: 22 kg/m^2) presents to her psychiatrist because of overwhelming anxiety and distress about her "fat" stomach. She frequently scrutinizes her appearance in the mirror and compares herself with other women. She now wears loose-fitting clothing to hide her abdomen, and she has stopped dating because of her conviction that potential partners would be "disgusted" by this defect. Which of the following would be the most appropriate diagnosis for this patient?

    A. Body dysmorphic disorder.
    B. Bulimia nervosa.
    C. Anorexia nervosa.
    D. Social anxiety disorder.

14.4   Which of the following represents the first-line intervention for a newly diagnosed patient with obsessive-compulsive disorder (OCD)?

A. Selective serotonin reuptake inhibitors (SSRIs).
B. Clomipramine.
C. Cognitive therapy.
D. Exposure and response prevention (ERP) therapy.

14.5   Which of the following statements accurately describes a way in which hoarding disorder differs from obsessive-compulsive disorder (OCD)?

A. Unlike OCD symptoms, hoarding disorder symptoms are typically chronic and unchanging over time.
B. Whereas clinically significant distress or impairment in important areas of functioning is required for a DSM-5 diagnosis of OCD, such distress or impairment is not required for a diagnosis of hoarding disorder.
C. Behavioral therapy is typically the first-line therapy for hoarding disorder, but not for OCD.
D. OCD has a strong heritable component, but hoarding disorder does not.

14.6   Which of the following neurostimulation therapies have been approved by the U.S. Food and Drug Administration (FDA) for use in the treatment of patients with intractable obsessive-compulsive disorder (OCD)?

A. Deep brain stimulation and repetitive transcranial magnetic stimulation.
B. Electroconvulsive therapy and deep brain stimulation.
C. Vagus nerve stimulation and deep brain stimulation.
D. Electroconvulsive therapy and repetitive transcranial magnetic stimulation.

14.7   A 13-year-old girl who regularly abuses marijuana and ecstasy told her mother that she believes her hair is "being contaminated from an external force" that is "infecting her brain," and she hears an external voice commanding her to "remove the hair," because otherwise she will "die of infection." Her mother has found large amounts of hair in her daughter's shower drain. The girl is missing eyelashes and patches of hair from her head. What is the appropriate DSM-5 diagnosis?

A. Trichotillomania (hair-pulling disorder).
B. Psychotic disorder.
C. Obsessive-compulsive disorder (OCD).
D. Body dysmorphic disorder (BDD).

14.8   Which of the following treatments for excoriation disorder was found to be *ineffective* in clinical trials?

A. Lamotrigine.
B. Fluoxetine.
C. *N*-acetylcysteine.
D. Habit-reversal therapy.

CHAPTER 15

Trauma- and Stressor-Related Disorders

15.1 An *increase* in which of the following physiological parameters is typically observed following the traumatic event in patients with posttraumatic stress disorder (PTSD)?

A. Serum cortisol levels.
B. Activity of the amygdala.
C. Activity of the ventromedial prefrontal cortex.
D. Heart rate variability.

15.2 Besides the requirement that the child has experienced extremes of social neglect or insufficient care that are presumed to have led to the child's disturbed behavior, what other diagnostic criterion is shared between the DSM-5 diagnoses of reactive attachment disorder (RAD) and disinhibited social engagement disorder (DSED)?

A. Attachment of the child to putative caregivers must be absent or grossly underdeveloped.
B. The diagnosis may not be made in children with autism spectrum disorder.
C. The disturbance in the child's behavior must be evident before 5 years of age.
D. The child must have a developmental age of at least 9 months.

15.3 Which of the following options best reflects the first-line treatment approach recommended by the 2010 American Academy of Child and Adolescent Psychiatry (AACAP) *Practice Parameter for the Assessment and Treatment of Children and Adolescents With Posttraumatic Stress Disorder (PTSD)*?

A. Start trauma-focused cognitive-behavioral therapy (CBT).
B. Start fluoxetine 10 mg/day.
C. Start lorazepam 0.5 mg at bedtime.
D. Start clonidine 0.05 mg at bedtime.

15.4   One week after presenting to the emergency department immediately following a reported sexual assault by a stranger, an 18-year-old woman is referred for follow-up with a health care provider. She reports multiple symptoms consistent with psychological trauma and screens positive on a brief instrument for acute stress disorder. Which of the following early posttrauma psychotherapeutic interventions has been shown to be *unhelpful* and *possibly harmful*?

A. Psychoeducation about typical trauma responses.
B. Psychological debriefing.
C. Brief trauma-focused supportive psychotherapy.
D. Multisession cognitive-behavioral therapy (CBT).

15.5   Along with prolonged exposure therapy, which of the following psychotherapy approaches possesses the best evidence for treating posttraumatic stress disorder (PTSD) symptoms?

A. Present-centered therapy.
B. Stress inoculation training.
C. Cognitive processing therapy.
D. Group cognitive-behavioral therapy.

15.6   A 28–year old man starts seeing a therapist several months after his father died suddenly of a heart attack at age 50 years. Since the days immediately following his father's death, the patient has suffered from profound distress over the loss, experiencing daily low mood, poor concentration, and fatigue, with a feeling of "heaviness" throughout his body. His performance at work suffers, and he ultimately quits his job. He dwells on memories of his father and has had frequent thoughts of death, wishing that he and his father could be reunited, although he denies active self-harm ideation or behaviors. These symptoms persist for a year; however, there is no evident increase in irritability or anger, hypervigilance, exaggerated startle, sleep disturbance, or avoidance behavior. What is the most appropriate DSM-5 diagnosis?

A. Acute stress disorder.
B. Posttraumatic stress disorder.
C. Adjustment disorder with depressed mood.
D. Other specified trauma- and stressor-related disorder.

15.7   Which of the following is a diagnostic criterion for DSM-5 acute stress disorder (ASD)?

A. At least three dissociative symptoms must be present.
B. Nine or more symptoms from any of five categories are required.
C. Symptoms must persist for at least 2 days after the trauma.
D. Symptoms may persist for up to 2 months after the trauma.

15.8 Which of the following specific cognitive-behavioral therapies (CBTs) for post-traumatic stress disorder (PTSD) recommended in the 2017 VA/DoD *Clinical Practice Guideline for Management of Post-Traumatic Stress* has been shown to be comparable in efficacy to prolonged exposure therapy?

A. Brief eclectic psychotherapy.
B. Narrative exposure therapy.
C. Written narrative exposure therapy.
D. Eye movement desensitization and reprocessing.

CHAPTER 16

Dissociative Disorders

16.1 Which of the following is an effective treatment option for dissociative identity disorder (DID)?

A. Antidepressants.
B. Benzodiazepines.
C. Antipsychotics.
D. Psychotherapy.

16.2 In addition to psychotherapy, which of the following has shown some efficacy in the reduction of depersonalization symptoms?

A. Antidepressants.
B. Psychostimulants.
C. Naltrexone.
D. Benzodiazepines.

16.3 Which of the following is the underlying disturbance in all dissociative disorders?

A. Poor reality testing.
B. Disturbance in the integration of mental contents.
C. Deficit in memory encoding and storage.
D. Disturbance in identity formation.

16.4 What is the hallmark characteristic of dissociative identity disorder (DID)?

A. Disordered perception.
B. Poor memory integration.
C. Fragmentation of identity.
D. Multiple personalities.

16.5 Which of the following is the most common dissociative disorder?

A. Dissociative identity disorder.
B. Dissociative amnesia.

C. Depersonalization/derealization.

D. Dissociative fugue.

16.6   Which of the following disorders is characterized by an inability to recall important personal information, usually of a traumatic or stressful nature, that cannot be explained by ordinary forgetfulness in the absence of overt brain pathology or substance use?

A. Dissociative identity disorder.

B. Acute stress disorder.

C. Dissociative amnesia.

D. Depersonalization/derealization.

16.7   Which of the following types of memory is most affected in dissociative amnesia?

A. Episodic memory.

B. Short-term memory.

C. Implicit memory.

D. Procedural memory.

16.8   A 33-year-old male veteran with a history of posttraumatic stress disorder presents with memory difficulties. Two weeks ago, the patient showed up to work and found out that he had quit his job the day before, despite having no recollection of it. The patient has also found new purchases in his home that he does not recall making. He has no history of traumatic brain injury, overt brain pathology, or substance use. What is the most likely diagnosis?

A. Dissociative identity disorder.

B. Depersonalization/derealization.

C. Dissociative amnesia.

D. Dissociative fugue.

16.9   Which of the following statements regarding the *dissociative subtype of posttraumatic stress disorder* (PTSD+DS) is accurate?

A. Functional magnetic resonance imaging (fMRI) research has shown lesser amygdala connectivity to regions involved in consciousness, awareness, and proprioception in PTSD+DS patients.

B. fMRI research has shown frontal hyperactivity and limbic hypoactivity in patients with PTSD+DS during exposure to trauma-related imagery.

C. fMRI research has shown frontal hypoactivity and limbic hyperactivity in patients with PTSD+DS during exposure to trauma-related imagery.

D. fMRI research has shown lesser amygdala functional connectivity to prefrontal regions involved in emotional regulation in PTSD+DS patients.

16.10 Which of the following statements accurately describes a way in which *dissociation* and *repression* differ?

A. The organizational structure of mental contents is horizontal in dissociation and vertical in repression.
B. In dissociation, the barrier preventing access to mental contents is dynamic conflict; in repression, the barrier is amnesia.
C. Retrieval of dissociated information often can be accomplished through interpretation, whereas retrieval of repressed information usually requires hypnosis.
D. Dissociation is a response to unwanted wishes and fears, whereas repression is often elicited as a defense against trauma.

CHAPTER 17

Somatic Symptom and Related Disorders

17.1   A 36-year-old man with a history of major depressive disorder, cerebral palsy, sei-
        zures, and multiple musculoskeletal injuries is psychiatrically hospitalized fol-
        lowing a self-aborted high-lethality suicide attempt. His depressive symptoms
        and suicidality occur in the setting of chronic pain and excessive worry related to
        his muscle injuries. His intense fear of future reinjury has led him to alternately
        engage in prolonged sedentary periods and periods of obsessive adherence to
        physical therapy exercise regimens, which often result in increased pain. In addi-
        tion to major depressive disorder, which psychiatric diagnosis best explains this
        patient's symptoms?

        A. Chronic pain secondary to cerebral palsy.
        B. Somatic symptom disorder.
        C. Obsessive-compulsive disorder.
        D. Illness anxiety disorder.

17.2   A 43-year-old woman with a history of anxiety and panic attacks has long-stand-
        ing symptoms of anxiety and a 2-year history of postprandial abdominal pain and
        dyspepsia. She thinks about these gastroenterological symptoms constantly. Con-
        sequently, she avoids eating, leading to a 50-pound weight loss. She has under-
        gone significant medical workup, including endoscopy, barium esophagram,
        esophageal manometry, and computed tomography of the abdomen and pelvis, as
        well as a small bacterial overgrowth study, all of which yielded normal findings.
        Which of the following would be the best initial step in this patient's treatment?

        A. Start sertraline 25 mg/day with plans to titrate to the maximum effective dos-
           age.
        B. Order a colonoscopy and further gastroenterological workup.
        C. Confront the patient about her negative workup.
        D. Start amitriptyline 10 mg/day and initiate a course of cognitive-behavioral
           therapy.

17.3   A 31-year-old woman with a history of generalized anxiety disorder that has been well managed on escitalopram presents to your office with significant concerns about having breast cancer. She has a family history of breast cancer in her mother. The patient reports that as a child, she had the traumatic experience of watching her mother go through chemotherapy and ultimately die. She is preoccupied with the thought that she could have breast cancer, examines her breasts daily, and makes frequent visits to her primary care physician. This preoccupation has affected her ability to fully attend to the needs of her child. Which of the following diagnoses best explains this patient's presentation?

   A. Adjustment disorder.
   B. Obsessive-compulsive disorder.
   C. Illness anxiety disorder.
   D. Somatic symptom disorder.

17.4   A 24-year-old woman who has a history of one major depressive episode that responded well to fluoxetine (which was subsequently discontinued) and who is currently in a long-term relationship with a boyfriend presents to her primary care physician with overwhelming concerns about having human papillomavirus (HPV). Despite having a negative Pap smear and no other symptoms consistent with infection with the virus (e.g., condylomas, evidence of cervical cancer), the patient continually worries about the prospect of having HPV. These worries have interfered with her ability to concentrate at work and to function appropriately in her social life. Which of the following would be the best treatment option for this patient?

   A. Have the primary care physician restart fluoxetine and continue with regular Pap smear screening at the recommended intervals.
   B. Provide reassurance that the patient shows no evidence of HPV and encourage her to make a follow-up appointment if she develops new symptoms.
   C. Refer the patient for cognitive-behavioral therapy without pharmacotherapeutic intervention.
   D. Make a psychiatric referral for cognitive-behavioral therapy, schedule regular office visits to provide support, and restart fluoxetine.

17.5   A 29-year-old woman with a medical history of partial complex seizures who is currently taking phenytoin (100 mg tid) presents to the emergency room 30 minutes after an episode of loss of consciousness and generalized limb shaking. Her boyfriend, who is accompanying her, states that this episode is similar to previous seizures and occurred immediately following a heated argument between the two of them. The patient, now awake and not experiencing residual symptoms but clearly in distress, states that she remembers falling on the floor with her eyes closed and her arms moving from side to side uncontrollably. Findings from her neurological examination and computed tomography (head without intravenous contrast) are within normal limits. Which of the following would be the best initial step in this patient's treatment?

A. Increase phenytoin to 100 mg qid, as her documented history of a seizure disorder indicates that she must be having epileptiform events.

B. Obtain a neurological consultation and order video electroencephalographic (vEEG) monitoring to capture a typical seizure event.

C. Obtain a psychiatric consultation, given the likely diagnosis of conversion disorder.

D. Confront the patient with the fact that her symptoms are inconsistent with the neurological examination findings and with known physiological presentations of seizures.

17.6 A 34-year-old woman with no significant medical history develops unilateral vision loss that becomes progressively worse over the course of 6 weeks, followed by difficulty walking due to right-sided weakness of the lower extremity. After these symptoms have persisted for several months, the woman presents to the emergency department at the urging of her family members. She is admitted to the neurological service with concerns for multiple sclerosis. Extensive workup, including a brain magnetic resonance imaging scan, yields unremarkable findings. In the absence of any neurophysiological explanation or findings, a diagnosis of conversion disorder is made by the consulting psychiatrist. Following a brief psychotherapeutic intervention, the patient's symptoms rapidly improve. When discharged, she has returned to her usual state of health. Which of the following features of this patient's profile may indicate a good prognosis?

A. Prompt resolution of the conversion symptoms.

B. Slow onset of symptoms.

C. Absence of clearly identifiable stress at the time of onset.

D. Long interval between onset of symptoms and institution of treatment.

17.7 A 42-year-old homeless man presents to the hospital complaining of fever and chills. He is febrile, hypotensive, and found to have *E. Coli* bacteremia. He is promptly started on intravenous (IV) antibiotics for treatment of sepsis. After initially demonstrating significant improvement, on day 3, the patient spikes a fever and decompensates. Shortly afterward, nursing staff discover numerous syringes filled with feces in the patient's backpack, leading the clinical staff to suspect that he has been injecting himself with them. Which of the following would be the best next step in the treatment of this patient?

A. Conduct regular room searches of all patient's belongings.

B. Confront the patient so that he can admit to his deception.

C. Continue with IV antibiotics and do not inform the patient of any change in treatment plan.

D. Involve the hospital administration and schedule regular treatment team meetings.

17.8   A 29-year old man with a history of type 1 diabetes mellitus is bought to the emergency room unconscious and is found to have a blood glucose level of 36 mg/dL. He is quickly stabilized with dextrose infusions, and after recovery, states that he "must not have eaten enough today." Soon afterward, the man's girlfriend arrives and discloses to the attending physician that the patient has been intentionally self-administering too much insulin, resulting in multiple recent hypoglycemic episodes requiring hospitalization. Exasperated, the girlfriend says she cannot understand why he would be doing such a thing. Which of the following diagnoses would be most appropriate for this patient?

A. Borderline personality disorder.
B. Somatic symptom disorder.
C. Factitious disorder.
D. Malingering.

17.9   A 27-year-old homeless man with an extensive history of high-risk sexual behavior and drug use is seen by a primary care physician for flu-like symptoms. The patients tests positive for HIV. He is referred to an HIV clinic and started on appropriate antiretroviral therapy. The patient, in denial of his diagnosis, continues to engage in regular unprotected sex, is nonadherent to his medications, and escalates his use of crystal methamphetamine. Several months later, the patient self-presents to the emergency room with paranoia and evidence of methamphetamine intoxication. His laboratory testing reveals a rapidly declining CD4 count and a high HIV viral load. Which of the following diagnoses best explains this patient's presentation?

A. Illness anxiety disorder.
B. Other specified mental disorder due to another medical condition.
C. Somatic symptom disorder.
D. Psychological factors affecting other medical conditions.

17.10 A 31-year-old woman, 16 weeks pregnant, has worried constantly about congenital illness and fetal malformations ever since she first learned she was pregnant. She has undergone all routine screening, including ultrasonography at appropriate intervals, but has not felt reassured by the lack of any abnormal findings. More recently, she has begun scheduling numerous urgent appointments to see her OB/GYN even though she is not experiencing any new physical symptoms. This anxiety has also begun to interfere with her sleep and has become a source of conflict between her and her partner. Which of the following diagnoses best explains this patient's symptoms?

A. Brief somatic symptom disorder.
B. Illness anxiety disorder without excessive health-related behaviors.
C. Brief illness anxiety disorder.
D. Pseudocyesis.

CHAPTER 18

Eating and Feeding Disorders

18.1 A 28-year-old woman (BMI: 16.8 kg/m^2) presents to a medical clinic at her family's insistence. When asked, she states that she does not feel there is any problem with her weight, although she admits to symptoms of disordered eating since she was a teenager. Her initial complaint is only of feeling anxious and depressed. She is highly preoccupied with her body shape, which she has always perceived to be "too fat" (causing persistent low self-esteem), and she diets and exercises excessively in order to counterbalance episodes of overeating during which she feels "out of control." What is the most appropriate diagnosis for this patient?

A. Bulimia nervosa.
B. Anorexia nervosa.
C. Major depressive episode.
D. Avoidant/restrictive food intake disorder.

18.2 A 24-year-old woman (BMI: 19.8 kg/m^2) comes in for help with her eating habits. She reports that over the past year, she has had repeated, uncontrollable overeating episodes at least twice weekly. She desperately fears "getting too heavy," and thus has begun inducing vomiting regularly after every such episode. You inform her that while all of the following medications have some data for efficacy in treating her condition, only one is U.S. Food and Drug Administration (FDA) approved for this purpose. What is this medication?

A. Nortriptyline.
B. Topiramate.
C. Selegiline.
D. Fluoxetine.

18.3   A 26-year-old woman (BMI: 34.2 kg/m^2) presents for evaluation for bariatric surgery. She reports episodes of rapid, excessive eating multiple times a week over the past 6 months, after which she feels overly full, and ashamed about the amount she has eaten. She denies overexercising, inducing vomiting, using diuretics, or engaging in any other compensatory weight-loss behavior, but she talks at length about how closely her self-esteem depends on her body image. She is worried that she may have bulimia nervosa. You tell her that you suspect she has binge-eating disorder (BED). What is the reason for your distinction?

A. She does not have anorexia nervosa.
B. Her binge-eating episodes do not occur every day.
C. She is not engaging in inappropriate behaviors to prevent weight gain.
D. She bases her self-esteem heavily on her body image.

18.4   The parents of a 12-year-old boy (weight: <5th percentile for age) report that since his early years, their son has had a rather anxious temperament and has been an exceptionally picky eater. He tends to rigidly stick to a handful of bland food options, rejecting all others because they "taste bad" or "feel weird when I eat them." The boy understands that his weight is low, but his efforts to gain weight have been stymied by significant anxiety around eating. Which of the following diagnoses best explains this patient's eating habits and struggles with low weight?

A. Anxiety disorder.
B. Avoidant-restrictive food intake disorder.
C. Normal childhood development.
D. Autism spectrum disorder.

18.5   A 13-year-old girl (weight: <5th percentile for age) is brought in to your clinic by her parents, who are concerned about her weight and recently decreased appetite. The patient denies any concerns about weight or body image, insisting that she is simply not hungry and has never had much interest in food. She appears generally downcast, although she does speak excitedly about upping her swim schedule to twice-daily practices in order to make the varsity team at her school. You speak to her parents alone, who convey that their daughter has seemed depressed over the past few months, and who tearfully report that they recently found extensively highlighted dieting magazines under her bed, along with myriad journal entries expressing her fears of "becoming heavy" and "looking too big." What diagnosis most likely explains this patient's new habits and weight loss?

A. Bulimia nervosa.
B. Anorexia nervosa.
C. Avoidant-restrictive food intake disorder.
D. Major depressive episode.

18.6 A 30-year-old obese man (BMI 36.4 kg/m^2) reports extremely low self-esteem from perceiving his body image to be "so overweight." He has tried exercising a bit, but finds it too painful on his joints. He has been suffering from low mood, anhedonia, avolition, and anergia over the past year or so. He blames his obesity on "these out-of-control episodes where I eat a ton and then feel horrible about it afterwards," which occur regularly. Because of other medical concerns, he is most interested in first stopping or decreasing the frequency of these episodes, rather than focusing on weight loss. Given this patient's current goal, which of the following is first-line treatment?

A. Cognitive-behavioral therapy or interpersonal therapy.
B. Lisdexamfetamine.
C. A selective serotonin reuptake inhibitor (SSRI).
D. Weight loss therapy.

18.7 Which of the following is a characteristic of rumination syndrome?

A. Effortful regurgitation of food.
B. Association with developmental disability.
C. Eating of nonnutritive substances.
D. Self-worth dependent on weight.

18.8 Which of the following evidence-based treatments for binge-eating disorder (BED) reduces both binge eating and weight?

A. Cognitive-behavioral therapy.
B. Selective serotonin reuptake inhibitors (SSRIs).
C. Interpersonal psychotherapy.
D. Lisdexamfetamine.

18.9 While recommending treatment for a 14-year-old girl with anorexia nervosa, you indicate that one intervention appears to be most effective for patients in her age group. What is this intervention?

A. Residential treatment.
B. Cognitive-behavioral therapy.
C. Adolescent-focused therapy.
D. Family-based treatment.

CHAPTER 19

Elimination Disorders

19.1 A 5-year-old boy with normal development stopped wetting his bed 6 months ago; however, 2 weeks ago, he began to wet the bed again (at a frequency of twice per week) after his family moved into a new house. He does not wet himself during the daytime. He is otherwise healthy and is not being treated with any medications. What is the most likely diagnosis?

A. Primary nocturnal enuresis.
B. Secondary enuresis.
C. Diurnal enuresis.
D. Retentive encopresis.

19.2 In comparison with children who have never had a period of sustained continence lasting at least 6 months, the patient described in question 19.1 is more likely to present with which of the following additional problems?

A. Urinary tract infection.
B. Diabetes insipidus.
C. Seizure disorder.
D. Comorbid psychiatric disorders.

19.3 Which of the following is a treatment for primary nocturnal enuresis that minimizes both side effects and relapse risk after treatment cessation, and therefore should generally be tried first?

A. Bell-and-pad method.
B. Oral imipramine.
C. Nasal desmopressin.
D. Punitive response.

19.4   A 4-year-old girl who had stopped wetting her bed for a month restarted bed wetting at a frequency of twice a week for the past month. Her developmental history
has otherwise been normal, and she is on no medications. She does not seem bothered by her bed wetting, but her parents are concerned about this possible "behavioral regression" and seek clinical evaluation. A maternal history of primary
nocturnal enuresis until age 6 years is noted. Her parents are coping with her bed
wetting, but are still concerned. Which of the following options would be the
most reasonable next step?

A. Start the patient on oral imipramine.
B. Refer the patient for cystoscopy.
C. Start the patient on nasal desmopressin.
D. Watch and wait.

19.5   A 6-year-old boy had soiled his undergarments three times in the past 3 months
while at school, and once placed fecal matter in his mother's purse. The mother
has found feces in a shoe box under her son's bed. The boy does not complain of
abdominal pain or constipation, and he continues to have regular bowel movements. He eats a normal diet and has a normal weight and height for his chronological age. Which of the following would be the best next step in a comprehensive
evaluation?

A. Bowel catharsis coupled with ongoing use of laxatives.
B. Fixed daily schedule of toileting.
C. Full psychological evaluation.
D. Watch and wait.

CHAPTER 20

Sleep–Wake Disorders

20.1 The normal onset of wakefulness is associated with which of the following patterns of hormonal changes and body temperature?

A. A fall in plasma melatonin and in body temperature.
B. A rise in plasma melatonin and in body temperature.
C. A rise in plasma cortisol and in body temperature.
D. A fall in plasma cortisol and in body temperature.

20.2 Older age is associated with which of the following changes (measured by electroencephalogram) in sleep latency, rapid eye movement (REM) sleep, and N3 (delta) non–REM (NREM) "deep sleep"?

A. Increased sleep latency and N3 NREM sleep and decreased REM sleep.
B. Decreased sleep latency, REM sleep, and N3 NREM sleep.
C. Decreased sleep latency and increased REM sleep and N3 NREM sleep.
D. Increased sleep latency and decreased REM sleep and N3 NREM sleep.

20.3 Which of the following is the strongest risk factor for obstructive sleep apnea (OSA)?

A. Hypothyroidism.
B. Prader-Willi syndrome.
C. Obesity.
D. Neuromuscular disease.

20.4 Which of the following medications does not cause or worsen restless legs syndrome (RLS)?

A. Bupropion.
B. Fluoxetine.
C. Amitriptyline.
D. Lithium.

20.5 Which of the following medications does not precipitate rapid eye movement (REM) sleep behavior disorder but treats it by reducing dream enactment?

A. Amitriptyline.
B. Phenelzine.
C. Clonazepam.
D. Fluoxetine.

CHAPTER 21

Sexual Dysfunctions

21.1   Which of the following statements best describes the direct role of cyclic guanosine monophosphate (cGMP) in physiological arousal in men?

A. cGMP relaxes smooth musculature of corpora cavernosa.
B. cGMP activates guanylate cyclase to increase stimulation of nitric oxide.
C. cGMP triggers emission of semen.
D. cGMP stimulates production of dopamine by the nucleus accumbens.

21.2   Which of the following has been found to be associated with erectile dysfunction?

A. Depression.
B. Personality traits of dominance.
C. High levels of physical activity.
D. Low levels of anxiety.

21.3   A 23-year-old man with a history of asthma, active nicotine use disorder, and anxiety disorder presents to a family medicine clinic for a routine checkup. He shares with his doctor that he's just recently started having sex and is worried that he may have erectile dysfunction. He is embarrassed that "most of the time" he has difficulty obtaining and maintaining an erection. What time duration and frequency of symptoms must be present to fulfill DSM-5 diagnostic criteria for erectile disorder?

A. Duration of at least 4 weeks, occurring more than 25% of the time.
B. Duration of at least 2 months, occurring more than 50% of the time.
C. Duration of at least 6 months, occurring more than 75% of the time.
D. No specific time duration is required, but the symptoms must have occurred every time penetrative sex has been attempted.

21.4 You are conducting an in-depth interview with a 35-year-old man with a medical history of Bechet's vasculitis and carotid stenosis who is experiencing new-onset erectile dysfunction. He denies low sexual desire. Which of the following would be the best initial step in terms of workup?

A. Nerve conduction studies.
B. Doppler ultrasound.
C. Serum free testosterone.
D. Lipid profile.

21.5 Which of the following antipsychotics is associated with the lowest incidence of delayed ejaculation?

A. Ziprasidone.
B. Risperidone.
C. Haloperidol.
D. Fluphenazine.

21.6 You are weighing the risks and benefits of prescribing tadalafil for your patient, a 63-year-old man with newly diagnosed erectile disorder and a history of coronary artery disease, diabetes, and benign prostatic hyperplasia. In regard to potential drug-drug interactions, which of the following medications, when taken in combination with a phosphodiesterase type 5 (PDE-5) inhibitor, can result in catastrophic hypotension?

A. Bupropion.
B. Nitroglycerin.
C. Amantadine.
D. Mirtazapine.

21.7 A 54-year-old man with type 2 diabetes mellitus and obstructive sleep apnea (OSA) has used a phosphodiesterase type 5 (PDE-5) to treat erectile dysfunction but finds the side effects too burdensome. Which of the following would be the next best intervention that is reversible?

A. Over-the-counter preparations for erectile disorder (e.g., L-arginine).
B. Penile prosthetic devices.
C. Vacuum pump with constriction ring.
D. Oral papaverine.

21.8 In regard to the etiology of female orgasmic disorder, approximately what percentage of the variability in frequency of orgasm during sexual contact is influenced by genetics?

A. 10%.
B. 20%.
C. 30%.
D. 40%.

21.9 Which of the following therapies has been approved by the U.S. Food and Drug Administration (FDA) for use in the treatment of DSM-IV hypoactive sexual desire disorder in premenopausal women?

A. L-arginine.
B. Testosterone patches.
C. Flibanserin.
D. Bupropion.

21.10 A 28-year-old woman presents to her primary care physician reporting chronic pain during sexual activity. Upon further questioning, she describes sharp, burning pain with penetration, including when she uses masturbatory aids and even when she tries to insert a tampon. She has read about various treatments and is motivated to "try anything at this point." Which of the following would be the best initial step in treatment?

A. Vulvar hygiene (i.e., milder soap, cotton underwear).
B. Systematic desensitization using vaginal dilators.
C. Gabapentin.
D. Topical lidocaine.

CHAPTER 22

Gender Dysphoria

22.1   A 40-year-old transgender woman presents to your outpatient practice for an initial evaluation. You have never received training in gender-affirming therapy and have not had significant experience treating gender-diverse individuals. You are unsure about your ability to treat her. What is the most appropriate next step?

   A. Invite the patient's friends and family to a session to provide collateral information.
   B. Assess for a mood disorder as the cause of the patient's gender dysphoria.
   C. Provide supportive interventions to help the patient process ambivalence and cope with the stressors of being transgender.
   D. Help guide the patient toward identifying long-term as male to minimize the risk of future distress and psychiatric symptoms.

22.2   Which of the following patient presentations would meet criteria for a DSM-5 gender dysphoria diagnosis?

   A. A patient who is biologically male but portrays themselves as female for sexual pleasure.
   B. A patient who is biologically male but for the past month has felt that they identify more as female.
   C. A patient who is biologically male but has experienced distress for several years because they strongly identify as female.
   D. A patient who is biologically male but does not identify as exclusively male or female in gender.

22.3   A 30-year-old woman of transgender experience presents to the psychiatric emergency room after a suicide attempt. On evaluation, she is found to have an extensive trauma history as well as a history of suicidality, interpersonal conflicts, and mood lability. She reports ongoing daily alcohol use and frequent cannabis use. On exam, the patient is irritable and continues to endorse suicidal ideation. What is the most appropriate diagnosis?

A. Borderline personality disorder.
B. Gender dysphoria secondary to a primary mood disorder.
C. Gender identity disorder.
D. Defer diagnosis and monitor longitudinally.

22.4 Which of the following statements regarding gender-affirming surgery is *correct*?

A. Patients who receive this surgery are at high risk of regretting their decision.
B. Insurance will not pay for any of the cost of the surgery.
C. Gender-affirming surgery is associated with positive mental health outcomes.
D. A high percentage of individuals who receive gender-affirming surgical procedures opt to "de-transition" and reverse the surgery.

22.5 Which of the following statements about hormone therapy is *true*?

A. The effects of hormones will be seen immediately.
B. Most individuals who take hormones are ultimately dissatisfied with the results.
C. There are no contraindications to hormone therapy.
D. Individuals who start hormone therapy often find that strangers are beginning to recognize and address them as their self-identified gender.

22.6 A 23-year-old patient presents to your office reporting symptoms of gender dysphoria and expressing a desire to transition. The patient discloses that his mother feels negatively about his desire to do so, and states she "does not understand" why he feels this way. How would you counsel this patient and his mother?

A. Gender-diverse individuals should try to portray themselves within cultural norms of masculinity and femininity.
B. Gender is assigned and constant from birth.
C. Masculinity and femininity are largely rooted in biological factors.
D. Gender exists on a continuum rather than as an either/or dichotomy.

22.7 Which of the following statements regarding gender diversity and gender-affirming care is *correct*?

A. The number of people seeking gender-affirming treatment is decreasing.
B. Individuals living outside traditional gender stereotypes is a relatively new social occurrence which only began in the past decade.
C. Gender-diverse people are more comfortable coming out and publicly expressing who they are.
D. There is no central leading authority that defines standards for gender-affirming care.

22.8   A 34-year-old gender-diverse patient who recently started hormone treatment, presents to your office reporting anxiety, depression, and intermittent suicidality. He discloses that his family remains unsupportive of his transition and that he feels hopeless about things ever improving. He also endorses feeling uncomfortable at work, where many of his colleagues have asked probing questions. Which of the following statements represents the most accurate understanding of this patient's symptoms?

   A. The patient should stop the hormones immediately, as anxiety and depression among transgender individuals is most commonly due to side effects of hormone treatment.
   B. Hostile environments, which many gender-diverse individuals are exposed to, can lead to the development of psychiatric symptoms.
   C. Although transgender individuals are exposed to heightened discrimination, rates of suicide do not differ compared with the general population.
   D. The patient's symptoms are likely to worsen over the course of his lifetime.

CHAPTER 23

Disruptive, Impulse-Control, and Conduct Disorders

23.1 A 6-year-old boy is brought to the doctor by his parents because of his persistently disruptive behavior over the past year. The patient's teacher reports that he frequently ends up in conflict with peers and refuses to follow along with class activities. At home, he refuses to do his assigned chores and instigates arguments with his siblings over his toys every night. His parents are worried that he will not be able to graduate to the next grade because of his constant disputes with others. This child's symptom profile suggests a potential future risk of developing which of the following disorders?

A. Major depressive disorder.
B. Attention-deficit/hyperactivity disorder (ADHD).
C. Conduct disorder.
D. Antisocial personality disorder.

23.2 An 8-year-old boy is brought to the doctor by his parents because of his persistently disruptive behavior over the past year. The boy's teacher reports that he has been generally irritable during class and becomes upset easily when teachers call on him. He lashes out when he feels that his peers are playing without him. The parents recall that their son was always a happy, easy-going child until the past year; however, he has become increasingly irritable, and lately, any small matter can cause him to explode into a tantrum. This child's symptom profile suggests a potential future risk of developing which of the following disorders?

A. Major depressive disorder.
B. Attention-deficit/hyperactivity disorder (ADHD).
C. Conduct disorder.
D. Antisocial personality disorder.

23.3   A 6-year-old boy is brought to the doctor by his parents because of his persistently disruptive behavior over the past year. The boy's teacher reports that he has been provoking his peers and getting in physical altercations several times a week. At home, his parents have noticed that he frequently lashes out vindictively. Last week, he intentionally threw his mother's favorite glass vase on the floor after being chastised for not doing his chores. This child's symptom profile suggests a potential future risk of developing which of the following disorders?

A. Major depressive disorder.
B. Attention-deficit/hyperactivity disorder (ADHD).
C. Conduct disorder.
D. Antisocial personality disorder.

23.4   A 10-year-old boy is brought to clinic by his mother because of frequent aggressive outbursts. His mother says that over the last several months, her son has been fighting with peers, is openly rude to his teachers, and actively ignores his parents' rules. She reports that he goes out of his way to bully his younger sister. A week ago, he stole his classmate's backpack. The classmate began crying, but her son did not return the backpack, apologize, or appear remorseful. The mother says she is worried that if this behavior continues, her son will soon be suspended from school. Which of the following traits displayed by this patient is more suggestive of a diagnosis of conduct disorder than of oppositional defiant disorder (ODD)?

A. Frequent verbal fights with peers.
B. Ignoring rules at home and at school.
C. Bullying of a younger sibling.
D. Lack of remorse over stolen backpack.

23.6   Which of the following strategies for the treatment of school-age children with oppositional defiant disorder (ODD) has the greatest amount of empirical support?

A. Group-based treatments.
B. Combining selective serotonin reuptake inhibitors (SSRIs) with individual cognitive-behavioral therapy (CBT).
C. Combining parent management training with individual CBT.
D. Combining a mood stabilizer with parent management training.

23.7   Multiple studies in patients with intermittent explosive disorder (IED) have found functional alterations in which of the following neurotransmitters?

A. Serotonin.
B. Dopamine.
C. Glutamate.
D. GABA.

23.8 Which of the following medications has been found to be effective in reducing aggression in patients with intermittent explosive disorder (IED) and comorbid Cluster B personality disorder features?

A. Fluoxetine.
B. Divalproex.
C. Phenytoin.
D. Risperidone.

23.9 A 15-year-old boy presents to the emergency department with his mother for treatment of smoke inhalation. According to his mother, he has recently become obsessed with fire after spending a week with his uncle, a firefighter. He has told his family he hopes to become a firefighter like his uncle. He spends his free time excitedly lighting various objects on fire, including pens, kitchen utensils, and most recently his father's watch. He accidentally set off a large fire on the stove top in the kitchen this morning. The patient does not appear particularly disturbed despite his mother's exasperation. He is otherwise a pleasant teenager. He has a few friends, and he does reasonably well in school. This patient's symptom profile is suggestive of which of the following disorders?

A. Pyromania.
B. Kleptomania.
C. Bipolar disorder.
D. Psychotic disorder.

23.10 Which of the following impulse-control disorders is more common in women than in men?

A. Pyromania.
B. Kleptomania.
C. Gambling disorder.
D. Intermittent explosive disorder.

23.11 Studies in patients with kleptomania have identified primary neurotransmitter alterations in which of the following brain areas?

A. Nucleus ambiguous.
B. Amygdala.
C. Nucleus accumbens.
D. Hippocampus.

CHAPTER 24

Substance-Related and Addictive Disorders

24.1   Which of the following substances produces its effects by increasing dopamine either through direct action or through disinhibition via GABAergic receptors?

A. Cocaine.
B. Opioids.
C. Stimulants.
D. Alcohol.

24.2   A patient comes to your office and says, "I'm considering cutting down on my drinking soon. Do you have any suggestions?" According to the Transtheoretical Model of Change, what is this patient's stage of change?

A. Precontemplation.
B. Contemplation.
C. Preparation.
D. Action.

24.3   An intoxicated patient presents to the emergency department with pupillary dilation, elevated blood pressure, psychomotor agitation, chest pain, and confusion. The patient appears quite thin. Which of the following substances is most likely the cause of these symptoms?

A. Cannabis.
B. Stimulant.
C. Opioid.
D. Phencyclidine.

24.4   A patient presents to your office reporting new-onset visual and auditory hallucinations over the past 24 hours. On examination you observe a bilateral hand
tremor and psychomotor agitation. Vitals are significant for tachycardia and hypertension. This patient is most likely experiencing withdrawal from which of the
following substances?

A. Cannabis.
B. Opioid.
C. Alcohol.
D. Stimulant.

24.5   Which of the following is a partial opioid agonist that can be administered to individuals with opioid use disorder for opioid maintenance treatment?

A. Buprenorphine.
B. Benzodiazepines.
C. Clonidine.
D. Methadone.

24.6   According to epidemiological data, which of the following is the most frequently
used illicit substance in the United States and around the world?

A. MDMA (3,4-methylenedioxymethamphetamine).
B. Cocaine.
C. Cannabis.
D. LSD (lysergic acid diethylamide).

24.7   Which of the following psychosocial treatments for substance-related and addictive disorders conceptualizes relapse as a process while improving the ability to
identify its warning signs?

A. Relapse prevention.
B. Cognitive-behavioral therapy.
C. Dialectical behavior therapy.
D. Contingency management.

24.8   Which of the following is a U.S. Food and Drug Administration (FDA)–approved
medication for treating opioid use disorder?

A. Acamprosate (Campral).
B. Varenicline (Chantix).
C. Bupropion (Wellbutrin, Zyban).
D. Naltrexone (ReVia, Vivitrol).

24.9   Which of the following is an aldehyde dehydrogenase inhibitor that is used to treat alcohol use disorder?

   A. Naltrexone (ReVia).
   B. Disulfiram (Antabuse).
   C. Acamprosate (Campral).
   D. Varenicline (Chantix).

24.10 Which of the following medications or medication classes is considered the main-stay treatment for alcohol withdrawal?

   A. Thiamine.
   B. Barbiturates.
   C. Clonidine.
   D. Benzodiazepines.

CHAPTER 25

Neurocognitive Disorders

25.1 A 47-year-old man has a remote past psychiatric history of depression treated with psychotherapy. He uses marijuana occasionally. His wife brings him for a psychiatric consultation because has been showing odd behavior, with worsening over the past 5 months. He has lost interest in spending time with his children, has been making sexually inappropriate comments, and has been eating large amounts of junk food. On examination, the patient denies any recent mood or behavioral change and exhibits a flat affect and indifference to his symptoms. His memory is intact, and he has a grasp reflex on physical exam. Urine toxicology is negative. What is the most likely diagnosis?

   A. Cannabis use disorder.
   B. Mild neurocognitive disorder.
   C. Frontotemporal lobar dementia.
   D. Alzheimer's disease.

25.2 Which of the following cognitive changes can be associated with normal aging?

   A. Decreased vocabulary.
   B. Decreased general knowledge.
   C. Decreased processing speed.
   D. Increased vocabulary.

25.3 Which of the following is the most appropriate initial medication regimen for a patient newly diagnosed with Alzheimer's disease in keeping with the standard of care for patients with moderate to severe Alzheimer's disease?

   A. An atypical antipsychotic.
   B. A cholinesterase inhibitor.
   C. An N-methyl-D-aspartate (NMDA) receptor antagonist.
   D. Combination of a cholinesterase inhibitor and an NMDA receptor antagonist.

25.4 A 75-year-old woman is brought to the emergency department (ED) by her husband because she is displaying confusion. He reports that for months, his wife has been talking about seeing "little animals" in their bedroom at night, has had difficulty walking, and has experienced sleep problems. She becomes agitated in the ED and is given an oral medication to calm her down. An hour later, she develops severe rigidity and tremor in her arms, as well as worsening mental status. Which of the following medications is most likely to have caused these symptoms?

A. Haloperidol.
B. Quetiapine.
C. Lorazepam.
D. Diphenhydramine.

25.5 Ms. C is an 80-year-old woman with a diagnosis of moderate neurocognitive disorder due to Alzheimer's disease. Her son, who is her caregiver, notices that although she is usually a very pleasant person, she has become more irritable out of frustration over her increasing limitations, such as inability to drive or cook for herself. She is occasionally agitated, and last week she yelled at him and stomped her foot. She complains of feeling "down" and "bored" at times, and has some trouble sleeping, but she denies persistent depressed mood. Which of the following would be the most appropriate first-line medication treatment for Ms. C's low mood and irritability?

A. Quetiapine.
B. Sertraline.
C. Clonazepam.
D. Valproic acid.

25.6 A 72-year-old man is hospitalized for cellulitis in his leg. Psychiatry is consulted because the man's daughter is worried that her father seems "a little off." On examination, the patient is well-appearing, alert, and attentive, with a euthymic reactive affect. He denies any complaints aside from leg pain. Although he is oriented to person, place, and month and year, he is unable to remember the exact date. He is able to recall only two out of three words on a short-term memory test. The patient's daughter notes that although her father lives independently, he has "slowed down a little" over the past few months and takes "a long time" to balance his checkbook, which surprises her because he worked as an accountant until a year ago. What is the most likely diagnosis?

A. Delirium.
B. Normal aging.
C. Mild neurocognitive disorder.
D. Major neurocognitive disorder.

25.7　A 65-year-old war veteran with a history of alcohol use was witnessed by his neighbor to fall down the stairs, sustaining a head strike but no loss of consciousness. In the emergency department, the patient's computed tomography head scan results are unremarkable, but X ray reveals a fracture in the left hip. Following hip surgery, the patient receives a single dose of alprazolam for sleep. He appears confused the following day and is not oriented to place (he believes he is in a hotel) or time (he states the year as 1898). In the following days, the patient is noted to show unusual eye movements. He tells nurses stories about himself that are inconsistent with information in the chart. He does not appear to remember the names of nurses or doctors or their directions regarding his activities. Neurological exam findings are otherwise nonfocal. Based on this patient's symptom profile, which of the following is the most likely underlying diagnosis?

A. Wernicke-Korsakoff syndrome.
B. Benzodiazepine-induced delirium.
C. Dissociative amnesia.
D. Postoperative cognitive dysfunction.

25.8　Which of the following strategies for the prevention of dementia has been shown to have cognitive benefits?

A. Physical exercise.
B. Vitamin E.
C. Nonsteroidal anti-inflammatory drugs (NSAIDs).
D. Cognitive exercises.

25.9　A 60-year-old woman is diagnosed with a nonfluent aphasia after a stroke. Which of the following tasks would present the *least* amount of difficulty for this patient?

A. Writing a sentence.
B. Repeating a phrase.
C. Following simple commands.
D. Reading aloud.

25.10　Which of the following positron emission tomography (PET) scan findings is most typical of Lewy body disease?

A. Reduced temporoparietal and posterior cingulate metabolism.
B. Reduced frontotemporal metabolism.
C. Reduced temporoparietal and occipital metabolism.
D. Reduced metabolism in the area of a prior stroke.

CHAPTER 26

Personality Pathology and Personality Disorders

26.1 Studies indicate that at least what percentage of patients evaluated in clinical settings have a personality disorder?

A. 15%.
B. 30%.
C. 50%.
D. 70%.

26.2 Section III of DSM-5 includes the Alternative DSM-5 Model for Personality Disorders (AMPD). Which of the following is included as a specific personality disorder in this model?

A. Schizotypal personality disorder.
B. Schizoid personality disorder.
C. Dependent personality disorder.
D. Histrionic personality disorder.

26.3 Which of the following statements about treatment of obsessive-compulsive personality disorder (OCPD) is *true*?

A. Patients with OCPD do not usually respond to any type of treatment.
B. Patients with OCPD often respond well to serotonin reuptake inhibitor medications.
C. Patients with OCPD often respond well to dialectical behavior therapy.
D. Patients with OCPD often respond well to psychoanalytic psychotherapy or psychoanalysis.

26.4 A 32-year-old man presents to your office for a consultation after being fired from his third job in 2 years. Evaluation reveals impulsivity, separation insecurity, emotional lability, hostility, and heightened anxiety. Which of the following diagnoses is suggested by this symptom profile?

A. Antisocial personality disorder.
B. Borderline personality disorder.
C. Narcissistic personality disorder.
D. Histrionic personality disorder.

26.5 Which of the following statements about diagnosing personality disorders in children and adolescents is *true*?

A. Personality disorders are usually diagnosed by late childhood or early adolescence, as personality traits remain stable over time.
B. Personality disorders should be diagnosed sparingly in children, whose personalities are still developing, but can be diagnosed in adolescents, whose personalities are fully formed.
C. Personality disorders should be diagnosed sparingly in children and adolescents, as their personalities are still developing.
D. Personality disorders should be diagnosed only in late adulthood, to ensure stability of symptoms over time prior to diagnosis.

26.6 What is the prevalence of personality disorders in the general population?

A. 7.5%.
B. 11%.
C. 22%.
D. 31%.

26.7 Which of the following personality disorders is most prevalent in the general population?

A. Borderline personality disorder.
B. Schizotypal personality disorder.
C. Antisocial personality disorder.
D. Obsessive-compulsive personality disorder.

CHAPTER 27

Paraphilic Disorders

27.1 A colleague asks your advice concerning a 20-year-old student who told her that a man had rubbed his genitals on her arm during a crowded bus ride. Your colleague notes that she has heard of similar incidents from other students and does not recall whether this behavior has a specific name. You reply that this behavior is most consistent with which of the following?

A. Fetishistic disorder.
B. Frotteuristic disorder.
C. Sexual masochism disorder.
D. Exhibitionistic disorder.

27.2 The mother of an 18-year-old man requests a consultation. She recently discovered that her son is in a consensual sexual relationship with a 16-year-old boy. She is employed as a court reporter and says she recently heard of a similar relationship where the older partner was convicted of a crime and labeled a "sexual offender" by the state. She shares her concern that her son might be a "pedophile" and requests an evaluation for him. Which of the following would be the most appropriate response?

A. Recommend that the son receive treatment for pedophilic disorder.
B. Suggest a phallometric assessment to gather more information.
C. Suggest visual reaction time testing with the Abel Assessment for Sexual Interest.
D. Advise the mother that an 18-year-old man's consensual sexual relationship with a 16-year-old partner does not meet criteria for any psychiatric disorder.

27.3 Which of the following statements regarding biological treatments of paraphilic disorders is *true*?

A. Surgical castration (orchiectomy) should be used for violent sexual offenders, because it is a permanent and irreversible treatment.
B. No medications on the market in the United States have been approved by the U.S. Food and Drug Administration (FDA) for treating paraphilic disorders or for reducing paraphilic fantasy and behavior.

C. Hormonal treatment should be used for all sexual offenders, given that these agents are effective and risk-free.

D. Hormonal treatment should be used only for sexual offenders who meet criteria for antisocial personality disorder.

27.4 A 23-year-old man comes to your office requesting treatment. He tells you that while vacationing in Europe, he visited a public beach where some women were topless, and he became sexually aroused. He noted that the beach was crowded and that other visitors did not seem surprised that the women were topless. He is worried that something may be wrong with him, and he has "diagnosed" himself with voyeuristic disorder after doing some research on the internet. After completing a full history, you decide which of the following?

A. He meets criteria for voyeuristic disorder.
B. He has an unspecified paraphilic disorder.
C. He meets criteria for exhibitionistic disorder.
D. Sexual arousal after incidental exposure to naked people in a public area is normal.

27.5 A mother brings in her 12-year-old son for an assessment. She explains that she recently found some printouts of photographs in her son's room that showed women in various states of undress. During the interview with the son, he adamantly denies any history of sexual activity. In documenting the case afterward, which of the following would be the best working diagnosis?

A. Pedophilic disorder.
B. Fetishistic disorder.
C. Pedophilic disorder, exclusive type.
D. Normal sexual interest.

27.6 A 55-year-old woman brings her 92-year-old father in for an evaluation. She is seeking advice because her father recently exposed himself to other patients and staff at the assisted living facility where he resides. During the patient evaluation, it is clear that the man shows a pattern of progressive memory loss over the last several years. More recently, he has been having difficulty performing some self-care tasks without assistance. There is no previous history of sexual inappropriateness. The woman is distraught, fearing that her father will be evicted from the facility if he exposes himself again. Which of the following statements represents the most accurate understanding of this patient's symptoms?

A. This patient has exhibitionistic disorder.
B. This patient's behavior may be the result of cognitive impairment and not represent a paraphilic disorder.
C. This patient should be prescribed hormonal treatment to lower his testosterone level.
D. This patient should be prescribed high-dosage selective serotonin reuptake inhibitor (SSRI) treatment.

27.7 A 23-year-old man is directed to your office by his parole officer. He shares that he has been arrested several times for theft of women's undergarments. During further review of his history, he shares that he has a difficult time achieving orgasm when masturbating unless he is looking at the undergarments. After completing a review of his sexual and psychiatric history, you establish a diagnosis of which of the following?

A. Transvestic disorder.
B. Fetishistic disorder.
C. Other specified paraphilic disorder.
D. Sexual sadism disorder.

27.8 You are asked by a local prosecutor to evaluate a 25-year-old man who was arrested and charged with a criminal offense after making several obscene telephone calls to a woman. The prosecutor explains that the patient was observed masturbating while peering through the window of the woman, who was changing at the time. While taking a sexual history, the man shares that since puberty he has been making similar phone calls, where he would repeatedly curse or graphically describe sexual practices. He explains he initially found the calls quite sexually arousing but has found that making these calls, while observing the recipient either undressing or engaged in sexual activity, is even more arousing. You establish a diagnosis of which of the following?

A. Sexual sadism disorder.
B. Exhibitionistic disorder.
C. Antisocial personality disorder.
D. Telephone scatologia with voyeuristic disorder.

27.9 While attending a conference, you have the opportunity to hear a lecture by a prominent forensic psychiatrist. During the lecture, he speaks about Jeffrey Dahmer, who at age 16 reported fantasies of attacking an unsuspecting runner, then having sex with the subdued victim. You learn that Mr. Dahmer eventually was arrested for serial murder and revealed that he would often masturbate while standing over the corpses of his victims. After the lecture concludes, you decide that Mr. Dahmer most likely had which of the following disorders?

A. Sexual masochism disorder.
B. Sexual sadism disorder.
C. Voyeuristic disorder.
D. Exhibitionistic disorder.

CHAPTER 28

Precision Psychiatry

28.1 What large-scale U.S. research project was the first to bridge the gap between scientific and technological advances and their clinical applications in the field of cardiology?

A. The Precision Medicine Initiative.
B. The BRAIN Initiative.
C. The Framingham study.
D. The Research Domain Criteria (RDoC) project.

28.2 Which of the following terms refers to the relationships among brain regions in the brain at rest?

A. Default mode.
B. Functional connectivity.
C. Biotype.
D. Stratified medicine.

28.3 High functional connectivity in which of the following intrinsic circuits is hypothesized to reflect maladaptive self-referential thoughts such as rumination and worry?

A. The attention circuit.
B. The default mode circuit.
C. The salience circuit.
D. The reward circuit.

28.4 Which of the following symptoms is associated with decreased activation in the ventral striatum?

A. Anhedonia.
B. Inattention.
C. Anxiety.
D. Rumination.

28.5 For which of the following disorders is there active pursuit of translation of genetic insights into genetic tests for screening and diagnosis?

A. Major depressive disorder.
B. Autism spectrum disorder.
C. Attention-deficit/hyperactivity disorder.
D. Bipolar disorder.

28.6 Which of the following variables was found to predict better response of depression to venlafaxine in the international Study to Predict Optimized Treatment for Depression (iSPOT-D) trial?

A. Early life stress.
B. High levels of anxious arousal.
C. More responsive threat circuitry.
D. Higher body mass index.

28.7 Which of the following biomarkers confers an increased risk of agranulocytosis in patients taking clozapine?

A. The *ABCB1* gene.
B. The *SLC6AF* gene.
C. The *HLA-DQB1* gene.
D. The *HTR2A* gene.

28.8 For which of the following tools in precision psychiatry is it more challenging to define normal functioning than it is to define abnormal functioning?

A. Genomic data.
B. Neuroimaging.
C. Cognitive testing.
D. Self-report scales.

28.9 Which of the following "re-purposed" medications is currently being evaluated for the treatment of bipolar disorder as a result of findings from genome-wide association studies?

A. Isradipine.
B. D-cycloserine.
C. Glucocorticoids.
D. Cannabinoids.

28.10 Which of the following is a potential beneficial social consequence of precision psychiatry?

   A. Quick dissemination of findings by researchers.
   B. Low costs and easy adoption by clinicians.
   C. Less stigmatizing discussions about psychiatry and mental health.
   D. Decreased disparities in health outcomes.

CHAPTER 29

Psychopharmacology

29.1   Which of the following statements accurately describes how drugs that are inducers of phase I metabolism by a specific cytochrome P450 (CYP) enzyme affect levels and rate of metabolism of that CYP enzyme?

A. Inducers increase CYP enzyme levels and rate of metabolism almost immediately.
B. Inducers decrease CYP enzyme levels and rate of metabolism almost immediately.
C. Inducers increase CYP enzyme levels and rate of metabolism over a period of weeks.
D. Inducers decrease CYP enzyme levels and rate of metabolism over a period of weeks.

29.2   Which of the following statements about pharmacodynamic drug interactions is *true*?

A. Pharmacodynamic interactions occur when drugs with similar or opposing effects are combined.
B. Pharmacodynamic interactions occur when an interacting substance alters a drug's concentration due to a change in cytochrome P450 (CYP)–mediated metabolism of the substrate drug by the interacting drug.
C. Pharmacodynamic interactions occur when an interacting substance alters a drug's concentration due to a change in drug protein binding.
D. Pharmacodynamic interactions occur when an interacting substance increases or decreases the oral bioavailability of a poorly bioavailable drug.

29.3   Which of the following statements accurately describes the appropriate use of oral antipsychotics in patients with impaired enteral absorption?

A. Patients with impaired enteral absorption can absorb oral antipsychotics normally, so this is not a concern.
B. Patients with impaired enteral absorption can absorb only orally dissolvable formulations of antipsychotics normally, and these must be used in place of normal formulations.

C. Patients with impaired enteral absorption can absorb only sublingual asenapine among oral antipsychotics because of its unique property of being bucally absorbed.

D. Patients with impaired enteral absorption must have all antipsychotics provided parenterally.

29.4 Which of the following statements accurately describes the effect of lithium on the kidneys?

A. Lithium causes sodium retention and free water diuresis secondary to the syndrome of inappropriate antidiuretic hormone (SIADH) secretion.

B. Lithium causes sodium and free water retention leading to oliguria.

C. Lithium causes free water retention and salt wasting.

D. Lithium causes free water and sodium diuresis and can lead to nephrogenic diabetes insipidus.

29.5 Which of the following statements accurately describes how carbamazepine and valproate affect lamotrigine levels?

A. Carbamazepine increases lamotrigine levels, whereas valproate does not affect lamotrigine levels.

B. Valproate increases lamotrigine levels, whereas carbamazepine decreases them.

C. Valproate decreases lamotrigine levels, whereas carbamazepine increases them.

D. Valproate decreases lamotrigine levels, whereas carbamazepine does not affect lamotrigine levels.

29.6 Which of the following statements most accurately describes the contribution of bupropion dosage and formulation to seizure risk?

A. Seizure risk is dose-dependent, and the immediate-release formulation of bupropion confers higher risk than the sustained-release formulation.

B. Seizure risk is idiosyncratic and dose-independent, and the immediate-release formulation of bupropion confers higher risk than the sustained-release formulation.

C. Seizure risk is dose-dependent, and the sustained-release formulation of bupropion confers higher risk than the immediate-release formulation.

D. Seizure risk is idiosyncratic and dose-independent, and the sustained-release formulation of bupropion confers higher risk than the immediate-release formulation.

29.7   Which of the following statements accurately describes how buspirone and benzodiazepines differ in their mechanism of action and effects?

A. Both buspirone and benzodiazepines affect GABA receptors, but buspirone
does not have the potential for abuse, tolerance, and withdrawal.
B. Buspirone is a 5-HT$_{1A}$ receptor partial agonist and does not have the potential
for abuse, tolerance, and withdrawal carried by benzodiazepines, which work
on GABA receptors.
C. Buspirone and benzodiazepines both work on GABA receptors, and both
carry a potential for abuse, tolerance, and withdrawal.
D. Although buspirone and benzodiazepines both have a potential for abuse, tolerance, and withdrawal, buspirone works as a 5-HT$_{1A}$ receptor partial agonist
whereas benzodiazepines work on the GABA receptor.

29.8   Which of the following antipsychotics has the lowest placental transfer?

A. Haloperidol.
B. Quetiapine.
C. Risperidone.
D. Olanzapine.

29.9   Which of the following statements about the combined use of memantine and a
cholinesterase inhibitor for treatment of Alzheimer's disease is *true*?

A. Memantine and cholinesterase inhibitors have dangerous effects on each
other's pharmacokinetics and should never be used in tandem.
B. Although memantine and cholinesterase inhibitors are safe to use together, no
clinical benefit is obtained from their combination.
C. Memantine and cholinesterase inhibitors used in tandem can significantly
slow the disease trajectory of Alzheimer's dementia and improve functional
performance.
D. Memantine and cholinesterase inhibitors do not interact pharmacokinetically;
used in tandem, they may modestly improve cognition and behavior, but not
functional performance.

29.10   An elderly patient has been taking metoprolol as part of her cardiac regimen. Her
psychiatrist prescribes paroxetine to treat a major depressive episode. Two weeks
after starting paroxetine, the patient returns to the office reporting dizziness and
is found to be bradycardic and hypotensive. Which of the following types of pharmacokinetic drug interaction is most likely responsible for this effect?

A. Drug absorption.
B. Drug distribution.
C. Drug metabolism.
D. Drug elimination.

29.11 What is the primary mechanism of action by which first-generation antipsychotics (FGAs) are thought to exert their therapeutic effects?

A. Antagonism of dopamine D_2 receptors.
B. Partial agonism of dopamine D_2 receptors.
C. Antagonism of serotonin 5-HT_{2A} receptors.
D. Partial agonism of 5-HT_{1A} receptors.

29.12 Which of the following potential side effects of clozapine prompted implementation of a federally mandated monitoring program for patients taking this drug?

A. Seizures.
B. Myocarditis.
C. Bowel obstruction.
D. Neutropenia.

29.13 Which of the following mood stabilizers is U.S. Food and Drug Administration (FDA) approved for both acute-phase and maintenance-phase treatment of bipolar disorder?

A. Lamotrigine.
B. Lithium.
C. Carbamazepine.
D. Valproate.

29.14 The presence of which of the following signs may help distinguish serotonin syndrome from neuroleptic malignant syndrome?

A. Rigidity.
B. Hyperreflexia.
C. Hyperthermia.
D. Autonomic disturbances.

29.15 Which of the following off-label uses of antipsychotics carries a U.S. Food and Drug Administration (FDA) black-box warning for increased mortality risk?

A. Adjunctive treatment for refractory obsessive-compulsive disorder (OCD).
B. Dementia-related psychosis.
C. Severe anxiety/agitation.
D. Delirium-related psychosis.

29.16 You are choosing an initial antidepressant for a healthy young man who is not taking any other medications. The patient notes that in the past he has had trouble remembering to take his medications every day. Which of the following antidepressants would be *least* likely to produce a withdrawal syndrome if a dose was missed?

A. Fluvoxamine.
B. Fluoxetine.
C. Paroxetine.
D. Venlafaxine.

29.17 Which of the following benzodiazepines does not undergo phase I oxidative metabolism and therefore may be safer to use in patients with liver disease?

A. Lorazepam.
B. Diazepam.
C. Clonazepam.
D. Alprazolam.

29.18 A 30-year-old woman with a history of bipolar disorder who is being maintained on lithium is planning to conceive. She asks you how to proceed with psychotropics during pregnancy. Which of the following statements best describes the relationship, in women with a previous mood disorder diagnosis, of risk of relapse with mood stabilizer use in pregnancy?

A. Continuation of mood stabilizers during pregnancy increases the risk of relapse.
B. Continuation of mood stabilizers during pregnancy does not change the risk of relapse.
C. Gradual tapering of mood stabilizers decreases the risk of relapse compared with abrupt cessation.
D. Gradual tapering of mood stabilizers increases the risk of relapse compared with abrupt cessation.

29.19 Which of the following has *not* been reported as a risk associated with maternal use of selective serotonin reuptake inhibitors (SSRIs) during pregnancy?

A. Increased rate of stillbirth.
B. Increased rate of pre-eclampsia.
C. Increased rates of persistent pulmonary hypertension in the newborn.
D. Increased rate of prematurity.

Brain Stimulation Therapies

30.1   Which of the following brain stimulation therapies predated the use of psychiatric medications?

A. Focused ultrasound.
B. Electroconvulsive therapy.
C. Epidural cortical stimulation.
D. Repetitive transcranial magnetic stimulation.

30.2   A patient with obsessive-compulsive disorder (OCD) spends all his waking hours cleaning despite having received adequate trials of clomipramine, sertraline, risperidone augmentation, and exposure and response prevention therapy. What brain stimulation therapy would be a U.S. Food and Drug Administration (FDA)–cleared next step in treatment?

A. Deep brain stimulation.
B. Epidural cortical stimulation.
C. Responsive neurostimulation.
D. Transcranial direct current stimulation.

30.3   Which of the following medications can improve outcomes in electroconvulsive therapy (ECT)?

A. Diazepam.
B. Clozapine.
C. Valproic acid.
D. Theophylline.

30.4   Which of the following repetitive transcranial magnetic stimulation (rTMS) targets is most commonly used in the treatment of major depressive disorder (MDD)?

A. The ventral striatum.
B. The frontopolar cortex.
C. The orbitofrontal cortex.
D. The dorsolateral prefrontal cortex.

30.5 A moderately depressed patient had no response to trials of sertraline (at a dosage of 200 mg/day for 3 months) and venlafaxine (at a dosage of 225 mg/day for 5 months). On the basis of research evidence for efficacy, which of the following interventions would be the best next step in treatment for this patient?

A. Deep brain stimulation (DBS).
B. Vagus nerve stimulation (VNS).
C. Switching to bupropion.
D. Repetitive transcranial magnetic stimulation (rTMS).

30.6 Subsequent repetitive transcranial magnetic stimulation (rTMS) treatments are most likely contraindicated after which of the following adverse events?

A. Seizure.
B. Syncope.
C. Headache.
D. Hearing loss.

30.7 For which of the following conditions has electroconvulsive therapy (ECT) been shown to achieve better remission rates than pharmacotherapy?

A. Social anxiety disorder.
B. Major depressive disorder.
C. Obsessive-compulsive disorder.
D. Borderline personality disorder.

30.8 A severely depressed patient whose symptoms have not responded to multiple medication trials and years of evidence-based psychotherapy asks if there are any U.S. Food and Drug Administration (FDA)–cleared stimulation treatments available. Which of the following treatments has demonstrated benefit for a patient with these characteristics but is unlikely to be covered by insurance?

A. Focused ultrasound.
B. Vagus nerve stimulation.
C. Responsive neurostimulation.
D. Repetitive transcranial magnetic stimulation.

30.9 Which of the following best explains the therapeutic mechanisms of brain stimulation therapies?

A. Effects on signaling of specific receptors.
B. Effects on functional networks of brain regions.
C. Effects on psychological processes.
D. Effects on individual brain regions.

30.10 Hypofunctioning of which of the following functional networks has been implicated in multiple psychiatric disorders based on neuroimaging data?

A. Visual network.
B. Salience network.
C. Ventral frontoparietal network.
D. Primary somatosensory network.

CHAPTER 31

Brief Psychotherapies

31.1   Which of the following is considered to be the key mechanism of change in short-term psychodynamic therapy?

A. Development of insight through interpretive comments.
B. Identification of patterns in defenses and interpersonal struggles through a focus on past experiences.
C. Active provision of corrective relational experiences within sessions.
D. The fostering of altered expectations in extratherapeutic relationships and experimentation with new patterns of communication.

31.2   A 31-year-old man presents to your clinic with recurrence of major depressive disorder after a recent breakup. His current symptoms include difficulty falling asleep, amotivation, social isolation, low self-esteem, and increased anxiety about meeting new people. He has been feeling lonely yet avoids going to social events. He is frequently self-critical and fears rejection. How would a provider using interpersonal therapy (IPT) conceptualize this patient's presenting problem?

A. The patient is experiencing a role transition resulting from an acute relational stressor (breakup) that exacerbates his preexisting vulnerability to avoidance and social isolation.
B. The patient has negative automatic thoughts (e.g., "no one will like me at the party") that are reinforced by cognitive distortions (e.g., catastrophizing) and driven by a self-critical core belief (e.g., "I'm unlovable").
C. The patient avoids social events and acts guardedly in an attempt to avoid rejection and abandonment, causing others to pull away from him.
D. The patient focuses excessively on his recent breakup, blinding him to his moments of success, including other fulfilling relationships.

31.3   What would be the role of a solution-focused therapist during sessions with the patient described in question 31.2?

A. Teach the patient specific skills and coach him to use these skills during behavioral exposures.
B. Build on the patient's prior experiences of success and apply them to the current situation.

C. Collaboratively work with the patient to problem-solve ways to manage relational challenges.

D. Create powerful emotional experiences during sessions to promote change.

31.4   Which of the following brief therapies is based on the biopsychosocial diathesis-stress model?

A. Interpersonal therapy.
B. Behavioral therapy.
C. Strategic therapy.
D. Short-term psychodynamic therapy.

31.5   Which of the following brief therapies conceptualizes presenting issues as the result of interactions between patients and their contexts, rather than as intrinsic to patients?

A. Behavioral therapy.
B. Strategic therapy.
C. Short-term psychodynamic therapy.
D. Interpersonal therapy.

31.6   A 44-year-old woman presents to your clinic with ruminative anxiety, insomnia, restlessness, and low energy after having found out that her spouse is having an affair and is requesting a divorce. She has been experiencing panic attacks about twice a month since this all began. Her symptoms have improved with a selective serotonin reuptake inhibitor, but she still finds it difficult to go on dates. She says dating triggers her anxiety, and "it feels hard to trust anyone." What would the therapist's role be if this patient were undergoing behavioral therapy?

A. Use Socratic questioning to challenge the patient's belief that "no one can be trusted" and replace it with more accurate and helpful thoughts.
B. Teach the patient skills to manage her anxiety and panic, then gradually expose her to triggers to provide her with direct experiences of mastery.
C. Find the exceptions to the patient's patterns of mistrust and social isolation, then use these exceptions to help her "do more of what is already working."
D. Act as a transference object, involving him- or herself in the patient's core relationship patterns.

31.7   In which of the following types of brief psychotherapy does the therapist specifically target the patient's current relationship challenges and communication patterns?

A. Strategic therapy.
B. Solution-focused therapy.
C. Long-term psychodynamic therapy.
D. Interpersonal therapy.

31.8   How would a short-term psychodynamic therapist manage a patient's resistance?

    A. Actively challenge and confront the resistance.
    B. Offer interpretive comments about the source of the resistance.
    C. Engage with patients in a highly collaborative manner to minimize resistance.
    D. Remain focused on patient's own goals to avoid resistance.

31.9   Which of the following statements about the existing research literature on brief therapies is *true*?

    A. Short-term psychodynamic and interpersonal therapies have been formally evaluated in only a limited number of studies.
    B. Study findings argue against providing maintenance sessions after a course of brief therapy.
    C. Research examining the dose-effect relationship in psychotherapy indicates that approximately 20% of patients experience significant improvement within 18–26 sessions of therapy.
    D. Studies suggest that patients with more chronic problems may not be appropriate for brief therapies.

31.10   Research findings highlight the importance of careful patient selection in the conduct of brief therapy. Which of the following patient characteristics would be predictive of a good outcome in time-limited therapy?

    A. Patients with weak social supports.
    B. Patients with simpler, less severe presenting problems.
    C. Patients with lower interpersonal functioning.
    D. Patients currently in the contemplative stage of change.

31.11   Which of the following brief therapies is generally the shortest in duration?

    A. Behavioral therapy.
    B. Interpersonal therapy.
    C. Solution-focused therapy.
    D. Strategic therapy.

CHAPTER 32

Psychodynamic Psychotherapy

32.1 The contemporary psychodynamic therapist is most likely to identify dominant issues from which of the following areas of patient focus?

A. Chief complaints.
B. Treatment satisfaction.
C. Psychiatric symptoms.
D. Early childhood experiences.

32.2 Which of the following represents an *expressive* psychodynamic intervention?

A. Advice.
B. Psychoeducation.
C. Empathic validation.
D. Clarification.

32.3 The most support for the efficacy of psychodynamic therapy is established in the treatment of which of the following disorders?

A. Bulimia nervosa.
B. Delusional disorder.
C. Avoidant personality disorder.
D. Obsessive-compulsive disorder.

32.4 Which of the following potential positive outcomes of psychodynamic therapy represents a *structural* change?

A. Improved interpersonal functioning.
B. Improved capacity for mentalization.
C. Improved self-esteem.
D. Improved management of aggression.

32.5 Which of the following change processes has demonstrated relatively consistent clinical utility and positive outcomes?

    A. Affective exploration.
    B. High-frequency interpretations.
    C. Minimal use of supportive interventions.
    D. A focus on isolated personal themes.

32.6 Which of the following statements regarding severe personality pathology and psychodynamic psychotherapy is *true*?

    A. Severe personality disorders are a contraindication to treatment with dynamic therapy.
    B. Longer dynamic treatments are preferred in this population.
    C. Transference work should ideally be minimized in this population.
    D. Countertransference work should ideally be minimized in this population.

CHAPTER 33

Cognitive-Behavioral Therapy

33.1 Which of the following patient interventions is a primary focus of cognitive-behavioral therapy (CBT) (as opposed to psychodynamic psychotherapy or interpersonal therapy)?

A. Cognitive appraisal and emotional responses to external events.
B. Relationship with the therapist.
C. Wishes, dreams, and fantasies.
D. Interpersonal communication patterns.

33.2 Which of the following types of pathological information processing is characteristic of both anxiety disorders and depressive disorder?

A. Fears of harm or danger.
B. Impaired performance on tasks requiring effort or abstract thinking.
C. Demoralization.
D. Overestimates of risk in situations.

33.3 Which of the following is one of the most frequently used techniques for identifying and modifying problematic cognitions in cognitive-behavioral therapy (CBT)?

A. Confrontation.
B. Direct guidance.
C. Socratic questioning.
D. Empathic validation.

33.4 Which of the following is one of the main behavioral techniques employed in cognitive-behavioral therapy (CBT) for anxiety disorders?

A. Examining the evidence.
B. Exposure.
C. Thought recording.
D. Cognitive rehearsal.

33.5 Research evidence supports use of cognitive-behavioral therapy (CBT) as a primary (first-line) intervention for which of the following disorders?

A. Schizophrenia.
B. Eating disorders.
C. Bipolar disorders.
D. Depression with psychotic features.

CHAPTER 34

Supportive Psychotherapy

34.1 Which of the following statements best describes the organizing goals of supportive psychotherapy?

A. To provide severely impaired patients with interventions aimed at improving ego functions, day-to-day coping, and self-esteem.
B. To change the patient's underlying personality structure.
C. To develop a supportive relationship between the therapist and the patient.
D. To utilize specifically definable techniques or interventions that are unique within the fields of psychiatry and psychology.

34.2 For which of the following diagnoses would supportive psychotherapy be contraindicated?

A. Acute bereavement.
B. Late-stage dementia.
C. Substance use disorder.
D. Pancreatic cancer.

34.3 Which of the following patients would be most likely to have a good outcome from supportive psychotherapy?

A. A patient with new-onset delirium secondary to electrolyte abnormalities.
B. A patient with an adjustment disorder after the loss of a loved one.
C. A patient with unremitting panic disorder and agoraphobia.
D. A patient with obsessive-compulsive disorder and contamination phobias.

34.4 Which of the following is one of the key strategies of supportive psychotherapy?

A. Promoting patient self-esteem.
B. Working primarily on conflict and instinctual issues with a focus on the past.
C. Self-disclosing to the patient in the interest of the therapist.
D. Questioning and directly confronting patient defenses.

34.5   Which of the following statements accurately describes the difference between a structural case formulation and a dynamic case formulation?

A. A *structural case formulation* attempts to capture the relatively fixed characteristics of an individual's personality, which are understood within a functional context; a *dynamic case formulation* focuses on conflicting wishes, needs, or feelings and on their meanings.

B. A *structural case formulation* focuses on conflicting wishes, needs, or feelings and on their meanings; a *dynamic case formulation* involves exploration of early development and life events that may help to explain an individual's current situation.

C. A *structural case formulation* addresses an individual's underlying psychological structure and the content of his or her thoughts; a *dynamic case formulation* attempts to capture the relatively fixed characteristics of an individual's personality, which are understood within a functional context.

D. A *structural case formulation* involves exploration of early development and life events that may help to explain an individual's current situation; a *dynamic case formulation* addresses an individual's underlying psychological structure and the content of his or her thoughts.

34.6   Which of the following best describes the communication style used in supportive psychotherapy?

A. There is a give-and-take exchange between patient and therapist.
B. Therapists typically ask patients challenging questions.
C. Patients are permitted extended periods of silence to reflect on their experiences.
D. Therapists often start questions with "Why."

34.7   Which of the following quoted therapist statements is an example of *clarification* in supportive psychotherapy?

A. "Most people with your condition improve."
B. "It's good that you can be so considerate of other people."
C. "Could it be that you got into the argument with them to avoid asking them for money?"
D. "It sounds like a lot of things are troubling you and you are feeling overwhelmed."

34.8   Historically, the components of the therapeutic relationship have been considered to be the transference–countertransference configuration, the real relationship, and the therapeutic alliance. Which of the following statements best describes the roles of transference and the real relationship in supportive psychotherapy?

A. In supportive psychotherapy, the therapist explores positive feelings and thoughts in the transference.
B. The real relationship is not a focus in supportive psychotherapy.

C. In supportive psychotherapy, the therapist must investigate negative transference reactions.

D. Supportive psychotherapy places more emphasis on the transference than on the real relationship.

34.9 Which of the following is a therapeutic intervention used in supportive psychotherapy?

A. Critical reflection.

B. Interpretation focused on the patient's past relationships.

C. Contradiction.

D. Exploration and interpretation of transference phenomena.

34.10 Which of the following statements accurately describes the role of the therapeutic alliance in supportive psychotherapy?

A. The therapeutic alliance tends to be more stable on the supportive psychotherapy side of the continuum.

B. The therapeutic alliance is a static process between patient and therapist.

C. The therapeutic alliance is a component of the transference.

D. Patients with limited capacity to form a therapeutic alliance should not receive supportive psychotherapy.

CHAPTER 35

Mentalizing
in Psychotherapy

35.1 Which of the following statements best characterizes implicit mentalizing (as opposed to explicit mentalizing)?

A. Implicit mentalizing is relatively automatic, procedural, and nonconscious.
B. Implicit mentalizing usually takes the form of a narrative.
C. Implicit mentalizing can be as simple as putting feelings into words.
D. Implicit mentalizing can be used to learn from past mistakes in the service of interacting more effectively in the future.

35.2 Which of the following is a characteristic of *external* mentalizing (as opposed to internal mentalizing)?

A. Intellectualizing.
B. Feeling emotions.
C. Responsiveness to observable aspects of behavior.
D. Requiring inference and imagination to understand the mental states conjoined with external behavior.

35.3 Which of the following is considered a hallmark of skillful mentalizing?

A. Focusing primarily on assumptions about others.
B. Mentalizing with high confidence in the accuracy of one's perceptions and interpretations of others.
C. Linking external behavior with internal mental states.
D. Mentalizing with the goal of benignly controlling others' thoughts or actions.

35.4 Mentalizing overlaps in some respects with *mindfulness*, a concept that has received considerable attention in recent years. Which of the following characteristics is exclusive to *mentalizing* and is not a focus of mindfulness?

A. Reflection and interpretation.
B. Problem-centered attention.
C. Attention to mental states in oneself or others.
D. A nonjudgmental attitude of acceptance, compassion, and curiosity.

35.5 Which of the following actions is characteristic of *mentalizing* (as opposed to *pre-mentalizing* or *nonmentalizing* modes of experience)?

A. Living in a mental state unmoored from reality.
B. Expressing mental states in goal-directed action.
C. Equating one's own mental states with reality.
D. Reflecting on the meaning of mental states.

35.6 In mentalization-based therapy for a patient in a state of *psychic equivalence*, which of the following would be the best initial approach for the therapist?

A. Point out logical inconsistencies in the patient's perspective.
B. Encourage the patient to imagine him- or herself as another person.
C. Attempt to see the situation through the eyes of the patient.
D. Introduce alternative perspectives to the patient.

35.7 Which of the following statements about the mentalizing approach is *true*?

A. Mentalizing is highly structured.
B. Mentalizing should be based on an explicit formulation.
C. Mentalizing is prescriptive.
D. Mentalizing is inherently freewheeling.

35.8 Which of the following statements best describes the relation of mentalizing to other therapeutic modalities?

A. Mentalizing is inherently limited in its scope of application.
B. Mentalizing is an integrative approach to psychotherapy.
C. Mentalizing is a new and groundbreaking therapeutic approach.
D. Because of its highly specialized techniques, mentalizing is compatible with only a few other therapies.

35.9 To which of the following patient problems would mentalizing-based treatment (MBT) be most applicable?

A. Deficits in social cognition in individuals with borderline personality disorder (BPD).
B. Psychotic disorders.

C. Problems in communication in individuals with autism spectrum disorder (ASD).

D. Impulsivity in individuals with attention-deficit/hyperactivity disorder (ADHD).

35.10 Which of the following is an outcome of trauma during the formation of attachment relationships?

A. Infant distress when separated from parent in the Strange Situation, followed by quick recovery when reunited with parent.

B. Secure attachment as measured in the Strange Situation.

C. Increased capacity for mentalization in adulthood.

D. Intergenerational transmission of impaired mentalizing capacity.

35.11 Randomized controlled trials examining the effectiveness of mentalization-based therapy (MBT) for treating borderline personality disorder (BPD) have reported which of the following findings?

A. Increased difficulty in interpersonal functioning.

B. Increased emergency room visits.

C. Decreased impulsivity and suicide attempts.

D. Increased inpatient psychiatric admissions.

CHAPTER 36

Hybrid Practitioners and Digital Treatments

36.1   Which of the following patient-referral options is available to a psychiatrist working in a traditional practice setting?

A. Arrange an in-person office consultation at a specialist psychiatry clinic.
B. Arrange an asynchronous telepsychiatry consultation for clinic or home.
C. Arrange a synchronous telepsychiatry consultation for clinic or home.
D. Arrange for a patient to be seen by a psychiatrist in the primary care clinic.

36.2   Which of the following is reduced in online psychotherapy?

A. Anxiety.
B. Safety in the virtual space.
C. Sense of self-control.
D. Option to engage.

36.3   A primary care clinic keeps track of patients who are maintained on antipsychotics. This patient roster is reviewed at regular intervals by a psychiatrist to ensure that appropriate metabolic screening is being completed. This arrangement is an example of which of the following clinical services?

A. E-consultations.
B. Direct consultation.
C. Evidence-based clinical reviews.
D. Patient registries.

36.4   Which of the following technology-based approaches has been reported to be potentially more effective than in-person treatment of children with attention-deficit/hyperactivity disorder and patients with posttraumatic stress disorder?

A. Telephony.
B. E-mail or secure messaging.

C. Videoconferencing.

D. Web-based applications.

36.5 Which of the following emergent technologies is used in mobile phones to detect the position of the device and estimate the activity of the user?

A. Virtual reality.

B. Virtual worlds.

C. GPS.

D. Social networking apps.

36.6 A patient wears wraparound three-dimensional goggles and body sensors while being immersed in a computer-generated environment for pain management. This scenario is an example of which of the following emergent technologies?

A. Virtual reality.

B. Virtual worlds.

C. GPS.

D. Social networking apps.

36.7 Which of the following technologies is routinely used by psychiatrists for clinical, administrative, and reimbursement purposes?

A. Videoconferencing.

B. Web-based applications.

C. Mobile devices.

D. Electronic medical records.

36.8 Asynchronous telepsychiatry consultations, while possibly involving no direct patient contact, may allow psychiatrists to potentially provide care for many more patients. In which of the following populations might psychiatrists find the largest number of potential patients for telepsychiatry?

A. Primary care patients.

B. Psychotic patients.

C. Highly anxious patients.

D. Patients on the autism spectrum.

36.9 Which of the following scenarios would constitute the only absolute contraindication to seeing a patient via videoconferencing?

A. The patient is engaging in behavior dangerous to him- or herself or others at the time of the interview.

B. The patient has paranoid ruminations about televisions or radios.

C. The patient suffers from severe anxiety that prevents him or her from leaving home.

D. The patient has a significant trauma history involving an "authority figure."

36.10 Which of the following types of clinical services uses "less intensive and less expensive interventions at the outset and gradually adds more intensive services if patients fail to improve"?

A. Evidence-based clinical reviews.
B. Patient registries.
C. Stepped models of care.
D. Online provider to online provider consultations.

CHAPTER 37

Complementary
and Integrative Psychiatry

37.1 A 30-year-old woman presents to your office to discuss pharmacological options for treatment of major depressive disorder (MDD). After discussion of the benefits, side effects, and alternatives to antidepressant medications, she asks if there are any vitamins or nutrients she could take instead. Which of the following nutrients has the strongest evidence of effectiveness as monotherapy for MDD?

A. Vitamin D$_3$.
B. L-methylfolate.
C. Vitamin B$_{12}$.
D. S-adenosylmethionine (SAMe).

37.2 A 70-year-old man diagnosed with major depressive disorder (MDD) with a seasonal pattern is still feeling depressed despite taking sertraline 200 mg/day for the past 3 months, over the winter. He follows a strict vegan diet. Although he would prefer to stop the sertraline, he is willing to continue taking it if advised. He asks whether there are any vitamins or nutrients he can take to supplement his treatment. Which of the following would be the best next step in managing this patient's depression?

A. Recommend that he take a daily multivitamin tablet containing vitamin B$_{12}$ and folic acid.
B. Check levels of vitamin B$_{12}$, folate, and 25-hydroxyvitamin D.
C. Recommend that he take vitamin D$_3$ at a dosage of 2,000 IU/day.
D. Recommend that he discontinue the sertraline and start L-methylfolate.

37.3 Which of the following statements regarding vitamin B$_{12}$ is *true*?

A. Adverse effects of vitamin B$_{12}$ have been noted at dosages of 8 mg/day.
B. The ability to absorb vitamin B$_{12}$ remains strong throughout the life span.
C. Supplementation with vitamin B$_{12}$ may help preserve cognitive function in geriatric patients.
D. There is evidence that vitamin B$_{12}$ can augment antidepressant treatment regardless of whether there is a deficiency.

37.4 Which of the following statements about omega-3 fatty acids is *true*?

A. α-Linoleic acid (ALA) is the omega-3 fatty acid best used by the body.
B. Fishy aftertaste can be avoided by freezing capsules before consuming.
C. Dosages above 3 g/day are optimal.
D. Docosahexaenoic acid (DHA) appears to have the main antidepressant effect.

37.5 A 75-year-old woman with a history of mild cognitive impairment and depression comes to your office stating that since she started taking a supplement, she has noticed improved mood and memory function, but has also noted foul-smelling urine and constipation. Which of the following supplements is the patient most likely taking?

A. Acetyl-L-carnitine.
B. Omega-3 fatty acids.
C. Kava (kava-kava, *Piper methysticum*).
D. St. John's wort (*Hypericum perforatum*).

37.6 A 37-year-old man returns to your office with increased difficulty maintaining an erection and decreased sexual performance since starting a selective serotonin reuptake inhibitor (SSRI) for anxiety. He also takes a benzodiazepine. Which adaptogenic herb is safe for this patient and may be used to mitigate symptoms of sexual dysfunction?

A. St. John's wort (*Hypericum perforatum*).
B. Maca (*Lepidium meyenii*).
C. American ginseng (*Panax quinquefolius*, Xi Yang Shen).
D. Kava (kava-kava, *Piper methysticum*).

37.7 A 29-year-old woman with schizophrenia and HIV (for which she is currently taking antiretroviral medication) asks if there are any natural treatments that she could add to her current antipsychotic regimen to help with her symptoms of psychosis, which include hallucinations and social withdrawal. Which of the following interventions may be helpful for this patient's symptoms?

A. Mindfulness.
B. Cannabis sativa.
C. Schizandra (*Schisandra chinensis*).
D. St. John's wort (*Hypericum perforatum*).

37.8 A 60-year-old man presents with depression. He has a history of hypertension and diabetes, and had a successful renal transplant several years ago. He takes maintenance immunosuppressive therapy consisting of cyclosporine, azathioprine, and prednisone. He is also takes an anticoagulant as he has paroxysmal atrial fibrillation. He does not want to add to his already long list of medications, and asks you about "natural products." Which of the following herbs is most likely to be safe and effective in treating this patient's depression?

A. St. John's wort (*Hypericum perforatum*).
B. Kava.
C. Arctic root (*Rhodiola rosea*).
D. Ginkgo biloba.

37.9   A 36-year-old pregnant woman presents with several weeks of low mood, poor sleep, decreased motivation, and decreased concentration. She has no history of manic symptoms. She does not want to take a conventional antidepressant, and is interested in taking an alternative treatment for her symptoms. Which of the following may be as effective as an antidepressant and would be safe for this patient?

A. s-adenosylmethionine (SAMe).
B. Ashwagandha (*Withania somnifera*).
C. Saffron (*Crocus sativus*).
D. St. John's wort (*Hypericum perforatum*).

37.10   Which of the following complementary and alternative treatments is considered to be a safe and possibly effective treatment for bipolar disorder?

A. Ashwagandha (*Withania somnifera*).
B. s-adenosylmethionine (SAMe).
C. Arctic root (*Rhodiola rosea*).
D. St. John's wort (*Hypericum perforatum*).

37.11   Which of the following effects can be produced by slow-breathing practices?

A. Decreased heart rate variability.
B. Decreased underactivity in prefrontal emotion regulatory centers.
C. Decreased levels of GABA (γ-aminobutyric acid).
D. Reduced overactivity in the amygdala.

37.12   An 81-year-old man with arthritis and a pacemaker presents with several years of gradually worsening memory, and a declining ability to care for himself. He is evaluated and subsequently diagnosed with major neurocognitive disorder. Which of the following interventions would be safe for this patient and has shown benefit for maintaining a stable clinical dementia rating over 5 months?

A. Qigong.
B. Yoga.
C. Cranial electrotherapy stimulation.
D. Vitamin E.

CHAPTER 38

Integrated and Collaborative Care

38.1 A 79-year-old woman with high cholesterol, diabetes complicated by retinopathy, peripheral arterial disease, and schizoaffective disorder lives in a rural area without public transportation and with limited numbers of mental health providers. Which of the following integrated treatment modalities would help this patient receive the care she needs?

    A. Colocated care.
    B. Collaborative care.
    C. Telepsychiatry.
    D. Medical care for psychiatric patients.

38.2 Which of the following collaborative care principles refers to an approach focused on a defined population, such as all individuals served by a particular primary care clinic, medical center, or health care system?

    A. Population-based care.
    B. Evidence-based care.
    C. Measurement-based treatment to target.
    D. Accountability.

38.3 Which of the following is an appropriate method for tracking progress toward a measurable treatment goal in the collaborative care model?

    A. Recording an increase in a patient's fluoxetine dosage from 20 mg/day to 60 mg/day.
    B. Recording a patient's "no-show" rate over a 3-month period.
    C. Reassessing a patient's symptom ratings on the Patient Health Questionnaire–9 (PHQ-9) during each appointment.
    D. Reviewing utilization of new coping skills with a patient.

38.4 In the collaborative care model, which of the following roles is primarily the responsibility of the psychiatrist?

A. Serving as the first contact for the patient.
B. Managing the details of patient care.
C. Providing brief, evidence-based psychotherapies.
D. Providing indirect consultation and recommendations for patients who are not improving.

38.5 Which of the following options describes an appropriate role for the psychiatrist in the collaborative care model?

A. Teaching the team how to identify hypomania in geriatric patients.
B. Spending 3 days per week providing short-term interpersonal therapy to patients in an outpatient setting.
C. Routinely working alongside the primary care provider during appointments to examine severely ill patients.
D. Exclusively providing direct, in-person patient care.

38.6 In the United States, approximately what percentage of people with psychiatric disorders see any mental health specialist?

A. 21%.
B. 2%.
C. 30%.
D. 65%.

38.7 Which of the following is a population-based model that uses systematic mental health screening of the clinic or health system population to identify patients for further diagnostic evaluation and evidence-based treatment?

A. Collaborative care model.
B. Colocated care model.
C. Telepsychiatry model.
D. Medical care for psychiatric patients model.

38.8 Which of the following terms refers to an approach that brings together mental health care and primary medical care to increase access to care and to improve mental health and medical outcomes for patients in a cost-effective manner?

A. Telepsychiatry.
B. Collaborative care.
C. Colocated care.
D. Integrated care.

38.9 Which of the following care models delivers treatment through a team consisting of the patient, a primary care provider, a care manager, and a psychiatric consultant?

A. Collaborative care model.
B. Telepsychiatry model.
C. Medical care for psychiatric patients model.
D. Colocated care model.

38.10 In the collaborative care model, which of the following practitioners is responsible for delivering evidence-based brief psychotherapy interventions to patients?

A. Care manager or behavioral health care provider.
B. Primary care provider.
C. Psychiatric consultant.
D. Any member of the team may be assigned responsibility for providing brief psychotherapy to patients.

38.11 Each of the various models of care delivery has advantages and limitations. Which of the following options describes a limitation of the *colocated care model*?

A. The requirement for specialized equipment.
B. The need for medical care providers to work within the mental health care setting.
C. The restriction that only patients who are specifically referred can be treated.
D. The requirement for many changes in the way providers usually practice.

38.12 A 24-year-old man with a medical history significant for schizophrenia is being followed by his primary care provider (PCP) at a collaborative care clinic. Over the past 4 months, the patient has had two separate episodes of increased paranoia, auditory hallucinations, and disorganized thinking that impaired his ability to maintain safety in the community. These episodes required treatment in an inpatient psychiatric unit. The PCP notes that the patient was most recently discharged on paliperidone 6 mg daily, quetiapine 150 mg at night, trazodone 100 mg at night, alprazolam 1 mg twice daily as needed for anxiety, benztropine 1 mg twice daily, and valproic acid 1,000 mg at night. Which of the following would be the most appropriate next step for the PCP?

A. Have the consulting psychiatrist schedule a series of in-person visits to examine the patient and provide treatment recommendations.
B. Have the care manager refer the patient to a specialty mental health care service and continue following the patient until care is established.
C. Schedule a "curbside consult" with the psychiatrist to discuss adjustment of the patient's current medication regimen.
D. Ask the care manager to increase the frequency of visits for psychodynamic therapy.

38.13 In which model of care would the psychiatric consultant most often provide indirect consultation to the patient without seeing the patient?

A. Collaborative care model.
B. Telepsychiatry model.
C. Medical care for psychiatric patients model.
D. Colocated care model.

CHAPTER 39

Standardized Assessment and Measurement-Based Care

39.1 Which of the following options correctly defines the term *measurement-based care*?

A. The process of making decisions by formulating, testing, and refining hypotheses based on clinical information that is often incomplete or inconsistent, often in the context of very brief clinical encounters.

B. The ongoing administration of validated measures throughout the course of treatment to track patient progress, and the use of those data to inform clinicians' and patients' decisions about clinical interventions.

C. The use of validated brief tools to enable improved detection and more accurate diagnosis of mental disorders in primary care.

D. The use of tests of behavior that assess people by rating their performance on standardized tasks.

39.2 What type of measure is the Alcohol Use Disorders Identification Test—Consumption (AUDIT-C)?

A. Broad symptom measure.

B. Scale of functioning or quality of life.

C. Screening tool.

D. Comprehensive self-report assessment battery.

39.3 A college student sees a psychiatrist for academic difficulties after minimal improvement with the help of an academic tutor. After assessment, the psychiatrist gives a diagnosis of attention-deficit/hyperactivity disorder (ADHD) and rules out other psychiatric disorders. After 3 months on a stimulant with improvements in attention, the student reports ongoing difficulty with testing performance and executive functioning tasks. What type of assessment would be most appropriate as a next step in differential diagnosis and treatment planning?

A. A comprehensive neuropsychiatric assessment using standardized measures.
B. A self-assessment personality questionnaire such as the Minnesota Multiphasic Personality Inventory.
C. A structured clinical interview such as the Mini International Neuropsychiatric Interview.
D. A projective personality test such as the Rorschach.

39.4   Which of the following statements describes a test that has high *validity*?

A. A test that yields consistent scores when administered to the same person under similar circumstances.
B. A test for which two interviewers assessing the same person arrive at similar results.
C. A test that measures the trait it is intended to measure.
D. A test that shows the same result on two different occasions.

39.5   For which of the following clinical purposes is a *structured interview* most useful?

A. Enabling detection of cognitive deficits and strengths that might not otherwise be immediately apparent.
B. Identification of people who may potentially have a psychiatric disorder who should be referred for further assessment.
C. Identification of stigmatizing problems such as substance use.
D. Informing treatment planning and differential diagnosis in complicated cases.

39.6   Which of the following standardized measures is designed to be administered by professionals in the primary care setting?

A. Morisky Medication Adherence Scale.
B. 24-Item Behavior and Symptom Identification Scale (BASIS-24).
C. Two-item Patient Health Questionnaire (PHQ-2).
D. Halstead-Reitan.

39.7   A 65-year-old man with depression has been your patient for 6 months and has tolerated a selective serotonin reuptake inhibitor (SSRI). As you review symptoms with the patient, you notice that he shows marked improvements in many of his depressive symptoms. When you comment on this, he says dejectedly, "I'm glad your checklist thinks I'm better." Which of the following standardized measures would be most appropriate as a next step?

A. Nine-item Patient Health Questionnaire (PHQ-9).
B. Generalized Anxiety Disorder seven-item scale (GAD-7).
C. 32-Item Behavior and Symptom Identification Scale (BASIS-32).
D. Alcohol Use Disorders Identification Test—Consumption (AUDIT-C).

39.8   Which of the following is considered a best practice for measurement-based care (MBC)?

A. Introduce MBC as a tool for increasing patients' control over their own treatment.
B. Streamline assessment protocols by limiting patient feedback.
C. Rely on standardized outcome data rather than resorting to collaborative decision making.
D. Provide concrete evidence to patients when they disagree with an assessment.

39.9   Which of the following statements best describes the function of actigraphy?

A. Recording of outcome data prior to appointments.
B. Detection of behavioral changes and disruptions in sleep that patients may not be aware of at the time.
C. Detection of changes in mood, thought process, and suicidality from social media postings and other patient writings.
D. Detection of mood or psychosis episodes on mobile phones prior to patients' or providers' awareness of a pending episode.

39.10 Which of the following changes is likely to result from implementation of Electronic Medical Record–embedded Measurement-Based Care (EMR-embedded MBC)?

A. Increased time spent in session to collect data.
B. Expanded need for additional data entry.
C. Improved overall quality of mental health care.
D. Reduced time waste during patient–provider discussions.

CHAPTER 40

Women

40.1 How do the presentations of women diagnosed with schizophrenia differ from those of men diagnosed with schizophrenia?

A. Women tend to have worse premorbid functioning.
B. Women are less likely to have a family history of schizophrenia.
C. Women are diagnosed earlier.
D. Women tend to have more mood symptoms.

40.2 In what phase of the menstrual cycle do the symptoms of premenstrual dysphoric disorder (PMDD) begin?

A. Early luteal phase.
B. Late luteal phase.
C. Early follicular phase.
D. Late follicular phase.

40.3 A 32-year-old woman is attempting to conceive, but wants to continue her antidepressant medications for depression and anxiety. Which of the following medications would pose the greatest risk of congenital malformation?

A. Paroxetine.
B. Fluoxetine.
C. Escitalopram.
D. Sertraline.

40.4 A patient who was started on sertraline 100 mg/day during the third trimester of her first pregnancy delivers a full-term baby. The newborn is found to be irritable and jittery, with poor muscle tone and a weak cry. Which of the following is the most likely diagnosis for this infant?

A. Cardiac malformation.
B. Persistent pulmonary hypertension of the newborn.
C. Neonatal adaptation syndrome.
D. Small-for-gestational-age infant.

40.5   A 25-year-old woman with bipolar disorder who was recently hospitalized for a severe manic episode and stabilized on valproate is interested in trying to conceive. What is the best initial recommendation for her mood stabilizer?

A. Discontinue valproate.
B. Continue valproate.
C. Cross-taper to carbamazepine.
D. Cross-taper to lithium.

40.6   Which of the following substances, when used by a mother during pregnancy, can cause a lifelong disabling condition in the offspring?

A. Alcohol.
B. Marijuana.
C. Cocaine.
D. Opioids.

40.7   You are following a 23-year-old woman with a history of major depressive disorder who gave birth 4 months ago. Her husband calls you with some concerns. He says that over the past few months, she has become increasingly isolative and irritable, taking poor care of herself and sleeping only 3–4 hours each night, and he has noticed that she has recently begun speaking to herself and making less sense. What is your initial recommendation?

A. Send a prescription for an antipsychotic and say you will follow up tomorrow.
B. Assess the patient over the phone and then schedule an office visit for the coming week.
C. Instruct the husband to bring the patient to your office tomorrow.
D. Tell the husband to bring the patient to the emergency room immediately for a full medical and psychiatric evaluation.

40.8   Which of the following is the most common postpartum psychopathology?

A. Postpartum "blues."
B. Postpartum depression.
C. Postpartum anxiety.
D. Postpartum psychosis.

CHAPTER 41

Children and Adolescents

41.1 A 12-year-old boy with a history of Tourette's disorder is brought by his parents to your office for evaluation of attention-deficit/hyperactivity disorder (ADHD) after scoring positive for ADHD on the Vanderbilt ADHD Diagnostic Rating Scales. He is not currently on any medications. The parents say that his tics are present throughout the day and feel that they inhibit his ability to focus on tasks such as schoolwork and household chores. Which of the following treatment strategies showed the greatest benefit for chronic tic disorders comorbid with ADHD in a randomized controlled trial?

A. Treatment of Tourette syndrome with aripiprazole.
B. Treatment of ADHD with clonidine.
C. Treatment of both disorders (ADHD and comorbid Tourette syndrome) with clonidine and methylphenidate.
D. Treatment of ADHD with methylphenidate.

41.2 A 16-year-old boy with a history of attention-deficit/hyperactivity disorder and epilepsy has received trials of multiple stimulants, but none have adequately controlled his symptoms. His parents therefore would like to switch him to the non-stimulant medication atomoxetine, given its more favorable risk–benefit profile. Which of the following statements correctly describes a U.S. Food and Drug Administration (FDA) bolded warning regarding atomoxetine?

A. Atomoxetine has been reported to prolong QTc and lead to arrhythmias.
B. Atomoxetine has been known to cause significant effects on growth (height and weight).
C. Atomoxetine has been shown to lower the seizure threshold.
D. Atomoxetine has been associated with severe liver injury in extremely rare cases.

41.3 Which of the following is the best first-line medication choice for treating pediatric mania?

A. Olanzapine.
B. Risperidone.

C. Lamotrigine.

D. Oxcarbazepine.

41.4 Which of the following is a first-line medication choice for treating adolescent depression?

A. Bupropion.

B. Venlafaxine.

C. Clomipramine.

D. Sertraline.

41.5 "PRIDE skills" are a component of parent–child interaction therapy. What does the acronym *PRIDE* stand for?

A. Playing with the child, Reflecting on appropriate talk, Imitating appropriate play, Describing appropriate behavior, and being Enthusiastic.

B. Playing with the child, Reflecting on appropriate talk, Imitating appropriate play, Describing appropriate behavior, and being Engaging.

C. Praising the child's appropriate behavior, Reflecting on appropriate talk, Imitating appropriate play, Describing appropriate behavior, and being Enthusiastic.

D. Praising the child's appropriate behavior, Reflecting on appropriate talk, Imitating appropriate play, Describing appropriate behavior, and being Engaging.

41.6 A depressed 17-year-old adolescent is struggling with new relationships and roles as he is transitioning to adult life. Which of the following therapy modalities would be most relevant for this patient?

A. Supportive therapy.

B. Interpersonal psychotherapy.

C. Cognitive-behavioral therapy.

D. Dialectical behavior therapy.

41.7 An 8-year-old boy has a history of attention-deficit/hyperactivity disorder (ADHD) and comorbid anxiety. He complains of insomnia, which has worsened since the start of school 2 weeks ago. The boy's parents have him get ready for bed at 9 P.M.; however, he is unable to fall asleep until midnight, despite having to wake up at 6 A.M. for school. Which of the following interventions should be *avoided* in the initial treatment of this child's insomnia?

A. Melatonin.

B. Benzodiazepines.

C. Sleep hygiene.

D. Clonidine.

CHAPTER 42

Lesbian, Gay, Bisexual, and Transgender Patients

42.1 What is the DSM-5 diagnosis given to an individual experiencing clinically significant distress or impairment due to a marked incongruence between their experienced gender and their assigned gender?

A. Gender incongruence.
B. Transsexualism.
C. Gender dysphoria.
D. Gender identity disorder.

42.2 To which of the following does the term *cisgender* refer?

A. Gender role.
B. Sexual orientation.
C. Gender expression.
D. Gender identity.

42.3 Epidemiological research indicates that sexual minority youth show which of the following trends in comparison with their heterosexual peers?

A. Lower rates of substance use disorders.
B. Lower rates of alcohol use and smoking.
C. Lower rates of depression and suicide attempts.
D. Higher rates of bullying and victimization.

42.4 During the course of a comprehensive sexual history, a 24-year-old male patient reports having experienced same-sex attraction since adolescence and engaging exclusively in sexual relationships with men. After this disclosure, he requests professional help in order to change his sexual orientation. This request reflects which of the following phenomena?

A. Gender dysphoria.
B. Outing.
C. Internalized homophobia.
D. Ego-dystonic homosexuality.

CHAPTER 43

Older Adults

43.1 A resident on her consultation-liaison psychiatry rotation receives a request for assistance in managing acute-onset agitation in a 79-year-old patient who received hip replacement surgery 5 days ago. The patient has no prior psychiatric history and up until the surgery has been living alone and fully functional. Upon entering the room, the resident observes a disheveled elderly woman who does not know where she is. When asked the date, the patient recites her birth date. She is unable to recite the months of the year in reverse, and nursing staff report that the patient spoke of visiting with a deceased family member earlier today. Nurses report that the patient was oriented to person, place, and time earlier in the day and until now has been calm and cooperative, with few needs other than pain control (for which she has been given scheduled morphine doses around the clock). Which of the following is the most likely diagnosis?

A. Neurocognitive disorder due to Alzheimer's disease.
B. Delirium.
C. Vascular neurocognitive disorder.
D. Very-late-onset schizophrenia.

43.2 Which of the following options is the most appropriate first step in managing behavioral disturbances associated with delirium?

A. Implementation of restraints and mittens.
B. Administration of haloperidol 0.5 mg PO.
C. Administration of lorazepam 0.5 mg IV.
D. Establishment of an adequate airway and close monitoring of vital signs.

43.3 What is the most common disorder contributing to memory loss?

A. Alzheimer's disease.
B. Parkinson's disease.
C. Alcohol use disorder.
D. Vascular disease.

43.4 A 73-year-old woman is brought to the physician by her children because she is becoming more forgetful. Until recently, she managed her finances independently and enjoyed cooking, but she has begun to receive overdue payment notices from her utility companies as well as from her landlord. She also is beginning to find it difficult to prepare balanced meals, having lost 4 kg in the past 5 months, and she recently left the water running in her bathtub, which flooded the apartment. When her children express their concerns, she becomes angry and resists their help. Lab tests reveal normal values for metabolic, hematological, and thyroid function. Which of the following would be the most appropriate next step in the diagnostic workup of this patient?

A. Genetic testing.
B. In-depth cognitive testing.
C. Mini-Mental State Examination.
D. Positron emission tomography.

43.5 Most pharmacological therapies for memory loss target the breakdown of a naturally occurring substance in the body. What is the name of this substance?

A. γ Secretase.
B. Acetylcholine.
C. N-methyl-D-aspartate (NMDA).
D. Estrogen.

43.6 A 65-year-old woman visits her primary care physician and complains of difficulty falling asleep, low energy during the day, difficulty concentrating, and low mood. On further questioning, the patient explains that every night after she gets into bed, she experiences leg discomfort for several hours before she can relax and fall asleep. Which of the following would be the most appropriate treatment for this patient?

A. Sertraline.
B. Polysomnography.
C. Quetiapine.
D. Ropinirole.

43.7 Which of the following effects may occur when benzodiazepines are prescribed to older persons?

A. Reduced levels of fatigue.
B. Memory improvement.
C. Confusion.
D. Decreased risk of falls.

43.8 Which of the following has been most closely linked to Alzheimer's disease?

A. Apolipoprotein E gene (ε2 allele).
B. Presenilin 1 gene.

C. Presenilin 2 gene.

D. Apolipoprotein E gene (ε4 allele).

43.9 An 84-year-old man with mild vascular neurocognitive disorder comes to his physician's office for a routine checkup. During the appointment, the patient discloses that his neighbor has been stealing his mail and spying on him, and because of this, he has been having trouble sleeping. The patient asks for "sleeping pills." What is the most appropriate next step?

A. Hospitalize the patient.

B. Confront the patient's delusion.

C. Interview family members of the patient.

D. Prescribe zolpidem 5 mg qhs.

43.10 A 74-year-old nursing home patient with dementia has been exhibiting many behavioral symptoms, such as frequently isolating in her room, becoming agitated when showering, losing weight, and is uninterested in participating in group activities she once enjoyed such as karaoke and bingo. She has told nursing home staff that she hears the voices of her children talking to her in her room when she is alone. The staff members are worried that the patient may be depressed. What is the best first step in the diagnostic workup?

A. Thyroid panel.

B. Psychological testing.

C. Magnetic resonance imaging (MRI).

D. Screening for HIV.

43.11 A 74-year-old woman visits her primary care physician and complains of worsened insomnia and anxiety over the past several months. The physician has been prescribing alprazolam for both of these symptoms for over a year, and the patient is distressed and frustrated that her symptoms have worsened. She admits that she has been taking more alprazolam than prescribed to relieve her worsening symptoms. She also admits to stealing her daughter's lorazepam when she runs out of her own medication and is feeling tremulous, sweaty, or anxious. Which of the following would be the best initial step in treating this patient?

A. Referral to a 12-step program.

B. Confrontation regarding her substance use.

C. Referral to a psychiatrist.

D. Detoxification.

CHAPTER 44

Culturally Diverse Patients

44.1 Which of the following best captures the DSM-5 definition of *culture*?

A. Systems of knowledge, concepts, rules, and practices that remain static over time.
B. Systems of knowledge, concepts, rules, and practices with minimal impact on an individual's identity.
C. Systems of knowledge, concepts, rules, and practices that are learned and transmitted across generations.
D. Systems of knowledge, concepts, rules, and practices that are easily intuited by a seasoned clinician.

44.2 You are conducting an evaluation for a new patient with a history of bipolar disorder. During the interview, the patient talks about a prior major depressive episode following the death of her grandmother, to whom she was very close. She later mentions that she still communicates with her deceased grandmother on occasion. Which of the following DSM-5 components would be most helpful in developing a case formulation for this patient?

A. The "Culture-Related Diagnostic Issues" subsection in the descriptive text for bipolar disorder.
B. The "Glossary of Cultural Concepts of Distress" in the DSM-5 Appendix.
C. The "Cultural Formulation Interview" in the "Cultural Formulation" chapter in DSM-5 Section III.
D. The "Cultural Issues" subsection of the DSM-5 Introduction.

44.3 Criteria for which of the following disorders were revised in DSM-5 to better accommodate cultural variation in psychiatric presentation?

A. Major depressive disorder.
B. Illness anxiety disorder.
C. Social anxiety disorder.
D. Bipolar disorder.

44.4   A relatively new patient presents to your office for a follow-up visit. He reports that he had an *"ataque de nervios"* last week. You explore the experience with him in session, but you are still puzzled by the term. Which of the following DSM-5 components would be most helpful for learning more about this phenomenon?

A. The "Glossary of Culture-Bound Syndromes."
B. The "Outline for Cultural Formulation."
C. The "Glossary of Cultural Concepts of Distress."
D. The "Cultural Formulation Interview."

44.5   Which of the following best defines the term *cultural competence* in health care settings?

A. A highly encouraged but optional component of a physician's career.
B. A theoretically useful strategy for reducing health disparities.
C. A form of political correctness that emerged during the civil rights era to promote care of diverse societies.
D. The ability of an individual or organization to provide effective and equitable care that is responsive to diverse cultural beliefs, practices, preferred languages, and communication needs of the patient.

44.6   In an effort to bridge the gap between formal theories of various psychotherapies and the cultural values of patients, mental health professionals have adapted interventions in multiple ways to increase their alignment and compatibility with patients' cultural perspectives and models. Which of the following cultural adaptations was shown in a peer-reviewed meta-analysis to have minimal benefit on treatment outcomes?

A. Matching race and ethnicity of provider and patient.
B. Substituting colloquial expressions for technical terms used in psychotherapy.
C. Making modifications that allow family members to participate in psychotherapy treatment.
D. Training therapists in local customs and metaphors to better facilitate communication with patients.

PART II

Answer Guide

CHAPTER 1

The Psychiatric Interview and Mental Status Examination

1.1   Which of the following statements could most appropriately be used as the chief complaint?

A. The patient was brought to the hospital by Emergency Medical Services after being found lying on the street surrounded by bottles.
B. "My brother seems more depressed and isolative recently."
C. Depression and suicide attempt.
D. "I'm not answering any of your questions."

The correct response is option D: "I'm not answering any of your questions."

The chief complaint is intended to be the patient's primary psychiatric concern and is generally written as a quotation (option D is correct). This brief section belongs to the patient. Quoting nonsensical or tangential responses can provide an excellent window into the patient's mental status, and clearly marking the patient's priority lays the groundwork for later adherence and an effective treatment plan. It is, therefore, not the spouse's or family's biggest complaint (option B is incorrect), the prior therapist's or treatment team's biggest concern (option A is incorrect), or the interviewer's assessment of what should be the chief complaint (option C is incorrect). **Chapter 1 (p. 20)**

1.2   When considering the biopsychosocial model, which of the following would be the most pertinent *social* contributor to a patient's clinical picture?

A. Ego defenses.
B. Comorbid medical diagnoses.
C. Race.
D. Medication adherence.

The correct response is option C: Race.

The "social" aspect of the biopsychosocial model refers to the sociological, religious, spiritual, ethnic, and racial issues that may be pertinent to the patient's current clinical picture (option C is correct). The "biological" aspect of the biopsychosocial model refers to the genetic, pharmacological, and comorbid medical conditions that may be pertinent to the patient's current clinical picture (options B and D are incorrect). The "psychological" aspect of the biopsychosocial model refers to the psychological understanding of patients, either via diagnostic descriptions (e.g., DSM-5 [American Psychiatric Association 2013] criteria) or narrative descriptions that are heavily informed by psychotherapeutic schools of thought (e.g., psychodynamics, cognitive-behavioral therapy [CBT], interpersonal therapy) (option A is incorrect). **Chapter 1 (pp. 4–7)**

1.3   Which of the following interviewer techniques or practices may be potentially *unhelpful* in the assessment of an agitated ("revved-up") patient?

A. Remain near the doorway during the interview.
B. Use open-ended questions.
C. Ensure that staff members and security guards are available during the interview.
D. Use a clear, gentle, and pleasantly firm tone of voice with the patient.

The correct response is option B: Use open-ended questions.

A focal concern in the evaluation of the revved-up patient is safety. Open-ended questions are generally not useful, and thus binary choices or direct questions are preferred (option B is correct). The interviewer might station him- or herself near the doorway to ensure a quick exit in case of a threat (option A is incorrect), and he might ensure the availability of helpful staff members (option C is incorrect), security guards, and sedating medications. Revved-up patients tend to calm down when talking to an interviewer who is clear, soft-spoken, and pleasantly firm (option D is incorrect). **Chapter 1 (pp. 16–17)**

1.4   During an emergency room psychiatric evaluation, which of the following represents the most important concern?

A. Accurate diagnosis.
B. Treatment strategy.
C. Safety assessment.
D. Patient disposition.

The correct response is option C: Safety assessment.

In the emergency room, the primary evaluation goals are always the same: *safety* (determining whether the patient is suicidal, homicidal, or unable to care for himself) and *triage* (considering whether the patient is to be admitted, discharged, transferred to medicine, or held overnight). Although all interviews in the emergency room aim to ascertain a safety assessment, differential diagnosis, treatment plan, and disposition, a safety assessment is the primary concern (option C is correct; options A, B, and D are incorrect). **Chapter 1 (pp. 14–15)**

1.5 A patient knowingly neglects to mention his recent escalating cocaine use when discussing his depression related to his wife leaving him. Which of the following terms best describes what causes the patient to leave out this information?

A. Conscious resistance.
B. Malingering.
C. Repression.
D. Factitious disorder.

The correct response is option A: Conscious resistance.

Resistance is anything that prevents the patient from talking openly to the interviewer. *Conscious resistance* occurs when the patient knowingly neglects, distorts, or makes things up (option A is correct). *Malingering* patients consciously lie about the presence or severity of an illness or disability in order to gain a reward or avoid an unpleasant outcome (option B is incorrect). Patients with factitious disorder know that they are creating an untrue story but do not know why (option D is incorrect). *Repression* is the result of underlying dynamic conflict, or motivated forgetting as a response to warded-off fears or wishes (option C is incorrect). **Chapter 1 (pp. 7, 18); see also Chapter 16 ("Dissociative Disorders"), Table 16–1 ("Differences between dissociation and repression," p. 440)**

1.6 Which of the following sample patient descriptions best fulfills the requirements for the *general appearance and behavior* component of the mental status examination (MSE)?

A. "Middle-aged man, appearing older than stated age, poor hygiene, numerous tattoos across his arms, uncooperative with interview."
B. "Elderly woman wearing hospital gown, disheveled, alert but psychomotor agitated and with loosening of associations."
C. "Young woman, unusually dressed, poor grooming, eye contact intense, psychomotor retarded, responding to internal stimuli."
D. "Adolescent boy, appearing younger than stated age, cooperative with interview, euthymic mood and congruent affect."

The correct response is option A: "Middle-aged man, appearing older than stated age, poor hygiene, numerous tattoos across his arms, uncooperative with interview."

In the MSE description of *appearance and behavior*, the interviewer notes the patient's level of consciousness, dress and grooming (including any idiosyncrasies), psychomotor status (i.e., agitation or retardation), and attitude toward the examiner (option A is correct). *Mood* and *affect* are not considered to be components of a patient's appearance and behavior (option D is incorrect). Thought process (option B is incorrect) and perceptions (option C is incorrect) are also not included under appearance and behavior; instead, these elements are addressed in separate sections of the MSE. **Chapter 1 (pp. 23–25; Table 1–6 [p. 24])**

1.7   Which of the following components of therapeutic interviewing is most helpful in encouraging patients to speak freely, particularly regarding potentially embarrassing or illegal activities?

A. Attentive listening.
B. Therapeutic alliance.
C. Confidentiality.
D. Therapeutic neutrality.

The correct response is option C: Confidentiality.

Confidentiality allows patients to speak more freely. Patients are more likely to reveal potentially shameful or illegal behaviors that may be contributing to their clinical picture if they are confident that there will not be legal or social repercussions (option C is correct). *Attentive listening* involves tactful eye contact and body language that demonstrate attention and help to indicate that the patient has been heard (option A is incorrect). *Neutrality* discourages the interviewer from moralizing, intellectualizing, or launching into prematurely zealous therapy (option D is incorrect). A *therapeutic alliance* develops as the patient and clinician work together to understand the presenting problem and create a treatment plan (option B is incorrect). Although attentive listening, a neutral therapeutic stance, and a strong therapeutic alliance are all important interviewing principles, ensuring confidentiality between the clinician and patient is most likely to yield information regarding potentially shameful or illegal activities. **Chapter 1 (pp. 12–13; Table 1–2 [p. 13])**

Reference

American Psychiatric Association: Diagnostic and Statistical Manual of Mental Disorders, 5th Edition. Arlington, VA, American Psychiatric Association, 2013

CHAPTER 2

DSM-5 as a Framework for Psychiatric Diagnosis

2.1   What U.S. organization currently oversees the process of making country-specific changes in the International Classification of Diseases (ICD)?

A. The World Health Organization.
B. The National Center for Health Statistics.
C. The American Psychiatric Association.
D. The U.S. Census Bureau.

The correct response is option B: The National Center for Health Statistics.

The ICD is developed and periodically revised by the World Health Organization (WHO). All member countries of WHO have the ability to make their own changes. In the United States, the National Center for Health Statistics (NCHS) oversees this process (option B is correct; option A is incorrect).

The NCHS collaborates with specialty organizations, such as the American Psychiatric Association (option C is incorrect), to incorporate diagnostic categories used in the United States.

The U.S. Census Bureau attempted to count people who had a mental disorder, but after 1890 abandoned its effort (option D is incorrect). **Chapter 2 (pp. 31–32, 37)**

2.2   Which of the following statements correctly describes how the DSM-5 Task Force attempted to address the imprecision in DSM-IV and earlier editions regarding the definition of *mental disorder*?

A. In DSM-5, the terms *distress* and *impairment* were eliminated from the definition of *mental disorder*.
B. In DSM-5, the definition of *mental disorder* specified a threshold for diagnosis.
C. DSM-5 introduced a new effort to apply dimensional measures to determine clinical significance.
D. DSM-5 no longer provides a definition for *mental disorder*.

The correct response is option C: DSM-5 introduced a new effort to apply dimensional measures to determine clinical significance.

The imprecision in describing diagnostic categories in DSM-IV and earlier DSM editions led critics to question how clinicians could distinguish mental disorders from reactions to normal life or problems in living. When there is no way to identify the causal factors or mechanisms of an illness, and the clinical presentation does not provide a clear division between normality and clinically relevant illness, specifying the point at which a syndrome crosses the boundary from normal to abnormal is one of the challenges for a classification system (Kendell and Jablensky 2003). In DSM-IV (American Psychiatric Association 1994), this challenge was met by requiring that a syndrome be associated with distress, impairment, or risk of other harmful outcomes. However, this pragmatic approach generated problems of its own. Terms such as *clinically significant* and *impairment* were not defined. Requiring impairment for diagnosis of a clinical disorder could preclude early intervention in preclinical phases of the disorder. Requiring that impairment be present could also complicate efforts to study the evolving relationship between the syndrome and any subsequent disability. Attempting to attribute distress or impairment to a particular disorder when more than one disorder is present would be difficult at best (Lehman et al. 2002; Sartorius 2009).

In DSM-5 (American Psychiatric Association 2013, p. 20), the definition of *mental disorder* is phrased in terms of dysfunctions and their underlying processes (option D is incorrect):

> A mental disorder is a syndrome characterized by clinically significant disturbance in an individual's cognition, emotion regulation, or behavior that reflects a dysfunction in the psychological, biological, or developmental processes underlying mental functioning. Mental disorders are usually associated with significant distress or disability in social, occupational, or other important activities.

This definition still does not provide operational guidance on specifying a threshold for diagnosis (option B is incorrect).

The difficulty in determining when a dysfunction has produced a change from normal variation to pathology has meant that the coupling of the definition of *mental disorder* to "significant distress or impairment" could not be removed completely (option A is incorrect).

This definition in DSM-5 serves mainly as a guidepost to the future. DSM-5 introduced a new effort to apply dimensional measures to determine clinical significance (option C is correct), to identify preclinical conditions, or to assess heterogeneity among cases. This dimensional approach anticipates a time when "dysfunction" can be measured and its underlying processes can be identified (Hyman 2010; Insel and Wang 2010). **Chapter 2 (pp. 34–35)**

2.3   In what year was the first DSM published?

A. 1917.
B. 1949.

C. 1952.
D. 1968.

The correct response is option C: 1952.

For clinicians, DSM-I (American Psychiatric Association 1952) presented a list of diagnostic terms, to serve as nomenclature (option C is correct). Although the terms could have been listed alphabetically, the list was presented according to the coding system in the then-current ICD-6 (World Health Organization 1949) (option B is incorrect). In 1917, the U.S. Census Bureau asked the precursor of the APA for assistance in developing a classification system for psychiatric illnesses (option A is incorrect). The APA's Committee on Nomenclature and Statistics produced DSM-II in 1968 (American Psychiatric Association 1968) (option D is incorrect). **Chapter 2 (pp. 35, 37–38)**

2.4   What were the initial goals of the DSM?

A. To be used in judicial proceedings and social welfare systems.
B. To provide extensive information beyond the criteria in an effort to help clinicians understand the disorder.
C. To provide a framework to record nondiagnostic data about a patient's condition and use five "axes" of diagnostic formulation.
D. To serve as a diagnostic manual and a guide to statistical reporting.

The correct response is option D: To serve as a diagnostic manual and a guide to statistical reporting.

From the manual's first publication in 1952, DSM was intended to serve as both a diagnostic manual for clinicians and a guide to statistical reporting useful for hospital and public health officials (option D is correct). The diagnostic system has been broadly used in judicial proceedings (e.g., to bolster a defense in a criminal trial) as well as in social welfare systems to justify claims for disability payments. However, DSM revisions have noted that diagnoses can only be made by well-trained clinicians, and DSM-5 reiterated that the presence of a mental disorder does not substitute for these other judgments (option A is incorrect). DSM-III (American Psychiatric Association 1980) provided extensive information beyond the criteria sets in an effort to help clinicians understand the disorder (option B is incorrect). Besides developing criteria for specific disorders, the task force also provided clinicians with a framework to record nondiagnostic data about a patient's condition. DSM-III recommended that each diagnostic formulation should include five types, or "axes," of information (option C is incorrect). **Chapter 2 (pp. 34–35, 39)**

2.5   What problems did DSM-5 Work Group members identify as they reviewed DSM-IV criteria?

A. Underutilization of the "not otherwise specified" (NOS) category.
B. Inappropriate characterization of distinct disorders as different presentations of a single disorder.
C. High rates of reported comorbidity.
D. Excessive coverage of clinical conditions so that no new disorders could be added.

The correct response is option C: High rates of reported comorbidity.

Work group members identified several types of problems as they reviewed DSM-IV (American Psychiatric Association 1994) criteria. Some diagnostic groups showed excessive use of the nonspecific residual category, labeled "not otherwise specified" (NOS) in DSM-IV (option A is incorrect). Some chapters had created distinct disorders in what may be better considered a single disorder with a range of presentations (option B is incorrect). Other chapters seemed to have gaps in coverage of clinical conditions, so that new disorders might need to be added to the classification (option D is incorrect). One problem for almost all of the conditions was determining proper diagnostic boundaries. The difficulty of setting boundaries had led to high rates of reported comorbidity (option C is correct). **Chapter 2 (p. 41)**

2.6   What change was made to substance use disorders in DSM-5?

A. Collapse of abuse and dependence categories.
B. Use of a categorical approach to grade severity.
C. Restriction of clinical assessment scope to a single diagnostic category.
D. Removal of withdrawal as a substance use disorder category.

The correct response is option A: Collapse of abuse and dependence categories.

For substance use disorders, the DSM-5 Task Force agreed to collapse the categories of substance abuse and dependence into a single category, substance use disorder (option A is correct).

The term *categorical* applies to a response that can be only one of two choices: yes or no. The term *dimensional* means that the individual differences between persons in expression of a disorder are reflected in one or more ordinal scales (e.g., level of relevant symptoms). In DSM-5, a dimensional approach is used to grade the severity of a substance use disorder (option B is incorrect).

An early focus of the effort to introduce dimensional measures in DSM-5 was on the assessment of important aspects of psychopathology that should be evaluated in an ongoing way with almost all patients. These measures cut across diagnostic boundaries; for example, substance use would be assessed in patients with any diagnosis (option C is incorrect).

DSM-5 provides diagnostic criteria for clinical presentations that are directly related to substance use, such as intoxication and withdrawal (option D is incorrect). **Chapter 2 (pp. 43, 45); see also Chapter 24 ("Substance-Related and Addictive Disorders"; p. 647)**

2.7   Which of the following was added in DSM-5 as an independent diagnosis?

A. Grief reaction.
B. Binge-eating disorder.
C. Asperger's disorder.
D. Somatoform disorder.

The correct response is option B: Binge-eating disorder.

Binge-eating disorder was listed in Appendix B of DSM-IV as a disorder that needed more study before being included in the list of Axis I disorders. In DSM-5, the disorder was formally moved into the new chapter "Feeding and Eating Disorders" (option B is correct).

One change to criteria that generated public concern was the decision to eliminate the so-called bereavement exclusion in the criteria for major depressive disorder. After concerns were expressed about appearing to "medicalize" normal life reactions, the DSM-5 Task Force provided language to clarify that grief reactions are not automatically considered evidence of a major depressive disorder (option A is incorrect).

In DSM-5, five disorders previously distinguished as separate categories were combined into a single autism spectrum disorder. This change prompted expressions of concern from advocacy groups, who feared that it would increase stigma for patients who had previously been diagnosed with Asperger's disorder, for example. However, the task force felt that stigma should be directly addressed as a problem on behalf of all of the patients with a condition in this spectrum (option C is incorrect).

In DSM-5, several of the DSM-IV somatoform disorders are now grouped into a single category, somatic symptom disorder, on the basis of their common features (option D is incorrect). **Chapter 2 (pp. 42–43)**

2.8   How is the *reliability* of a given diagnosis defined?

A. Accuracy of the criteria in making a diagnosis.
B. Demonstration of a clear etiology and pathogenic mechanism.
C. Agreement between raters that a disorder is or is not present.
D. Percentage of total variance specifically from the signal.

The correct response is option C: Agreement between raters that a disorder is or is not present.

The *reliability* of a diagnosis is the property of agreement between raters that a disorder is or is not present (option C is correct). *Validity* reflects whether the criteria for a disorder provide the basis for making an accurate diagnosis (option A is incorrect). Determining the validity of the disorder could rest, in the simplest model, on demonstrating a clear etiology and a straightforward pathogenic mechanism (option B is incorrect). In the absence of a definitive cause and mechanism, one proposal for validity is to show that a disorder has clear boundaries from other disorders and from normal variation. For any diagnosis, categorical or dimensional, the total variance (i.e., individual difference among subjects) comprises three nonoverlapping parts: signal, interference, and noise. The reliability of a measure is the percent of total variance free of noise and validity is the percentage specifically from the signal, free of both noise and interference (option D is incorrect). **Chapter 2 (pp. 46–47)**

2.9   Which of the following diagnoses is addressed most differently between DSM-5 and ICD-11?

A. Binge-eating disorder.
B. Personality disorder.
C. Autism spectrum disorder.
D. Schizoaffective disorder.

The correct response is option B: Personality disorder.

ICD-11 (World Health Organization 2018) eliminated the categories and criteria for individual personality disorders and adopted a dimensional approach. Clinicians will use the overall definition to establish whether a personality disorder is present and will rate it by severity. The DSM-5 Personality and Personality Disorders Work Group considered revising the DSM-5 approach to personality disorders by adopting a hybrid system that combined the traditional categorical model with a new model that used quantitative ratings of personality domains and traits. However, the peer review committees felt that this approach was not well enough established to be incorporated into the manual for routine clinical use, and that removing any personality disorders was premature (option B is correct).

Other proposed changes to ICD-11—such as introducing binge-eating disorder, collapsing disorders into an autism spectrum, and dropping the subtypes of schizophrenia (options A, C, and D are incorrect)—reflected the same reasoning used by the DSM-5 Task Force. **Chapter 2 (pp. 44, 51)**

2.10   Which of the following options best describes the Research Domain Criteria (RDoC) approach to investigating mental disorders?

A. A "bottom-up" strategy to examine basic cognitive, psychological, social, or biological processes and then determine how any dysfunctions in them are expressed clinically.
B. A "top-down" approach that uses the prespecified disorder in a classification like DSM or ICD as the starting point for an investigation.
C. A diagnostic system meant to help develop a precision medicine approach to mental disorders.
D. A simplified organizational framework for the definition of mental disorders that reduces time and funding needs.

The correct response is option A: A "bottom-up" strategy to examine basic cognitive, psychological, social, or biological processes and then determine how any dysfunctions in them are expressed clinically.

Since 1980, each revision of DSM has had the goal of basing changes on the best evidence available. However, few studies have conducted formal comparisons of different sets of criteria. The prevailing research strategy for understanding mental disorders has been to examine associated characteristics, such as risk factors, familial patterns, treatment response, or biological markers. This "top-down" approach uses the prespecified disorder in a classification like DSM or ICD as the starting point for an investigation (option B is incorrect). That approach has not led to breakthroughs in identifying biomarkers or other validating factors for the disorders; instead, this routine application of pre-established criteria can lead to a reification of the existing categories (Cuthbert 2014; Hyman 2010).

A more open-ended approach would be to examine basic cognitive, psychological, social, or biological processes and then determine how any dysfunctions in them are expressed clinically. This "bottom-up" strategy might lead to new paradigms for specifying and classifying clinical disorders. In 2010, the Research Domain Criteria (RDoC) project announced its intention to use this approach as an organizational framework for studying and classifying the features of mental disorders (Insel et al. 2010) (option A is correct). Such an ambitious undertaking fits with the definition of mental disorder in DSM-5 but will require much time and funding (option D is incorrect).

National Institute of Mental Health leaders have acknowledged that RDoC is currently only a way to guide research and catalog findings: "At this point…, RDoC is not a diagnostic system, it's merely a framework for organizing research. It begins with the humble realization that we do not know enough to develop a precision medicine approach to mental disorders" (Insel 2014, p. 396) (option C is incorrect). **Chapter 2 (pp. 51–52)**

References

American Psychiatric Association: Diagnostic and Statistical Manual: Mental Disorders. Washington, DC, American Psychiatric Association, 1952
American Psychiatric Association: Diagnostic and Statistical Manual of Mental Disorders, 2nd Edition. Washington, DC, American Psychiatric Association, 1968
American Psychiatric Association: Diagnostic and Statistical Manual of Mental Disorders, 3rd Edition. Washington, DC, American Psychiatric Association, 1980
American Psychiatric Association: Diagnostic and Statistical Manual of Mental Disorders, 3rd Edition, Revised. Washington, DC, American Psychiatric Association, 1987
American Psychiatric Association: Diagnostic and Statistical Manual of Mental Disorders, 4th Edition. Washington, DC, American Psychiatric Association, 1994
American Psychiatric Association: Diagnostic and Statistical Manual of Mental Disorders, 5th Edition. Arlington, VA, American Psychiatric Association, 2013
Cuthbert BN: The RDoC framework: facilitating transition from ICD/DSM to dimensional approaches that integrate neuroscience and psychopathology. World Psychiatry 13(1):28–35, 2014 24497240

Hyman SE: The diagnosis of mental disorders: the problem of reification. Annu Rev Clin Psychol 6:155–179, 2010 17716032

Insel TR: The NIMH Research Domain Criteria (RDoC) Project: precision medicine for psychiatry. Am J Psychiatry 171(4):395–397, 2014 24687194

Insel TR, Wang PS: Rethinking mental illness. JAMA 303(19):1970–1971, 2010 20483974

Insel TR, Cuthbert B, Garvey M, et al: Research domain criteria (RDoC): toward a new classification framework for research on mental disorders. Am J Psychiatry 167(7):748–751, 2010 20595427

Kendell R, Jablensky A: Distinguishing between the validity and utility of psychiatric diagnoses. Am J Psychiatry 160(1):4–12, 2003 12505793

Lehman AF, Alexopoulos GS, Goldman H, et al: Mental disorders and disability: time to reevaluate the relationship? in A Research Agenda for DSM-5. Edited by Kupfer DJ, First MB, Regier DA. Washington, DC, American Psychiatric Association, 2002, pp 201–218

Sartorius N: Disability and mental illness are different entities and should be assessed separately. World Psychiatry 8(2):86, 2009 19516925

World Health Organization: Manual of the International Statistical Classification of Diseases, Injuries, and Causes of Death, 6th Revision. Geneva, Switzerland, World Health Organization, 1949

World Health Organization: International Statistical Classification of Diseases and Related Health Problems, 11th Edition (ICD-11), Draft Version. Geneva, World Health Organization, June 18, 2018. Available at: http://www.who.int/classifications/icd/en/. Accessed October 17, 2018.

CHAPTER 3

Normal Child and Adolescent Development

3.1   How does family systems theory define the term *attractor states*?

A. Attractor states provide coherence and social meaning to the individual narrative.
B. Attractor states are phases that are recognizable but infinitely variable and often unevenly achieved in any individual child at any given moment.
C. Attractor states arise from the interaction between emerging ego capacities, the interpersonal world, unconscious fantasy, and the pull toward the next level of mental organization.
D. Attractor states form the basis of the autobiographical narrative that is part of everyone's mental life, whether conscious or unconscious.

The correct response is option B: Attractor states are phases that are recognizable but infinitely variable and often unevenly achieved in any individual child at any given moment.

The interaction of multiple systems, ranging from tangible physical maturation all the way to the intangible development of unconscious fantasy, produces infinite variations of the superficially identifiable (albeit profoundly individualized) phases traversed as children progress through life in a given society. Across the wide swath of cultural conditions, these phases seem to emerge and, in the language of systems theory, represent *attractor states*—that is, novel configurations individually and idiosyncratically composed out of multiple interacting systems but nonetheless recognizable across individuals in similar societies (option B is correct).

Indeed, the evolution of the individual narrative "that provides coherence and social meaning" is considered an important treatment outcome (Hammack and Toolis 2014, p. 43) (option A is incorrect).

Development can be defined as the interface between physical maturation, emerging ego capacities, mental structure, the unconscious mind and its drives, and the interpersonal (and, more recently, the computer-mediated) world, as represented by and filtered through the family early in life and gradually including the society at large (option C is incorrect).

Finally, the subjective experience of development forms the basis of the autobiographical narrative that is part of everyone's mental life, whether conscious or unconscious (option D is incorrect). **Chapter 3 (pp. 60–61)**

3.2   A father with a 6-month-old baby makes a sad face when his infant son cries, and accurately identifies a dirty diaper. He stays calm but responds immediately and alleviates the baby's distress. The father also shows excitement when the baby is enjoying a new toy, and the two share a big laugh together. This reciprocal relationship between father and baby is most likely to help the infant achieve which of the following tasks?

A. Moving toward psychological differentiation and individuation from parents.
B. Develop foundation for identity consolidation.
C. Achieve an objective and separate sense of self, with rudimentary grasp of gender distinctions.
D. Manifest beginning self-regulatory capacities as representations of shifting psychosomatic states.

The correct response is option D: Manifest beginning self-regulatory capacities as representations of shifting psychosomatic states.

Manifesting beginning self-regulatory capacities as representations of shifting psychosomatic states is a task of infancy (option D is correct). Moving toward psychological differentiation and individuation from parents is a task of adolescence (option A is incorrect). Developing a foundation for identity consolidation is a task of adolescence (option B is incorrect). Achieving an objective and separate sense of self, with a rudimentary grasp of gender distinctions, is a task of toddlerhood (option C is incorrect). **Chapter 3 (Table 3–2 [p. 66], Table 3–3 [p. 69], Table 3–7 [p. 82])**

3.3   A 13-year-old boy has noticed his body starting to change. As he looks in the mirror, he thinks about whether his classmates in his all-male school will make comments. He contemplates what it would be like to go to a coed school after his parents have "the talk" with him. He knows it is time to ask for a later curfew and decides to communicate this to his parents. What underlying factor is propelling this boy's current developmental process?

A. Ego capacities.
B. Physical maturation.
C. Environmental effects.
D. A false sense of identity.

The correct response is option B: Physical maturation.

The anticipation of physical transformation, the associated intensification of drives, and the new psychological agenda of adolescence begin to preoccupy children as latency draws to a close. Wide variations in the timing and pace of development notwithstanding, both preadolescents and the adults around them are keenly aware that this momentous decade will take them from obedient childhood, in which parents both rule and protect them, to the status of adulthood (or emerging adulthood), hopefully accompanied by achievements in the arenas of autonomy, personal identity, sexuality, self-determined values, and professional aspirations (option B is correct).

The concept of ego capacities includes aspects of cognition, self-regulation, defenses, emotional repertoire, object relations, and self-reflection that emerge in a roughly invariant (although highly individualized) program, provided that the environment offers the essential nutriment required for their appearance. The impact of the environment on developmental experience and outcome is so idiosyncratic and variable that it is difficult to theorize, but nonetheless it is profound and far-reaching. On the larger scale, every society, from developing nations to fully digitalized cultures, produces a paced and sequential set of expectations as the individual matures and enters that specific society's form of adulthood. Three major intrapsychic developments are central to the adolescent experience: integration of the sexual self and romantic longings into the self-representation, the second individuation (Blos 1967), and the identity crisis (Erikson 1968). Sexuality, gender identity, romantic love, individuation, and resolution of the adolescent identity crisis rely on new relationships, require new opportunities for growth, and are deeply shaped by the nature of the environmental context, demands, and responses. Thus, while ego capacities, the environment, and intrapsychic developments are involved here, they are not the main propelling factor (options A, C, and D are incorrect). **Chapter 3 (pp. 61, 76–78)**

3.4   A new mother with postpartum depression is experiencing sleep deprivation and is feeling completely overwhelmed. When she hears her baby crying, she huddles in bed, covering her ears, and is unable to respond appropriately to the infant's distress. Which of the following infant developmental tasks would likely be most affected as a result of this mother's depression?

A. Self-regulation.
B. Joint attention.
C. Rapprochement.
D. Object constancy.

The correct response is option A: Self-regulation.

Preverbal infants signal distress largely by fussing and crying; when contingent responses—caretaking behaviors that closely match the baby's signals and actions—are consistently received, the parent's comforting presence and interventions are gradually internalized. Over time, the infant's enhanced social and cognitive apparatus, along with the parent's reliable reactions, contribute to increasingly complex, organized representations of tension-reducing parent–child interactions. The result is a greater internal tolerance for momentary distress and a dawning capacity for self-regulation (option A is correct).

The infant engages in joint attention, gazing back and forth from the mother's face to an object of mutual focus, for the first time at 8–10 months (option B is incorrect).

A physical ability to move farther from the parents and a growing awareness of the separate "self" gives rise to a sense of personal smallness, powerlessness, and vulnerability. Such realizations often lead to an upsurge of separation anxiety and renewed efforts to reestablish the proximity of infancy. At the same time, the toddler is vigorously motivated toward autonomy, exploration, and mastery. These competing urges cause the child unfamiliar internal discomfort and confusion, often expressed via moodiness and tantrums; noting the toddler's intensified need for parental reassurance, Mahler referred to this period of relative negativity and contradictory behaviors (e.g., shadowing the parent and then darting away) as the rapprochement crisis (Mahler 1972) (option C is incorrect).

Object constancy—a stable, internalized image of the self and others that is not vulnerable to shifting moods and situations—is a major accomplishment of early childhood (option D is incorrect). **Chapter 3 (pp. 63–64, 67)**

3.5   As a 4-year-old boy, Mike got into trouble with his parents and preschool teacher for pulling wings off insects and plucking hairs off cats. What process best explains his becoming a veterinarian as an adult?

A. Internal conflict.
B. Rapprochement crisis.
C. Object constancy.
D. Oedipal complex.

The correct response is option A: Internal conflict.

Once the adult's expectations are known and internalized, the young child's opposing desires—for example, to touch forbidden objects, pinch a sibling, or urinate on the floor—create *internal conflict*. Although painful, the toddler's inner discomfort, dread of shaming, and fears of parental irritation powerfully motivate him or her toward better self-control and emotional self-regulation (option A is correct).

A physical ability to move farther from the parents and a growing awareness of the separate self give rise to a sense of personal smallness, powerlessness, and vulnerability. Such realizations often lead to an upsurge of separation anxiety and renewed efforts to reestablish the proximity of infancy. At the same time, the toddler is vigorously motivated toward autonomy, exploration, and mastery. These competing urges cause the child unfamiliar internal discomfort and confusion, often expressed via moodiness and tantrums; noting the toddler's intensified need for parental reassurance, Mahler referred to this period of relative negativity and contradictory behaviors (e.g., shadowing the parent and then darting away) as the *rapprochement crisis* (Mahler 1972) (option B is incorrect).

Object constancy refers to a stable, internalized image of the self and others that is not vulnerable to shifting moods and situations (option C is incorrect).

The variations of the oedipal configuration are infinite. It is nonetheless usually possible to recognize components of the classical "positive" configuration—the child's longings for the opposite-sex parent (daughter for father, son for mother) and rivalry with the same-sex parent—as well as elements of the so-called negative oedipal complex (son longing for father, daughter for mother; rivalry with the opposite-sex parent) (option D is incorrect). **Chapter 3 (pp. 67–68, 71)**

3.6   A 5-year-old boy places potatoes inside a cookie jar and says, "Mom is going to be tricked because she will think there are cookies in there." Which of the following developmental concepts is illustrated by this child's actions?

A. Theory of mind.
B. Superego precursors.
C. Formal operations.
D. Hatching.

The correct response is option A: Theory of mind.

The acquisition of a *theory of mind*, or understanding of mental states, is a transformational process in development demonstrable by the age of 4 years. Once children achieve this cognitive-social-emotional capacity, they begin to grasp the difference between inner life and outer reality, the notion that people possess unique subjectivities, and the link between internal states and behavior (Fonagy and Target 1996) (option A is correct).

The toddler's capacity for self-aware emotions and increased grasp of self–other boundaries and the novel pressure of parental discipline all contribute to the formation of *superego precursors* or internalizations of the parents' expectations and attitudes (option B is incorrect).

Entering the cognitive period of *formal operations*, to begin to think more abstractly about intellectual problems and social dilemmas, is a task of preadolescence (option C is incorrect).

By the middle of the first year of life, the infant begins to emerge from the parent–child "cocoon" and become increasingly aware of the world just beyond the dyad. Mahler refers to this emergence as the process of *hatching,* wherein the baby begins to realize that the parent and the self are separate, differentiated individuals (Mahler 1972) (option D is incorrect). **Chapter 3 (pp. 64, 67–68, 70, 82; Table 3–6 [p. 79])**

3.7   Which of the following stages of normal development is best characterized by an inward drive toward independence along with a newfound sense of vulnerability?

A. Infancy.
B. Toddlerhood.
C. Oedipal phase.
D. Emerging adulthood.

The correct response is option B: Toddlerhood.

Toddlerhood (ages 1–3 years) commences with the baby's upright mobility, increased self-awareness, and emerging sense of separateness from the parent. An inward drive toward independence and exploration conflicts with a newfound sense of vulnerability, leading to ambivalence and negative moods (option B is correct).

Developing a greater awareness of self–other differentiation (hatching), fueled by cognitive and motor milestones, is a task of *infancy* and is not characterized by a drive toward independence (option A is incorrect).

Major achievements of the *oedipal phase* include managing the new emotion of guilt around moral transgressions, a manifestation of a functioning superego, and achieving the following crucial symbolic capacities: narrative building, fantasy, imaginative play, and mentalization (theory of mind). This phase does not include a strong drive for independence with newfound vulnerability (option C is incorrect).

Determining the personal importance of traditional adult milestones, including autonomous living, is an important part of *emerging adulthood*. However, this phase is focused on renegotiating family relationships toward equality, rather than solely independence (option D is incorrect). **Chapter 3 (pp. 66, 74, 84–85)**

3.8   Which of the following tasks is associated with toddlerhood?

A. Establishment of peer relationships and pursuit of group activities.
B. Acquisition of basic concepts of the world through sensorimotor practice.
C. Use of sublimation to deal with feelings and impulses.
D. Begin the process of socialization via the establishment of superego precursors.

The correct response is option D: Begin the process of socialization via the establishment of superego precursors.

The process of socialization (e.g., toilet training) begins via the establishment of superego precursors during toddlerhood (option D is correct).

During this time, expected standards of behavior for toddlers by their parents are established by means of the powerful shaping influence of adult approval. Establishment of peer relationships and pursuit of group activities, as well as use of sublimation to deal with feelings and impulses, is seen during the *latency* period (options A and C are incorrect).

Infants, not toddlers, acquire basic concepts of the world through sensorimotor practice (option B is incorrect). **Chapter 3 (pp. 66, 69, 77)**

3.9   A 4-year-old girl picks up a tennis ball and "hops" it along the surface of a table while saying, "This is Mister Kangaroo, we are going to find all of the other kangaroos!" Which of the following developmental tasks is this child's behavior illustrating?

A. Fantasy play.
B. Rudimentary understanding of gender distinctions.
C. Formal operations and abstract thinking.
D. Hatching.

The correct response is option A: Fantasy play.

The oedipal phase (ages 3–6) is characterized in part by the capacity for fantasy play, narrative building, and imaginative play (option A is correct).

Achieving an objective and separate sense of self, with a rudimentary grasp of gender distinctions, occurs during toddlerhood (option B is incorrect).

Entering the cognitive period of formal operations, preadolescents begin to think more abstractly about intellectual problems and social dilemmas. A 4-year-old would not have this cognitive capacity (option C is incorrect).

By the middle of the first year of life, the infant begins to emerge from the parent–child "cocoon" and become increasingly aware of the world just beyond the dyad. Mahler referred to this emergence as the process of *hatching*, wherein the baby begins to realize that the parent and the self are separate, differentiated individuals (Mahler 1972) (option D is incorrect). **Chapter 3 (pp. 64, 69, 74, 79)**

3.10   Which of the following terms is used to describe the coalescence of a child's sexual and aggressive drives with feelings of jealousy and rivalry?

A. Internal conflict.
B. Object constancy.
C. Sublimation.
D. Oedipal complex.

The correct response is option D: Oedipal complex.

Oedipal complex is a term used to designate the coalescence of the child's expanding object relations, emotions, and sexual and aggressive drives into recurrent triadic dramas involving the family: love, desire, rivalry, murderous aggression, and narcissistic mortification are all part of this tumultuous period. The advance of the superego, in addition to the development of other systems, facilitates the gradual quiescence and repression of this force field, although its impact is evident in personality development going forward (option D is correct).

Once the adult's expectations are known and internalized, the young child's opposing desires—for example, to touch forbidden objects, pinch a sibling, or urinate on the floor—create *internal conflict*. Although painful, the toddler's inner discomfort, dread of shaming, and fears of parental irritation powerfully motivate him or her toward better self-control and emotional self-regulation (option A is incorrect).

Object constancy refers to a stable, internalized image of the self and others that is not vulnerable to shifting moods and situations (option B is incorrect).

Sublimation, as seen during the latency period, involves transforming socially unacceptable impulses and feelings into structured activities such as academics and competitive sports (option C is incorrect). **Chapter 3 (pp. 67–68, 73, 85)**

3.11 In normal childhood development, *preadolescence* is most strongly associated with which of the following tasks?

A. Entering the cognitive period of preoperational thinking.
B. Entering the cognitive period of concrete operations.
C. Entering the cognitive period of formal operations.
D. Entering the cognitive phase of acquiring an understanding of triadic relationships.

The correct response is option C: Entering the cognitive period of formal operations.

Formal operations describe the ability to think more abstractly about intellectual problems and social dilemmas, which begins to develop during the *preadolescence* stage (option C is correct).

Preoperational thinking describes the phase of cognitive development that starts in *toddlerhood* and is marked by acquisition of object permanence and more abstract symbolic functions (option A is incorrect).

In *latency*, children enter the cognitive period of concrete operations and begin to master multiple intellectual skills and an enormous fund of academic information (option B is incorrect).

Triadic relationships—the complex emotions flourishing in the family context—are first grasped during the *oedipal phase* of development, as the child experiences ambivalence and learns to tolerate and modulate rivalry, jealousy, narcissistic mortification, excitement and desire, and hatred and love (option D is incorrect). **Chapter 3 (pp. 69, 74, 77, 79)**

3.12 Robin, as an irrepressible 7-year-old, loved to spend her evenings talking with her father about her day, but as she grew older, she became less inclined to engage in these conversations. She would often call from school asking if she could sleep over at a friend's house or "hang out" at the mall. She would frequently shut the door to her room to call classmates, often spending her evenings on the phone. Which of the following developmental tasks of preadolescence is illustrated in Robin's changing behavior?

A. Turning away from parental intimacy and toward peer socialization.
B. Integration of the sexual self and romantic longings into the self-representation.
C. Adjustment to the subjective experience of bodily changes.
D. Development of the capacity to love.

The correct response is option A: Turning away from parental intimacy and toward peer socialization.

A task of preadolescence is to turn more powerfully away from parental intimacy and toward peer socialization (option A is correct). Three major intrapsychic developments are central to the experience of *adolescence*: integration of the sexual self and romantic longings into the self-representation, the second individuation (Blos 1967), and the identity crisis (Erikson 1968) (option B is incorrect). Adjusting to the subjective experience of heightened hormonal pressures and changing bodies is indeed a task of preadolescence, but it does not best identify what the parent is describing (option C is incorrect). Developing the capacity to love, commit to, and depend on a significant other is associated with *emerging adulthood* (option D is incorrect). **Chapter 3 (pp. 78–79, 84)**

3.13   At age 11, Katie had a crush on a popular boy named Austin. She liked his "skater boy" clothing and style. At age 16, in her photography class, Katie was paired with a 17-year-old senior named Patrick. They had never interacted much before, but after an hour it was clear that while they were both very different, they recognized and appreciated each other's quirks. They soon became inseparable. Their common interests in books, music, and photography connected them deeply. The differences in Katie's romantic interests demonstrate which developmental change in adolescence?

A. Solidifying of the gender identity.
B. The "midadolescence shift" toward romance.
C. Demonstrating the ability to commit to and depend on a significant other outside of familial relations.
D. Completing identity exploration to achieve a role in contemporary society.

The correct response is option B: The "midadolescence shift" toward romance.

A "midadolescence shift" toward romance has been described: teens ages 15–17 years begin to choose partners based on personal compatibility as opposed to the conventional status features (e.g., clothing, looks, or possessions [Collins 2003]) more typical of middle schoolers (option B is correct). Midadolescents are still seeking to define their own version of their identified gender; the meaning of gender and sexuality continues to evolve at this stage (option A is incorrect). Demonstrating the capacity to love, commit to, and depend on a significant other is a task of *emerging adulthood*, not adolescence (option C is incorrect). Completing identity exploration to achieve a role in contemporary society is a task of *emerging adulthood* (option D is incorrect). **Chapter 3 (pp. 78, 80, 84)**

3.14   Gideon started college as a freshman and moved into a 1-bedroom apartment with a junior named Gus. He idealized Gus's charm, intelligence, and ability to easily navigate a world that to Gideon was still overwhelming and novel. He emulated Gus's mannerisms and aspired to be as successful as Gus. The influence of Gus in Gideon's life at this developmental stage illustrates_____, which largely occurs in_____?

A. The revision of the superego; late adolescence.
B. Gender identity; late adolescence.
C. Rejection of infantile ties; middle adolescence.
D. Risky behaviors; early to middle adolescence.

The correct response is option A: The revision of the superego; late adolescence.

The coalescence of superego precursors into the relatively coherent mental agency that emerges toward the end of the oedipal phase requires contributions from a range of other developing systems, including receptive and expressive language, affect elaboration and affect tolerance, new defenses such as internalization, reaction formation and identification with the aggressor, the new capacity to mentalize, and a new cognitive organization of preoperational thinking. These developments all contribute to the relatively stable and coherent organization of superego activities, primarily *direction giving*, *limiting*, and *punishing/rewarding functions*. The search for self-selected "new developmental objects" (i.e., adults available for idealization and identification) such as a mentor facilitates the gradual revision of the superego that is the work of late adolescence. The grip of parental values diminishes as the older adolescent is exposed to a vastly expanded world; new identifications develop that are at least in part directed by self-selected interests and ideals. Of course, these identifications are both conscious and unconscious; the college student may actively strive to emulate an admired professor and, out of awareness, be deeply influenced by a charismatic roommate or the contemporary cultural idol. The development of such identifications occurs primarily in late adolescence (option A is correct).

By around the age of 2 years, most children begin to acquire a gendered sense of self. They accurately label themselves as boy or girl; positive and negative self-feelings accrue to the toddler's notion of male and female. However, a full understanding of gender concepts—that is, of the link between one's sex and genitalia, the stability of one's sex, and the idiosyncratic but shared meanings of gender—is not grasped until several years later, toward the close of the oedipal phase, 3–6 years (de Marneffe 1997) (option B is incorrect).

In preadolescence, an urgent push toward independence, a rejection of infantile ties and dependency, and a powerful turn to the peer group propel the child out into the world beyond the family (option C is incorrect).

Middle adolescence is a peak conflictual moment in parent–child relationships as teenagers' increasing independence makes the task of knowing how and when to intervene, set limits, and guide behavior a tremendous challenge for parents.

This tension corresponds to adolescents' ongoing intrapsychic process of disengaging from parental values and morals, which leaves them more susceptible to peer and media influences and more prone to risky behaviors (option D is incorrect). **Chapter 3 (pp. 67, 72, 78, 80–81)**

3.15   Jared, a 26-year-old man, had a strife-filled relationship with his father and mother while growing up. As a young adult first starting out, he had minimal communication with them; however, after working at a steady job for a few years, he felt more open to reengaging with his parents. To his surprise, he and his parents were able to successfully interact, both feeling more equipped to navigate the complexity of the past, and remaining respectful of each other's boundaries. Which of the following tasks of emerging adulthood (ages 22 or 23 years through 30 years) does Jared's newfound ability to interact with his parents illustrate?

A.   Renegotiating family relationships toward equality.
B.   Achieving formal operations.
C.   Integrating sexuality.
D.   Transformation of self-representation.

The correct response is option A: Renegotiating family relationships toward equality.

Renegotiating family relationships toward equality is an important task of emerging adulthood (22 or 23 years through 30 years). Determining the personal importance of traditional adult milestones, including autonomous living, career, marriage, and child rearing is also an important task of emerging adulthood (option A is correct).

Entering the cognitive period of formal operations is a task of *preadolescence* (10–12 years) (option B is incorrect).

Integration of sexuality, gender identity, ideas on romantic love, and self-individuation occurs during *adolescence* and does not represent the change in dynamics described here (option C is incorrect).

Managing the transformation of the body and self-representation, especially in relation to peers, occurs in *adolescence* and does not describe the change in family dynamics (option D is incorrect). **Chapter 3 (pp. 78–79; Table 3–6 [p. 79], Table 3–7 [p. 82], Table 3–8 [p. 84])**

References

Blos P: The second individuation process of adolescence. Psychoanal Study Child 22:162–186, 1967 5590064

Collins WA: More than myth: the developmental significance of romantic relationships during adolescence. Journal of Research on Adolescence 13(1):1–24, 2003

de Marneffe D: Bodies and words: a study of young children's genital and gender knowledge. Gender and Psychoanalysis 2:3–33, 1997

Erikson E: Identity: Youth and Crisis. New York, WW Norton, 1968

Fonagy P, Target M: Playing with reality, I: theory of mind and the normal development of psychic reality. Int J Psychoanal 77(Pt 2):217–233, 1996 8771375

Hammack PL, Toolis E: Narrative and the social construction of childhood, in Rereading Personal Narrative and Life Course: New Directions in Child and Adolescent Development, No 145. Edited by Schiff B. San Francisco, CA, Wiley Periodicals, 2014, pp 43–56

Mahler MS: On the first three subphases of the separation-individuation process. Int J Psychoanal 53(Pt 3):333–338, 1972 4499978

CHAPTER 4

Assessment of Suicide Risk

4.1   A psychiatry resident is evaluating a patient who was brought to the hospital after she told a coworker that she was hearing voices and having suicidal thoughts. The resident begins the interview by asking questions about the patient's thoughts. He observes that the patient is responding in short phrases and is not answering his questions about hallucinations and suicidal ideation. Which of the following actions would be the best initial approach for the resident to take?

A. Ask if the patient has access to a firearm.
B. Address the patient's fear of answering questions as understandable and offer basic information about suicidal thoughts.
C. Ask the patient if she had taken objective or preparatory steps to act on her suicidal thoughts.
D. Consider that the patient may be experiencing perceptual disturbances and ask about auditory hallucinations.

The correct response is option B: Address the patient's fear of answering questions as understandable and offer basic information about suicidal thoughts.

Feelings of fear or shame are perhaps most salient in the care of a person newly experiencing suicidal thoughts and having an initial encounter with a psychiatrist or other mental health professional. A young college student with first-episode psychosis, for example, may be scared of the voices or intrusive thoughts he is experiencing. He may be worried that others will reject him or "lock him up," and because of these fears, his thoughts of suicide may intensify. In this situation, it is ideal if the psychiatrist can first reassure the patient, address his fears as natural under the circumstances, offer nonjudgmental support, and introduce some basic information about mental disorders and the system of care (option B is correct; option D is incorrect).

The clinician may then, as the second goal, be able to turn to the task of assessing more deeply the differential diagnosis, precipitating factors, and the student's context, strengths, relevant safety issues, and resources (options A and C are incorrect). **Chapter 4 (p. 93)**

4.2   A patient is experiencing increasing severity of suicidal thoughts. He states that he is going through a divorce and has been struggling to find a job. He admits to feeling like he has no future. Which of the following, if communicated by the patient, would indicate a higher risk of suicide?

A. He reports having increased thoughts about what death is like.
B. He reports that he has been seeing a supportive therapist weekly over the past 4 months.
C. He discloses that he has been feeling consistently hopeless for the past 3 weeks.
D. He states that he has been having a difficult time talking to his children.

The correct response is option C: He discloses that he has been feeling consistently hopeless for the past 3 weeks.

Hopelessness has been found in clinical and through empirical evidence to have great salience for suicidal intent. It is not just the presence or absence of hopelessness that is important, but also the duration and severity of hopelessness. Patients who report enduring hopelessness are at greater risk for suicide both acutely and chronically (option C is correct).

Differentiating among suicidal thoughts, morbid ruminations, and thoughts of self-harm is important for the patient and the clinician. Knowing that having thoughts about death is not the same as being actively suicidal may ease the anxiety of a patient with morbid ruminations (option A is incorrect).

Most identifiable precipitants and stressors can be understood as losses. The clinician should suspend his or her own view of the precipitant or stressor and instead seek to evaluate the precipitant or stressor according the mindset of the suicidal individual. The clinician needs to weigh acute and chronic health problems, along with acute family challenges associated with displacement, divorce, death of a loved one, or other disruptions (option D is incorrect).

In considering suicide risk, social support represents an important protective factor. Signs of social support should not be vague or remote; social support needs to be both available and accessible (option B is incorrect). **Chapter 4 (pp. 95–97, 104–106)**

4.3   A 28-year-old woman with major depressive disorder was brought to the hospital after taking 24 pills of her duloxetine 90 mg/day prescription. She was found by her sister, who called the ambulance. Which of the following factors, if disclosed by or discovered about this patient, would place her at highest risk of suicide?

A. She has a coping card in her bag.
B. She was discharged from inpatient hospitalization 3 weeks ago.
C. She confides that her sister is her own main reason for living.
D. She reports having thoughts that life is not worth living for many years.

The correct response is option B: She was discharged from inpatient hospitalization 3 weeks ago.

Recent discharge from inpatient psychiatric treatment is associated with increased risk within the first year of release; risk is highest during the first month after discharge (option B is correct).

An imbalance between identified reasons for living and reasons for dying provides a metric for either intent or ambivalence (e.g., many reasons for dying and few reasons for living may signify that the intent is more heavily weighted toward death). On the other hand, reasons for living may be few but powerful, such as family relationships, cultural values, or religious beliefs (option C is incorrect).

The presence of a coping card may be indicative of previous suicidal behavior. However, carrying such a card is not necessarily indicative of acute risk; it is not unusual for patients with chronic or intermittent suicidal thoughts to carry a coping card with them in their backpack, purse, or wallet (option A is incorrect).

A patient may have been having suicidal thoughts for decades—the mere presence or absence of suicidal thinking is thus, in this case, not a particularly helpful indicator of escalating risk. Some patients may think about suicide intermittently but without intent. Other patients may think about suicide with sincere intent very often, yet not act on the cognition (option D is incorrect). **Chapter 4 (pp. 101–104)**

4.4   A 54-year-old woman who was referred to your outpatient clinic for depression reports that she has been experiencing low mood, anhedonia, and insomnia for the past 6 weeks. She becomes tearful, stating that she has been feeling worthless and that "life has been tough to tolerate lately." What approach should you take when raising the issue of this patient's suicidal thoughts?

A. Approach questioning of the patient more broadly rather than focusing solely on the suicidal thoughts.
B. Refrain from asking directly about suicidal thoughts, because direct questioning increases the risk of the patient committing suicide.
C. Ask detailed and explicit questions about the patient's suicidal thoughts.
D. Avoid addressing any ambivalence expressed by the patient regarding suicide.

The correct response is option C: Ask detailed and explicit questions about the patient's suicidal thoughts.

Careful and fine-grained, highly specific questions, when offered in a gentle and supportive manner, facilitate a good therapeutic connection with the patient. Detailed questioning can communicate positive therapeutic intent and support for the patient's efforts in being fully open and detailed with the clinician (option C is correct; option A is incorrect).

The clinician should clarify that the goal of the interview is to help the patient recover a sense of personal agency, safety, control, and hope. If the patient has been contemplating suicide for a while, it is helpful to positively acknowledge any ambivalence and to express support for whatever efforts the patient has made in self-care and in staying alive (option D is incorrect).

If the patient gives the clinician an opening, the clinician can take a few minutes to explore reasons for the patient to stay alive. The clinician can acknowledge the patient's distress, comment on how the patient's symptoms are influencing the patient's feelings, and clarify that his or her intent is to collaborate with the patient toward a safe solution. Providing accurate information about how suicidal feelings can be managed and how mental health issues can be addressed will help to establish trust and may serve to inspire hope for the distressed patient contemplating self-harm (option B is incorrect). **Chapter 4 (p. 93)**

4.5 A 60-year-old woman discloses that she has been depressed for the past 6 months, ever since her husband died. She reports staying in bed most days and having little motivation to do the things she used to enjoy. She also describes having thoughts about wishing she were dead and about what her family would do if she died. Which of the following statements best characterizes this patient's thoughts?

A. The patient is having active suicidal thoughts.
B. The patient's thoughts are focused on self-harm.
C. The patient's thoughts express an intention to end her own life.
D. The patient's thoughts represent morbid rumination.

The correct response is option D: The patient's thoughts represent morbid rumination.

It is important to differentiate among three constructs of suicidal cognitions: suicidal thoughts, morbid ruminations, and thoughts of self-harm. *Suicidal thoughts* are thoughts of intentionally ending one's life—of killing oneself (options A and C are incorrect).

Morbid ruminations are thoughts about death, dying, or ending up dead, or nonexistence, without active thoughts about killing oneself (option D is correct).

Thoughts of self-harm may have little to do with a desire to die and are typically motivated as a strategy for emotional regulation and problem solving, or for a reason other than seeking death, such as avoiding embarrassment, feelings of unrelenting guilt, dealing with a stigmatizing event, or managing serious interpersonal conflict (option B is incorrect). **Chapter 4 (p. 95)**

4.6 While exploring a patient's history, you learn that she has made suicide attempts in the past. You attempt to learn the details and the overall pattern of the patient's behavior. Which of the following features of the patient's past suicide attempts would provide the most useful information about her current risk?

A. The patient's emotional response to each previous attempt.
B. The method most often used in past attempts.
C. The overall presence of chronic suicidality.
D. The first attempt and the most serious of past attempts.

The correct response is option D: The first attempt and the most serious of past attempts.

A thorough exploration of all past suicide attempts may require several encounters (3–5 sessions) before the clinician makes a collaborative decision with the patient about providing ongoing care and treatment. In the initial interview, current risk can be understood with good accuracy by exploring the first attempt and the most serious of the past attempts (Joiner et al. 2003), with the patient identifying the most serious or "worst" attempt subjectively (option D is correct).

If the clinical setting does not permit a longitudinal evaluation, the clinician should document the situation, deferring historical review to the next encounter. The clinician should be certain to explore whether the patient has been thinking about more than one method of suicide and about access to means for each method. The clinician must direct the interview to achieve saturation; the clinician should continue to ask the patient about possible methods and access until the patient says no other methods have been considered. Until questioned thoroughly, patients will sometimes withhold their most ready or accessible means (option B is incorrect).

With chronic suicidality, simple comments or notes in the chart about the presence or absence of suicidal thoughts are insufficient. A patient may have been having suicidal thoughts for decades—the mere presence or absence of suicidal thinking is thus, in this case, not a particularly helpful indicator of escalating risk (option C is incorrect).

The patient's emotional reactions to previous attempts can help the clinician to identify the persistence of what has been called "residual intent" (e.g., patient answers such as "I learned that next time I need to use a gun") (Rudd 2006). While exploring residual intent is important for a comprehensive suicide assessment, it is not as indicative of a patient's current risk as the details of the most serious past attempts (option A is incorrect). **Chapter 4 (pp. 98–99, 100, 101)**

4.7   You are interviewing a 45-year-old man with a history of major depressive disorder (diagnosed when he was in his twenties). He reports that he had done well for almost a decade without being in treatment; however, over the past 4 weeks, his depressive symptoms have returned and have been progressing. He discloses that at times he has been having thoughts of wanting to end his life. Which of the following domains would be most important for you to inquire about during the interview with this patient?

A. Family history of completed suicide.
B. Previous history of morbid rumination.
C. History of scratching his thigh when feeling overwhelmed.
D. Access to bottles of medications.

The correct response is option D: Access to bottles of medications.

In assessing intent, the clinician needs to again determine how specific the patient's thinking and behavior are in relation to suicide. The clinician should ask about frequency, intensity, and duration of suicidal thoughts; about when and where the patient has thought about committing suicide; and about access to means (option D is correct).

Time constraints are usually a big factor in initial psychiatric evaluations and may affect subsequent care in many systems. It is essential that the clinician take responsibility for pacing the discussion with the patient. When necessary, the clinician may have to defer detailed history taking regarding previous crises or suicide attempts to later sessions (option B is incorrect).

Thoughts of self-harm may have little to do with a desire to die and are typically motivated as a strategy for emotional regulation and problem solving, or for a reason other than seeking death, such as avoiding embarrassment, feelings of unrelenting guilt, dealing with a stigmatizing event, or managing serious interpersonal conflict (option C is incorrect).

There are a number of empirically supported domains essential to accurate assessment of suicide risk (Rudd et al. 2004). One approach to assessing each of the risk assessment domains involves moving in sequential fashion from the precipitating event to the patient's current situation and symptoms (Rudd 2012). This approach to the interview represents a strategic clinical intervention that serves to reduce anxiety about disclosing difficult material to the clinician. Figure 4–1 (from Rudd 2012) illustrates this approach to the overall interview (including family history of suicide). Such hierarchical questioning may not be needed if suicidal thoughts and behaviors led to the clinical encounter (option A is incorrect). **Chapter 4 (pp. 97–100; Table 4–2 [pp. 103–104]; Figure 4–2 [p. 105])**

4.8   You are assessing a 16-year-old Native American girl who was sent in from her school after a teacher noticed multiple scratch marks on her arms. The patient discloses that she has been struggling in school, and her grades have dropped. Her father has been traveling more for work, and she reports that her father's absence has been hard on her mother and siblings. The girl is close to her mother, and they both are active in their local church. She reports depressed mood, insomnia, and a 5-pound weight loss. When asked about suicidal thoughts, the patient becomes quiet. Which of the following factors in this patient's profile may place her at greater risk of suicide?

A.   The patient is a Native American teenager.
B.   The patient is female.
C.   The patient has a close relationship with her mother.
D.   The patient is active in her local church.

The correct response is option A: The patient is a Native American teenager.

Evidence suggests that there is heightened risk among certain subpopulations (e.g., Native American adolescents, physically ill elders, transgender or gender-nonconforming individuals) and during certain sensitive time periods (e.g., first-episode psychosis, recent discharge from an inpatient psychiatric unit, divorce or widowhood). Individuals in these subpopulations or in these specific sensitive time periods may feel especially isolated or untrusting of the health care system and accurate risk assessment can be very difficult to attain (option A is correct).

Male gender confers a greater risk of suicidal behavior than does female gender (option B is incorrect).

Precipitant: *Is there anything in particular that happened that triggered thoughts about suicide?*

Symptomatic presentation: *Tell me about how you've been feeling lately. It sounds like you've been feeling depressed. Have you been feeling anxious, nervous, or panicky? Have you been down, low, or blue lately? Have you had trouble sleeping [additional symptoms of depression and anxiety]?*

Hopelessness: *It's not unusual for someone who's been feeling depressed to feel hopeless, like things won't change or get any better. Do you ever feel that way?*

Morbid ruminations: *It's not unusual when you're feeling depressed and hopeless to have thoughts about death and dying. Do you ever think about death or dying?*

Suicidal thinking: *It's not unusual when feeling depressed, hopeless, and having thoughts about death and dying to have thoughts about suicide. Have you ever thought about suicide?*

FIGURE 4–1.   Hierarchical approach to the interview as a whole: an example.

Source.   Reprinted from Rudd MD: "The Clinical Risk Assessment Interview," in *The American Psychiatric Publishing Textbook of Suicide Assessment and Management*, 2nd Edition. Edited by Simon RI, Hales RE. Washington, DC, American Psychiatric Publishing, 2012, pp 57–74. © 2012 American Psychiatric Publishing. Used with permission.

Resilience and the presence (or absence) of protective factors are increasingly recognized for their importance in suicidality and in the patient's ability to cope in life despite suicidal cognitions and behaviors. In considering suicide risk, social support represents an important protective factor (options C and D are incorrect). **Chapter 4 (pp. 102, 106; Table 4–2 [pp. 103–104])**

4.9   Before a clinician begins a patient evaluation, it can be helpful to communicate the purpose of the interview to the patient. Which of the following best expresses the goal of the initial interview of a patient with new suicidal thoughts?

A. To obtain a thorough report regarding the events leading up to the patient's presentation.
B. To develop a deep understanding of the patient's psychiatric history.
C. To help the patient recover a sense of personal agency, safety, and hope.
D. To point out the patient's unrealistic thinking about suicide.

The correct response is option C: To help the patient recover a sense of personal agency, safety, and hope.

The clinician should clarify that the goal of the interview is to help the patient recover a sense of personal agency, safety, control, and hope (option C is correct).

The clinician can acknowledge the patient's distress, comment on how the patient's symptoms are influencing the patient's feelings, and clarify that his or her intent is to collaborate with the patient toward a safe solution. It is ideal if the psychiatrist can first reassure the patient, offer nonjudgmental support, and introduce some basic information about mental disorders and the system of care. The clinician may then be able to turn to the task of assessing more deeply the differential diagnosis, precipitating factors, and the patient's context, strengths, relevant safety issues, and resources (options A and B are incorrect). Because fear and shame may dominate the thinking of suicidal individuals (Rudd et al. 2004), the clinician must avoid comments that may be experienced as threatening or judgmental (option D is incorrect). **Chapter 4 (p. 93)**

References

Joiner TE Jr, Steer RA, Brown G, et al: Worst-point suicidal plans: a dimension of suicidality predictive of past suicide attempts and eventual death by suicide. Behav Res Ther 41(12):1469–1480, 2003 14583414

Rudd MD: The Assessment and Management of Suicidality. Sarasota, FL, Professional Resource Exchange, 2006

Rudd MD: The clinical risk assessment interview, in The American Psychiatric Publishing Textbook of Suicide Assessment and Management, 2nd Edition. Edited by Simon RI, Hales RE. Washington, DC, American Psychiatric Association Publishing, 2012, pp 57–74

Rudd MD, Joiner TE, Rajab H: Treating Suicidal Behavior. New York, Guilford, 2004

CHAPTER 5

Laboratory Testing and Neuroimaging Studies in Psychiatry

5.1   A 51-year-old patient with a prior history of alcohol use disorder is brought to the emergency room for evaluation for danger to self and is being considered for psychiatric admission. The complete blood count (CBC) and comprehensive metabolic panel (CMP) were unremarkable, the chest X ray was normal, and the blood alcohol level (BAL) was 0.03%. Which of the following statements accurately describes the clinical utility of an electrocardiogram (ECG) for medical clearance prior to psychiatric admission of this patient?

A. ECG screening for prolonged QT interval is cost-effective in reducing the risk of sudden cardiac death in patients admitted to psychiatric hospitals.
B. This patient's BAL is low and does not indicate increased risk of an acute cardiac event.
C. Because this patient is younger than 60 years, he is at low risk of a cardiac event and does not need an ECG.
D. A normal chest X ray is an appropriate substitute for an ECG.

The correct response is option A: ECG screening for prolonged QT interval is cost-effective in reducing the risk of sudden cardiac death in patients admitted to psychiatric hospitals.

ECG screening for prolonged QT interval is cost-effective in reducing the risk of sudden cardiac death in patients admitted to psychiatric hospitals. A study employing a decision analytic model found that ECG screening for prolonged QT interval for all patients on admission to psychiatric hospitals was cost-effective in reducing the rate of sudden cardiac death (Poncet et al. 2015) (option A is correct).

In one study among patients with alcohol dependence, the adjusted risk ratio for sudden cardiac death was found to be 16.97 ($P<0.019$) (Wu et al. 2015), and the fact that this patient has any alcohol in his system indicates that his use is active (option B incorrect).

Because this patient has alcohol use disorder and is being psychiatrically admitted, he is already considered to be at elevated risk of sudden cardiac death and therefore warrants a screening ECG regardless of age (option C incorrect).

Chest X rays (option D incorrect) are appropriately performed for patients with suspected acute or unstable chronic cardiopulmonary disease and for some elderly patients, while ECGs can be used to identify ischemia, infarction, cardiac hypertrophy, conduction delays, the source of abnormal rhythms, and tissue inflammation such as pericarditis. **Chapter 5 (pp. 121–125)**

5.2 A multiple sleep latency test (MSLT) demonstrated that a patient's average time to sleep onset was 12 minutes, and three sleep-onset rapid eye movement (REM) periods were observed. The baseline electrocardiogram (EEG) was within normal limits. Which of the following disorders can be diagnosed on the basis of these findings?

A. Narcolepsy without cataplexy.
B. Hypersomnolence.
C. Delirium.
D. Subacute sclerosing panencephalitis.

The correct response is option A: Narcolepsy without cataplexy.

The MSLT is indicated to confirm the diagnosis of primary hypersomnia (narcolepsy) and to determine the effectiveness of treatment for this condition. The average time to sleep onset for patients without daytime hypersomnolence (option B is incorrect) is 10–20 minutes (Rack et al. 2005), so this patient is in the normal range.

If the average time to sleep onset were less than 8 minutes, the test would be considered positive for hypersomnolence. If more than two sleep-onset REM periods are observed, narcolepsy without cataplexy could be diagnosed (Rack et al. 2005) (option A is correct).

An EEG can be useful in the diagnosis of delirium; however, it typically shows generalized slow-wave activity in the delta and theta ranges, slowing of the posterior dominant frequency, disorganization of the background rhythm, and loss of reactivity to eye opening and closing (Jacobson and Jerrier 2000) (option C is incorrect).

The EEG in subacute sclerosing panencephalitis is not normal (option D is incorrect); rather, it shows periodic complexes consisting of 2–4 high-amplitude delta waves, usually bisynchronous and symmetrical, repeated every 5–7 seconds. **Chapter 5 (pp. 129, 132–134)**

5.3 Which of the following imaging modalities detects cerebrospinal fluid (CSF) with high-intensity (white) signal?

A. Computed tomography.
B. Proton density–weighted magnetic resonance imaging.
C. T1-weighted magnetic resonance imaging.
D. T2-weighted magnetic resonance imaging.

The correct response is option D: T2-weighted magnetic resonance imaging.

Computed tomography (CT) generates a two-dimensional grayscale map of the brain, with bone appearing most radiopaque (white) and air the least radiopaque (black). CSF is mostly water and has an intermediate level of radiopacity on a CT scan (option A is incorrect).

Descriptors for CT images predominantly use the terms *density* (hypodense, isodense, hyperdense) and *attenuation* (hypoattenuation, hyperattenuation), whereas magnetic resonance imaging (MRI) descriptors focus on *intensities*. Proton density–weighted MRI images typically have intermediate to low signal from CSF (option B is incorrect); T1-weighted images show CSF as hypointense dark areas (option C is incorrect); and T2-weighted images show CSF as hyperintense white areas (option D is correct). **Chapter 5 (pp. 140, 141 [Table 5–12])**

5.4   Which of the following imaging modalities would be most effective for detecting damage to the structural integrity of white matter tracts?

A. Magnetic resonance spectroscopy (MRS).
B. Magnetoencephalography.
C. Diffusion tensor imaging (DTI).
D. Functional magnetic resonance imaging (fMRI).

The correct response is option C: Diffusion tensor imaging (DTI).

MRS and DTI are structural imaging modalities, while magnetoencephalography and fMRI are functional imaging modalities (options B and D are incorrect).

MRS provides information about neuronal injury by measuring several markers of cellular integrity and function and has been used to assess pharmacokinetics and pharmacodynamics of various psychotropic medications (option A is incorrect).

DTI measures the diffusion of water in brain tissues, allowing quantification of orientation and structure via metrics such as fractional anisotropy and mean diffusivity, as well as qualitative aspects of white matter tracts via tractography (option C is correct). **Chapter 5 (pp. 141–148)**

5.5   A 44-year-old woman with a history of alcohol use disorder presents to the emergency room. She has a blood alcohol level (BAL) that is below the threshold of detection. A laboratory test of which of the following would provide the most reliable indicator of recent alcohol consumption in this patient?

A. Aspartate transaminase.
B. Gamma-glutamyltransferase.
C. Alkaline phosphatase.
D. Alcohol breath analysis.

The correct response is option B: Gamma-glutamyltransferase.

Aspartate transaminase (AST) (option A is incorrect) should be used in combination with other laboratory measurements (such as the AST/alanine aminotransferase [ALT] ratio) to support a diagnosis of alcohol use disorder.

A low BAL suggests that this patient has already metabolized any ethanol in her system; thus, ethanol would be unlikely to show up on a breath analysis (option D is incorrect).

In males, measurement of the liver enzyme gamma-glutamyltransferase (GGT) and percentage carbohydrate-deficient transferrin (%CDT) together provides the most reliable indicator of recent drinking. However in females, measurement of GGT alone (option B is correct) better correlates with recent drinking (Rinck et al. 2007).

GGT elevations of >25 U/L in women is consistent with 4+ drinks daily for 4 weeks or more. Alkaline phosphatase can be helpful in distinguishing etiologies of liver injury (option C is incorrect). **Chapter 5 (pp. 114, 154–155)**

5.6   Which of the following is a commonly observed laboratory abnormality in patients with alcohol use disorder?

A. Low magnesium.
B. Elevated phosphate.
C. Low mean corpuscular volume.
D. Low serum total homocysteine.

The correct response is option A: Low magnesium.

Patients with alcohol use disorder often are found to have blood lab abnormalities, including low magnesium, low phosphate, low blood sugar, anemia, low platelets, and abnormal blood clotting times (Magarian et al. 1992) (option A is correct; option B is incorrect). Mean corpuscular volume and serum total homocysteine are *elevated*, not decreased, in alcohol use disorder (options C and D are incorrect). **Chapter 5 (pp. 154–155; Table 5–17 [p. 155])**

5.7   Which of the following statements about single photon emission computed tomography (SPECT) is *true*?

A. SPECT measures cerebral glucose metabolism.
B. SPECT is typically more expensive than positron emission tomography (PET).
C. SPECT uses a radiotracer that is attached to a drug.
D. SPECT provides higher structural anatomic visualization than magnetic resonance imaging (MRI).

The correct response is option C: SPECT uses a radiotracer that is attached to a drug.

SPECT provides images of cerebral blood flow and brain activity. The technique involves the injection of a radioactive tracer attached to a drug (option C is correct) such as technetium-99m-hexamethylpropyleneamine oxime (HMPAO) or technetium-99m-ethyl cysteinate dimer (ECD), lipophilic drugs that are able to diffuse across the blood–brain barrier and into neurons.

Cerebral glucose metabolism can be measured with PET (option A is incorrect), and PET is more expensive than SPECT (option B is incorrect).

Compared with MRI, SPECT provides limited structural anatomic visualization (option D is incorrect). **Chapter 5 (pp. 144–147)**

5.8   A patient has abnormal liver function test findings on a comprehensive metabolic panel (CMP) after initiation of chlorpromazine. Which of the following, if elevated to more than three times the upper limit of normal, would point to a cholestatic drug reaction?

A. Aspartate transaminase (AST).
B. Alanine aminotransferase (ALT).
C. Alkaline phosphatase.
D. Bilirubin.

The correct response is option C: Alkaline phosphatase.

One of the most important uses of the CMP is the identification of drug-induced hepatobiliary injury. A cholestatic drug reaction is suspected when alkaline phosphatase is more than three times the upper limit of normal (option C is correct) and AST and ALT levels are normal or only minimally elevated (options A and B are incorrect).

A hepatotoxic drug reaction is suspected when AST or ALT are three or more times the upper limit of normal, bilirubin is two or more times the upper limit of normal (option D is incorrect), alkaline phosphatase is two or less than three times the upper limit of normal, and there is no other known reason for liver injury. **Chapter 5 (p. 114)**

5.9   A patient with low thyroid-stimulating hormone (TSH) and normal free thyroxine (T_4) is most likely to have which of the following conditions?

A. Hypothyroidism.
B. Subclinical hypothyroidism.
C. Hyperthyroidism.
D. Subclinical hyperthyroidism.

The correct response is option D: Subclinical hyperthyroidism.

High TSH is associated with hypothyroidism and subclinical hypothyroidism, although hypothyroidism is also associated with low T_4 (options A and B are incorrect). Low TSH is associated with hyperthyroidism, subclinical hyperthyroidism, and a nonthyroidal illness. Subclinical hypothyroidism is associated with a normal free T_4 (option D is correct), while high free T_4 is associated with hyperthyroidism (option C is incorrect) and low free T_4 is associated with nonthyroidal illness. **Chapter 5 (pp. 119–120)**

5.10 Which of the following findings on an electroencephalogram (EEG) would be most consistent with delirium?

A. Alpha power highest over occipital areas.
B. Generalized slow-wave activity.
C. Reactivity to eye opening and closure.
D. Periodic complexes consisting of 2–4 high-amplitude delta waves repeated every 5–7 seconds.

The correct response is option B: Generalized slow-wave activity.

An EEG of a delirious patient typically shows generalized slow-wave activity in the delta and theta ranges (option B is correct), slowing of the posterior dominant frequency, disorganization of the background rhythm, and loss of reactivity to eye opening and closing (option C is incorrect) (Jacobson and Jerrier 2000). Alpha power that is highest over the occipital areas is a normal EEG finding (option A is incorrect). EEG in patients with subacute sclerosing panencephalitis can show periodic complexes consisting of 2–4 high amplitude delta waves, usually bisynchronous and symmetrical, repeated every 5–7 seconds (option D is incorrect). **Chapter 5 (pp. 129–133)**

References

Jacobson SA, Jerrier H: EEG in delirium. Semin Clin Neuropsychiatry 5(2):86–92, 2000 10837097
Magarian GJ, Lucas LM, Kumar KL: Clinical significance in alcoholic patients of commonly encountered laboratory test results. West J Med 156(3):287–294, 1992 1595246
Poncet A, Gencer B, Blondon M, et al: Electrocardiographic screening for prolonged QT interval to reduce sudden cardiac death in psychiatric patients: a cost-effectiveness analysis. PLoS One 10(6):e0127213, 2015 26070071
Rack M, Davis J, Roffwarg HP, et al: The multiple sleep latency test in the diagnosis of narcolepsy. Am J Psychiatry 162(11):2198–2199, author reply 2199, 2005 16263876
Rinck D, Frieling H, Freitag A, et al: Combinations of carbohydrate-deficient transferrin, mean corpuscular erythrocyte volume, gamma-glutamyltransferase, homocysteine and folate increase the significance of biological markers in alcohol dependent patients. Drug Alcohol Depend 89(1):60–65, 2007 17234365
Wu SI, Tsai SY, Huang MC, et al: Risk factors for sudden cardiac death among patients with alcohol dependence: a nested case-control study. Alcohol Clin Exp Res 39(9):1797–1804, 2015 26207644

CHAPTER 6

The Social Determinants of Mental Health

6.1 As described by scholars of public health and global health, what are *social determinants of mental health*?

    A. Aspects of daily socialization with friends, family, and coworkers that affect an individual's mental health.

    B. The impact of religious and cultural traditions on how mental health symptoms are expressed within a given society.

    C. Environmental, societal, and economic conditions that affect mental health outcomes at a population level.

    D. Legal, psychiatric, and medical consensus definitions of psychiatric disorders, used mainly by social service entities.

The correct response is option C: Environmental, societal, and economic conditions that affect mental health outcomes at a population level.

The concept of social determinants of health is used within the public and global health spheres to refer to the fact that social variables (including a person's gender, race, economic status, physical environment, and other factors) can have significant impacts on people's health outcomes (Braveman et al. 2011b; Centers for Disease Control and Prevention 2018). Similarly, within the behavioral health sphere, environmental, societal, and economic factors have been found to have population-level impacts on mental health outcomes. These factors are referred to as *social determinants of mental health* (option C is correct).

    Social determinants of health are thought to be largely responsible for existing disparities and inequities in mental health service access, quality, and outcomes seen within and between population groups. Social determinants of mental health exert their impact at a population level, although not necessarily at an individual level (option A is incorrect).

    Several adverse social determinants of mental health have been identified, including discrimination, adverse early-life experiences, poor education, poverty, job and food insecurity, and unstable housing (Compton and Shim 2015). Although legal, medical, and cultural ways of describing psychiatric illness are certainly relevant to patients' experiences, these are not among the social determinants of mental health that have been thus far characterized (options B and D are incorrect). **Chapter 6 (pp. 163–165)**

6.2   As used in public health and public policy contexts, what does the term *health inequities* mean?

    A. Disparities in health that result from unjust and avoidable social and economic policies.
    B. Marked interpersonal variations in health that result entirely from genetic risk factors.
    C. Observed health differences between segments of the population, which have many causes.
    D. Discrepancies in how behavioral health care and medical care are covered by insurance.

The correct response is option A: Disparities in health that result from unjust and avoidable social and economic policies.

Health inequities are differences in health status resulting from systemic, avoidable, and unjust social and economic policies and practices that create barriers to opportunity (option A is correct).

The concept of health inequities refers specifically to disparities occurring as a result of unfair policies, rather than other causes of health differences such as genetics (options B and C are incorrect).

Health inequities exist within the related but broader concept of health disparities. Health disparities are differences in health status among segments of the population, including differences that occur by gender, race or ethnicity, education or income, disability status, or geographic area. Health inequities and disparities most often adversely affect socially disadvantaged groups. The elimination of health disparities was a goal proposed by the *Healthy People 2020* initiative issued by the United States Department of Health and Human Services (Braveman et al. 2011b). Many public health researchers situate the concepts of health disparities and health equity and inequity within broader contexts of human rights and social justice. Although health insurance coverage of behavioral health versus medical claims is certainly important, it is not necessarily related to health inequuities (option D is incorrect). **Chapter 6 (p. 164)**

6.3   You are working as an embedded psychiatrist in a primary care clinic. You are asked to evaluate an 18-year-old who recently immigrated from Ecuador who was referred to you by her primary care physician for a major depressive episode. This patient was born biologically male and currently identifies as female. She is living with family members who are critical of her gender identity and presentation. While at her workplace, she has experienced derogatory comments regarding her gender identity and immigration status. Which of the following adverse social determinants of health would be of greatest relevance to you, the psychiatrist, in considering the best approach to caring for this patient?

A. Hormonal treatment should be encouraged for this patient, because untreated gender dysphoria increases the likelihood that the patient's depressive symptoms will worsen.

B. Psychiatric care is stigmatized in immigrant communities; thus, it would most likely be preferable for this patient's depression to be treated by her primary care physician.

C. Depressive symptoms arising in the context of psychosocial stressors are likely to self-resolve and do not require medication.

D. Experiences of discrimination are associated with adverse mental health symptoms, placing this patient at increased risk for depression.

The correct response is option D: Experiences of discrimination are associated with adverse mental health symptoms, placing this patient at increased risk for depression.

Discrimination and social exclusion are among the social determinants of mental health. Discrimination based on multiple characteristics (including race/ethnicity, gender, religion, sexual orientation, immigration status, and social class) has been linked to adverse mental health outcomes in studies conducted with multiple patient populations that experience discrimination (Krieger 2014; Viruell-Fuentes et al. 2012). Adverse mental health outcomes associated with discrimination include depressive symptoms, anxiety disorders, and substance use disorders, among others. For example, there are high rates of posttraumatic stress disorder, anxiety, and depression among American Indians, a population that has experienced significant discrimination (Walters et al. 2011). As a recent immigrant and transgender person experiencing discrimination, the patient in this case is at elevated risk for adverse mental health outcomes (option D is correct).

Of note, about 40% of male-to-female transgender persons experience significant discrimination (Krieger 2014). Transgender patients should not be pressured to begin hormone therapy, as each transgender person's interest in hormonal or surgical options may vary (option A is incorrect).

It should not be assumed that this patient would not want to interact with a psychiatrist (option B is incorrect). Depressive episodes precipitated by psychosocial stressors will not necessarily resolve, and standard-of-care medication should still be offered (option C is incorrect). **Chapter 6 (p. 166)**

6.4 You are a community psychiatrist who receives a referral of an 18-year-old woman who is aging out of a local child psychiatry clinic, where she is being treated for persistent depressive disorder (dysthymia). The evaluation provided by the clinic comments that this patient is at increased risk for poor mental health outcomes based on her multiple "adverse childhood experiences." You recognize *adverse childhood experiences* as a term from the public psychiatry literature. To what does this term refer?

A. Childhood experiences of interpersonal abuse or neglect.

B. Childhood experiences of displacement or forced migration.

C. Childhood experiences of school-based bullying or exclusion.

D. Childhood experiences of being adopted or in foster care.

The correct response is option A: Childhood experiences of interpersonal abuse or neglect.

The term *adverse childhood experiences* became widely known as a result of the Adverse Childhood Experiences (ACE) Study, which surveyed thousands of adult men and women about whether they had experienced so-called "adverse childhood experiences" or ACEs (Dube et al. 2001). ACEs include abuse (emotional, physical, or sexual), witnessing of domestic violence at home, exposure to alcohol or drug abuse at home, having a parent with psychiatric illness, having divorced or separated parents, and having a household member who was incarcerated (option A is correct).

Each participant received a score based on the number of ACEs they had been exposed to. Higher ACE scores were found to be strongly associated with a higher likelihood of attempting suicide (Dube et al. 2001). Higher ACE scores were also associated with increased risk of depression, alcohol use disorder, and recreational drug abuse (Felitti et al. 1998). Subsequent studies have replicated these associations and identified additional associations, including between ACEs and anxiety (Mersky et al. 2013). Although it is certainly likely that other potentially stressful childhood experiences (including forced migration, bullying, adoption, or placement in foster care) can negatively impact a person's mental health, these types of experiences are not covered by the term *adverse childhood experiences* as used in the public psychiatry literature (options B, C, and D are incorrect). **Chapter 6 (p. 166)**

6.5   You recently started working at a community psychiatry clinic. You are wondering what approach to use for patients who are affected by adverse determinants of mental health. What would a public psychiatry expert most likely recommend that you do?

A. Avoid asking new patients about childhood abuse or neglect, as such questions may trigger traumatic memories.

B. Educate patients that concerns about employment would be best shared with a social worker.

C. Screen patients routinely for food insecurity, and provide them with lists of local resources.

D. Encourage patients who are victims of discrimination to find a provider with a similar background.

The correct response is option C: Screen patients routinely for food insecurity, and provide them with lists of local resources.

The authors of this chapter encourage psychiatrists to try to improve adverse social determinants of mental health within their practice and community. In order to do this, psychiatrists can advocate against social norms or public policies that result in, for instance, social exclusion or discrimination. The authors of this chapter also recommend that psychiatrists implement concrete strategies in their clinical settings that can help provide immediate assistance to patients and community members. Such strategies can include screening for adverse social determinants of mental health, including childhood abuse or neglect (option A is incorrect).

Several additional interventions are suggested, including adding evening or weekend appointment times to increase access to care, offering supported employment positions within the practice or clinic, and creating lists of local resources (e.g., food banks, public assistance programs) (option C is correct).

While it may be helpful to partner with a social worker, it is still important for psychiatrists to understand and attempt to improve their patients' psychosocial circumstances, as these factors significantly impact mental health (option B is incorrect).

Community psychiatrists should ideally make their services as accessible as possible, and thus it is likely counterproductive for providers to assume that they should not work with certain patient populations due to socioeconomic, racial, gender, or other differences (option D is incorrect). **Chapter 6 (pp. 170–171)**

References

Braveman P, Egerter S, Williams DR: The social determinants of health: coming of age. Annu Rev Public Health 32:381–398, 2011a 21091195

Braveman PA, Kumanyika S, Fielding J, et al: Health disparities and health equity: the issue is justice. Am J Public Health 101 (suppl 1):S149–S155, 2011b 21551385

Centers for Disease Control and Prevention: Social Determinants of Health. Last updated December 9, 2018. Available at: https://www.healthypeople.gov/2020/topics-objectives/topic/social-determinants-of-health. Accessed December 9, 2018.

Compton MT, Shim RS (eds): The Social Determinants of Mental Health. Washington, DC, American Psychiatric Publishing, 2015

Dube SR, Anda RF, Felitti VJ, et al: Childhood abuse, household dysfunction, and the risk of attempted suicide throughout the life span: findings from the Adverse Childhood Experiences Study. JAMA 286(24):3089–3096, 2001 11754674

Felitti VJ, Anda RF, Nordenberg D, et al: Relationship of childhood abuse and household dysfunction to many of the leading causes of death in adults. The Adverse Childhood Experiences (ACE) Study. Am J Prev Med 14(4):245–258, 1998 9635069

Krieger N: Discrimination and health inequities. Int J Health Serv 44(4):643–710, 2014 25626224

Mersky JP, Topitzes J, Reynolds AJ: Impacts of adverse childhood experiences on health, mental health, and substance use in early adulthood: a cohort study of an urban, minority sample in the U.S. Child Abuse Negl 37(11):917–925, 2013 23978575

Viruell-Fuentes EA, Miranda PY, Abdulrahim S: More than culture: structural racism, intersectionality theory, and immigrant health. Soc Sci Med 75(12):2099–2106, 2012 22386617

Walters KL, Mohammed SA, Evans-Campbell T, et al: Bodies don't just tell stories, they tell histories: embodiment of historical trauma among American Indians and Alaska Natives. Du Bois Review: Social Science Research on Race 8:179–189, 2011

CHAPTER 7

Ethical Considerations in Psychiatry

7.1   A 45-year-old woman with a history of schizophrenia and end-stage renal disease on hemodialysis is admitted to the hospital for acute psychotic decompensation. She is disheveled, and her thinking is disorganized. She denies suicidal/homicidal ideation. She is alert and can tell you why she gets hemodialysis, although in very simple, concrete terms. She scores 20/30 on the Montreal Cognitive Assessment. Since her admission, she has been adamantly and consistently refusing hemodialysis, because she believes that the admitting medical team is trying to "poison the blood" with the dialysis machine. She cannot tell you the medical consequences of refusing this treatment. What are the conflicting ethical considerations in this situation?

A. Clinical indications and patient preferences.
B. Clinical indications and patient quality of life.
C. Contextual influences and patient preferences.
D. Patient quality of life and contextual influences.

The correct response is option A: Clinical indications and patient preferences.

In the clinical setting, a widely used approach to ethical problem solving is the "four-topics method" described by Jonsen et al. (2006). This method entails gathering and evaluating information about 1) clinical indications, 2) patient preferences, 3) patient quality of life, and 4) contextual or external influences on the ethical decision-making process. Many ethical dilemmas in clinical care involve a conflict between the first two topics of the four-topics method—*clinical indications* and *patient preferences* (option A is correct). Examples of such dilemmas include a depressed cancer patient who refuses life-prolonging chemotherapy and a young person undergoing a "first psychotic break" who is brought to a hospital for treatment against his or her will. In each of these situations, the preferences of the patient are at odds with what is medically beneficial, creating a conflict for the physician between the duties of beneficence and respecting patient autonomy.

The most fundamental goal of medical care is the improvement of *quality of life* for all those who need and seek care. Patients and their physicians must determine what quality of life is desirable, how it is to be attained, and what risks and disadvantages are associated with the desired quality, including the long-term consequences of accepting or refusing a recommendation for medical intervention. In this scenario, the patient has not disclosed her decision to refuse treatment as a reflection of her desired quality of life (options B and D are incorrect).

Contextual features address the social, legal, economic, and institutional circumstances in which a particular case of patient care occurs. Although contextual features are present in almost all clinical circumstances to some degree, no mention is made of a contextual influence affecting the patient's preference or her quality of life in this scenario (options C and D are incorrect). **Chapter 7 (pp. 180–181)**

7.2   A 65-year-old woman with Stage IV breast cancer with metastasis to the brain has decided she does not want to pursue chemotherapy. She is cachectic appearing and reports to be in a lot of pain. She can tell you details of her diagnosis, which treatment is recommended and why. She demonstrates an understanding of the consequences of refusing treatment, which could include death. On examination, she is alert throughout and able to attend to the interview. She has mild cognitive impairment on formal testing, with a Montreal Cognitive Assessment score of 22/30. She denies suicidal ideation but she expresses pessimism that treatment would help to improve her quality of life or extend her survival. A psychiatrist has been asked to perform a decisional capacity evaluation to determine this patient's capacity to refuse proposed treatment. The psychiatrist happens to be a friend of the patient's intimate partner. Which essential ethical skills must the psychiatrist make particular use of when evaluating this patient?

A. The ability to identify ethical dilemmas, to understand how one's personal biases may affect one's care of patients, and to know one's own scope of clinical competence and be willing to work within those boundaries.
B. The ability to identify ethical dilemmas, to anticipate ethically high-risk situations, and to understand how one's personal biases may affect one's care of patients.
C. The ability to identify ethical dilemmas and to know one's own scope of clinical competence and be willing to work within those boundaries.
D. The ability to understand how one's personal biases may affect one's care of patients, to anticipate ethically high-risk situations, and to seek information and consultation and make use of advice received when faced with difficult situations.

The correct response is option B: The ability to identify ethical dilemmas, to anticipate ethically high-risk situations, and to understand how one's personal biases may affect one's care of patients.

Psychiatrists whose work embodies the highest ethical standards tend to rely on a set of core "ethics skills" that are learned during or before medical training and are continually practiced and refined during their career (Roberts 2016; Roberts and Dyer 2004). The first of these core skills is *the ability to identify ethical issues as they arise*. For some, this identification will be an intuitive insight (e.g., an internal sense that "something is not right"). The second skill is *the ability to understand how one's personal values, beliefs, and sense of self may affect one's care of patients*. For instance, a psychiatrist who is emotionally invested in his or her ability to "do good" as a healer should recognize that this emotional investment may subtly influence his or her judgment when evaluating the decisional capacity of a patient who refuses medically necessary treatments (option B is correct).

The third key ethics skill is *an awareness of the limits of one's medical knowledge and expertise and a willingness to practice within those limits*. Providing competent care within the scope of one's expertise fulfills both the positive ethical duty of doing good and the obligation to "do no harm." There is no indication that the psychiatrist is not competent to answer the clinical question of decisional capacity (options A and C are incorrect).

The fourth skill is *the ability to recognize high-risk situations in which ethical problems are likely to arise*. Ethically high-risk situations may be obvious, such as in circumstances in which a psychiatrist must step out of the usual treatment relationship to protect the patient or others from harm. Some are harder to recognize—for example, providing clinical care to people with whom one has other relationships (e.g., friends or relatives)—but may create vulnerability for poor decision making, as in this case (option B is correct).

The fifth skill is *the willingness to seek information and consultation when faced with an ethically or clinically difficult situation and the ability to make use of offered guidance*. Again, there is no indication that the psychiatrist requires further consultation for this clinical question (option D is incorrect).

The final essential ethics skill is *the ability to build appropriate ethical safeguards into one's work*. For example, a psychiatrist who treats children and adolescents would be wise to routinely inform new patients and their parents, at the onset of treatment, about the limits of confidentiality and the physician's legal mandate to report child abuse. **Chapter 7 (pp. 178–180; Table 7–1 [p. 179])**

7.3   A psychiatrist working in a private practice of three psychiatrists notices that her colleague has not shown up to work twice this week and also noticed that he was stumbling toward his car after work one day. She is unaware of any adverse patient outcomes based on these observed behaviors. What is the appropriate action to be taken by the psychiatrist?

A. Respect her colleague's confidentiality and keep this information private.
B. Do nothing until she has enough information to make a definitive judgment about whether or not the colleague is practicing competently.
C. Wait until her colleague confides in her that he has a substance use disorder.
D. Report her colleague to the appropriate professional bodies.

The correct response is option D: Report her colleague to the appropriate professional bodies.

Intervening in and reporting colleague misconduct or impairment are some of the most difficult ethical imperatives of the conscientious psychiatrist. When psychiatrists bring legitimate cases of physician misconduct to light, they fulfill the ideals of beneficence and nonmaleficence by protecting the physician's current and future patients. Nevertheless, a number of psychological barriers to reporting colleague impairment have been identified, including overidentification with the impaired physician, collusion with the colleague's denial and minimization, and a tendency to overvalue confidentiality and protect the colleague's reputation and career at the expense of safety (Roberts and Miller 2004). To help psychiatrists overcome their reluctance to report problem behavior, Overstreet (2001) suggested a useful four-step procedure for working through the issue. First, the psychiatrist should become informed about the reporting requirements of his or her state. In some localities, physicians may experience legal penalties if they fail to report physician impairment. Second, the psychiatrist should seek to more fully understand the situation, including how his or her own feelings may complicate the ability both to observe the colleague's behavior objectively and to report it. Third, all of the options that fulfill the duty to "strive to expose" the misconduct should be considered (options A and C are incorrect).

Just as there is a range of physician misbehaviors, there can be a range of appropriate responses. These may include speaking privately with the colleague, informing the colleague's supervisor or administrative chief, filing an ethics complaint with the district American Psychiatric Association branch, and/or notifying the state licensing board (option D is correct).

Finally, the psychiatrist should choose the most appropriate option or options as a first step (Overstreet 2001). It is important to note that the reporting physician is not expected to make a definitive judgment about whether or not a colleague is practicing competently (option B is incorrect). **Chapter 7 (pp. 190–191)**

7.4   A patient with bipolar disorder is admitted to the hospital due to shortness of breath and found to have an acute coronary syndrome requiring cardiac catheterization. On exam, he is intermittently hypotensive and somnolent. He is not able to tell you why he is in the hospital. His Montreal Cognitive Assessment score is 8/30. When informed of his medical diagnosis and the proposed treatment, the patient decides he does not want a cardiac catheterization. You are asked to assess the patient's decisional capacity to refuse the procedure. A judgment of decisional capacity is based primarily on which of the following?

A. The judgment depends on whether the procedure is deemed high risk or low risk.
B. The judgment depends on the psychiatric diagnosis of the patient.
C. The judgment is based on an assessment of the adequacy of the patient's understanding, appreciation, reasoning, and indication of a choice regarding the proposed intervention.
D. The judgment is determined on the basis of whether the patient has a severe mental illness such as schizophrenia.

The correct response is option C: The judgment is based on an assessment of the adequacy of the patient's understanding, appreciation, reasoning, and indication of a choice regarding the proposed intervention.

The phrase *decision-making capacity* differs from the term *competency* in that competency to perform a specific function or competency in a particular life domain is a legal determination made through a judicial or other legal process. Legal jurisdictions have differing standards for establishing competency (Appelbaum and Grisso 1995). Psychiatrists are often called upon to make determinations of the decisional capacity. A detailed understanding of the concept of decisional capacity is therefore important for all psychiatrists and is especially crucial for those who perform consultation-liaison work and for those involved in the care of patients with disorders characterized by cognitive impairment (Bourgeois et al. 2017). *Decisional capacity* refers to a determination made by a clinical professional. A patient who refuses treatment but whose understanding, appreciation, reasoning, and indication of a choice are adequate has the right to refuse treatment (option C is correct).

Although there is no clear index for deciding how stringent the standard for consent should be, a general rule of thumb is to use a "sliding scale" approach (Appelbaum 2007). Decisions involving higher risks or greater risk–benefit ratios generally require a more stringent standard for decisional capacity, whereas more routine, lower-risk decisions generally require a less rigorous standard for decisional capacity (option A is incorrect). For example, the standard for understanding the procedure, risks, benefits, and alternatives related to an invasive treatment (such as deep brain stimulation) should be substantially higher than the standard for a relatively low-risk treatment (such as selective serotonin reuptake inhibitor treatment).

Crucially, a judgment of capacity is independent of the patient's diagnosis (option B is incorrect) and the severity of the illness (option D is incorrect). This is a key point to reemphasize to nonpsychiatric colleagues, who may assume that patients with psychiatric disorders lack capacity de facto. Patients with schizophrenia, bipolar disorder, mania, severe depression, or any other mental illness may possess or lack decisional capacity to accept or refuse a variety of procedures and treatments. Although disease process, age, and cognitive functioning may substantially impair patients' abilities to make a fully informed, meaningful choice about treatment, empirical evidence suggests that many people with severe mental illness commonly have adequate ability to make treatment decisions (Okai et al. 2007). **Chapter 7 (pp. 186–187)**

7.5   A third-year medical student often works long hours and spends his weekends studying for exams. Despite this busy schedule, he enjoys spending his free time volunteering at a child advocacy center, where he helps to organize fundraising events and cook meals for families. Which of the following ethical principles is this man practicing by his participation in such volunteer activity?

A. Fidelity.
B. Autonomy.
C. Integrity.
D. Beneficence.

The correct response is option D: Beneficence.

Fidelity is the virtue of promise keeping (option A is incorrect). *Autonomy* is the principle honoring the individual's capacity to make decisions for him- or herself and to act on the basis of such decisions (option B is incorrect). *Integrity* is the virtue of coherence, and of adherence to professionalism, in intention and action (option C is incorrect). *Beneficence* is the principle of engaging in actions to bring about good for others (option D is correct). **Chapter 7 (p. 179)**

7.6   A 65-year-old man with diabetes mellitus type 2, chronic obstructive pulmonary disease (COPD), congestive heart failure (CHF), and schizophrenia is admitted to the medical floor for cellulitis. His COPD and CHF are end stage, with an estimated 6-month survival. He is not actively psychotic and does not need medication adjustments. His Montreal Cognitive Assessment score is 27/30. In the discussion of code status, his understanding of his systemic illnesses and prognosis is adequate, and after the discussion, he chooses to be listed as DNR/DNI (Do Not Resuscitate/Do Not Intubate). Which of the following statements most accurately describes the ethical basis of the informed consent process for a decisionally intact patient to exercise his/her autonomy regarding a code status decision?

A. Given that the patient has schizophrenia, the philosophical basis for informed consent resides in what the clinician thinks would be the best treatment decision for the patient.
B. Promoting autonomy alone creates an environment for true informed consent that enhances a patient's meaningful decision making.
C. The clinician must also appraise whether the patient has the opportunity to make a choice consistent with the preferences of his or her family and friends.
D. Informed consent is the process by which individuals make free, knowledgeable decisions about whether to accept a proposed plan for assessment and/ or treatment.

The correct response is option D: Informed consent is a process by which individuals make free, knowledgeable decisions about whether to accept a proposed plan for assessment and/or treatment.

Informed consent is the process by which individuals make free, knowledgeable decisions about whether to accept a proposed plan for assessment and/or treatment (option D is correct).

Informed consent is a cornerstone of ethical practice. The philosophical basis for informed consent is found in our societal and cultural respect for individual persons and affirmation of individuals' freedom of self-determination (option A is incorrect).

An adequate process of informed consent reflects and promotes the ethical principle of autonomy. Promoting autonomy alone without incorporating other ethical principles, however, fails to create an environment for true informed consent that enhances a patient's meaningful decision making (option B is incorrect).

The principle of beneficence is also crucial to the informed consent process. The clinician must thoroughly appraise to what degree the consent process meets the patient's need for information. The clinician must also appraise whether the patient has the opportunity to make a choice consistent with his or her authentic preferences and values (option C is incorrect) (Roberts 2002). **Chapter 7 (p. 186)**

7.7   Which of the following statements regarding decisional capacity and competency is *true*?

A. Legal jurisdictions have differing standards for establishing decisional capacity.
B. *Decisional capacity* refers to a determination made by a clinical professional, and *competency* is a legal determination.
C. *Competency* refers to a determination made by a clinical professional, and *decisional capacity* in a particular life domain is a legal determination.
D. A decisional capacity assessment must be performed by a psychiatrist.

The correct response is option B: *Decisional capacity* **refers to a determination made by a clinical professional, and** *competency* **is a legal determination.**

The phrase *decision-making capacity* differs from the term *competency* in that competency to perform a specific function or competency in a particular life domain is a legal determination made through a judicial or other legal process, whereas decisional capacity refers to a determination made by a clinical professional (option B is correct; option C is incorrect).

Legal jurisdictions have differing standards for establishing *competency* (Appelbaum and Grisso 1995) (option A is incorrect).

Psychiatrists are often called upon to make determinations of the decisional capacity of nonpsychiatric patients. Although psychiatrists are usually consulted in these cases, any clinical professional can make this determination (option D is incorrect). A detailed understanding of the concept of decisional capacity is important for all psychiatrists and is especially crucial for those who perform consultation-liaison work and for those involved in the care of patients with disorders characterized by cognitive impairment (Bourgeois et al. 2017). Moreover, being able to explain and teach standards and strategies for assessing capacity to nonpsychiatric colleagues is a critical skill, as many clinicians have not been adequately trained to do even basic screening for capacity (Armontrout et al. 2016). **Chapter 7 (p. 186)**

7.8   Dr. Jones is a first-year resident, working more than 80 hours per week and sleeping, at most, 5 hours each night. She is not involved in health-promoting recreation or exercise and is often isolated from family and friends. She has finished a particularly long day of work and is exhausted. She is sitting down to chart and notices after reviewing her patient list that she ordered laboratory work on the wrong patient, a medical error. Other than increasing the likelihood of medical error, which of the following is an additional negative consequence of diminished physician well-being?

A. Substance use.
B. Delivering high-quality care.
C. Improved health and service outcomes.
D. Increased empathy and engagement.

The correct response is option A: Substance use.

Caring for patients is a great privilege and a source of fulfillment for health professionals, yet it is increasingly recognized that the sustained, intensive work effort and personal sacrifice involved in being a physician or physician-in-training can take their toll on physician well-being over time (Gengoux and Roberts 2018). Negative consequences of diminished physician well-being are serious and have been well documented. Consequences may include emotional exhaustion; greater likelihood of medical mistakes and boundary violations; lack of empathy and engagement (option D is incorrect); lessened overall resilience; substance use (option A is correct); greater vulnerability to mental health issues and relationship issues; occupational, functional, or social impairment; the emergence of suicidality; and decisions to drop out of medical training or depart early from the profession of medicine (Brown et al. 2009; Shanafelt et al. 2010). More positively, it is increasingly recognized that physicians who proactively take care of their own health are more likely to support the preventive health practices of their patients, to experience joy in their work, to deliver high-quality care (option B is incorrect), and to see improved health or service outcomes (option C is incorrect) (Schrijver et al. 2016). **Chapter 7 (p. 181)**

References

Appelbaum PS: Clinical practice. Assessment of patients' competence to consent to treatment. N Engl J Med 357(18):1834–1840, 2007 17978292
Appelbaum PS, Grisso T: The MacArthur Competence Study, III: abilities of patients to consent to psychiatric and medical treatments. Law Hum Behav 19(2):149–174, 1995 11660292
Armontrout J, Gitlin D, Gutheil T: Do consultation psychiatrists, forensic psychiatrists, psychiatry trainees, and health care lawyers differ in opinion on gray area decision-making capacity cases? A vignette-based survey. Psychosomatics 57(5):472–479, 2016 27400660
Bourgeois JA, Cohen MA, Erickson JM, et al: Decisional and dispositional capacity determinations: neuropsychiatric illness and an integrated clinical paradigm. Psychosomatics 58(6):565–573, 2017 28734555

Brown SD, Goske MJ, Johnson CM: Beyond substance abuse: stress, burnout, and depression as causes of physician impairment and disruptive behavior. J Am Coll Radiol 6(7):479–485, 2009 19560063

Gengoux GW, Roberts LW: Enhancing wellness and engagement among healthcare professionals. Acad Psychiatry 42(1):1–4, 2018 29297148

Jonsen AR, Siegler M, Winslade WJ: Clinical Ethics, 6th Edition. New York, McGraw-Hill, 2006

Okai D, Owen G, McGuire H, et al: Mental capacity in psychiatric patients: systematic review. Br J Psychiatry 191(4):291–297, 2007 17906238

Overstreet MM: Duty to report colleagues who engage in fraud or deception, in Ethics Primer of the American Psychiatric Association. Washington, DC, American Psychiatric Association, 2001, pp 51–56

Roberts LW: Informed consent and the capacity for voluntarism. Am J Psychiatry 159(5):705–712, 2002 11986120

Roberts LW: A Clinical Guide to Psychiatric Ethics. Arlington, VA, American Psychiatric Publishing, 2016

Roberts LW, Dyer AR: Concise Guide to Ethics in Mental Health Care. Washington, DC, American Psychiatric Publishing, 2004

Roberts LW, Miller MN: Ethical issues in clinician health, in Concise Guide to Ethics in Mental Health Care. Edited by Roberts LW, Dyer AR. Washington, DC, American Psychiatric Publishing, 2004, pp 233–242

Schrijver I, Brady KJ, Trockel M: An exploration of key issues and potential solutions that impact physician wellbeing and professional fulfillment at an academic center. Peer J 4:e1783, 2016 26989621

Shanafelt TD, Balch CM, Bechamps G, et al: Burnout and medical errors among American surgeons. Ann Surg 251(6):995–1000, 2010 19934755

CHAPTER 8

Legal Considerations in Psychiatry

8.1   Which of the following legal terms refers to the concept of "guilty mind"?

A. *Actus reus.*
B. *Mens rea.*
C. *Voir dire.*
D. *Pro se.*

The correct response is option B: *Mens rea.*

Mens rea literally translates from the Latin as "guilty mind" (option B is correct). This term refers to the Western notion of criminal intent (in other words, the intention of wrongdoing related to the commission of an illegal act). *Actus reus* is a distinct Latin term that translates to the "guilty act" and refers to the physical act of committing a crime (option A is incorrect). The concept of *mens rea* can still have a profound impact on whether the *actus reus* is mitigated or voided. For example, if a court determines that a criminal defendant's psychiatric illness impacted his state of mind at the time he committed a crime, it might lessen or even set aside the charges. *Voir dire* is the process by which the court determines an expert witness's expertise and qualifications prior to receiving his or her testimony (option C is incorrect). *Pro se* refers to situations in which defendants choose to represent themselves in court (option D is incorrect). **Chapter 8 (pp. 201–202, 222)**

8.2   Which of the following legal rulings has served as the basis for many state sanity statutes, by which a legal defendant may claim that he did not know right from wrong because of a mental illness?

A. *Tarasoff.*
B. *M'Naghten.*
C. *Cruzan.*
D. *Jaffee.*

The correct response is option B: *M'Naghten.*

Under the "M'Naghten standard" (*M'Naghten's Case* 1843), a mentally ill defendant may demonstrate insanity by meeting at least one of two criteria. First, a defendant may be unable to know the nature and quality of the act (e.g., someone is so disorganized that they are unaware of their actions). Alternately, a mentally ill defendant may argue that because of a mental illness, he or she was unable to distinguish right from wrong (option B is correct).

Tarasoff refers to a mental health practitioner's duty to protect a potential victim from foreseeable danger (option A is incorrect). Specifically, after a series of lengthy legal battles, the California Supreme Court ruled in *Tarasoff v Regents of the University of California* (1976) that a therapist has a duty to protect a potential victim from foreseeable danger.

Cruzan v Director of Missouri Department of Health (1990) involved a family's request to remove their daughter from life support after she had been in a persistent vegetative state for some time (option C is incorrect).

In the case of *Jaffee v Redmond* (1996), the U.S. Supreme Court was tasked to decide whether federal courts should uphold psychotherapist–patient privilege (option D is incorrect). **Chapter 8 (pp. 201–203, 206, 211–212)**

8.3   Three weeks after being discharged from an inpatient psychiatric unit, a 40-year-old female patient commits suicide. Dr. Jones had treated the patient during a 10-day voluntary hospitalization for a major depressive episode. The patient came to the hospital on her own to seek help and had specifically asked Dr. Jones not to tell her family members about her diagnosis and hospitalization. In the days prior to discharge, Dr. Jones completed a competent suicide risk assessment. The patient adamantly denied any thoughts of self-harm, including intent or plan to commit suicide. Which of the following elements must the patient's family prove by a preponderance of the evidence to win a malpractice claim against Dr. Jones?

A. Dr. Jones should have been able to predict that a patient suffering from a major depressive episode would have attempted suicide after leaving the hospital.
B. The patient's suicide occurred as a direct result of Dr. Jones's actions during the patient's treatment.
C. In letting the patient leave the hospital without completing a "no-harm contract," Dr. Jones violated his duty of care.
D. The patient's family suffered psychic harm damages as a result of the patient's death.

The correct response is option B: The patient's suicide occurred as a direct result of Dr. Jones's actions during the patient's treatment.

In professional malpractice cases, a plaintiff bringing suit must demonstrate, by a preponderance of the evidence (i.e., more likely than not), each aspect of the "four D's"—duty of care (e.g., the doctor–patient relationship), dereliction of duty (e.g., failing to meet an accepted standard of care), direct cause (e.g., the injury to patient occurred as a direct result of the physician's actions), and damages (e.g., personal injury, psychic harm, or death). For their claim to prevail, the family in this case example must prove that the injury to the patient occurred as a direct result of Dr. Jones's actions (option B is correct).

Courts do not expect that psychiatrists will be able to predict whether a patient will attempt or complete suicide. Standard of care necessitates that psychiatrists perform and document a competent suicide risk assessment, which was completed by Dr. Jones in this case (option A is incorrect).

A "no-harm contract" is not considered to be part of a psychiatrist's duty of care to a patient and does not need to be completed prior to patient discharge (option C is incorrect).

While plaintiffs need to prove some type of damages in order to win a malpractice claim against the physician, those damages can include, but are not limited to, personal injury, psychic harm (i.e., emotional distress), or death. Thus, even if the family did not suffer psychic harm damages, they might be able to demonstrate other damages that were sustained as a result of the patient's death (option D is incorrect). **Chapter 8 (pp. 203, 204, 216–217)**

8.4   Which of the following is an accurate characterization of patient confidentiality under the Health Insurance Portability and Accountability Act of 1996 (HIPAA)?

A. Before HIPAA was implemented, there were no guidelines governing the scope of patient confidentiality with regard to the therapist–patient relationship.
B. Following HIPAA's implementation, psychotherapy notes cannot be released without explicit authorization from the patient even if they are stored with the remainder of a patient's medical records.
C. Under HIPAA, a patient's psychiatric symptoms, treatment plan, and prognosis cannot be released without explicit authorization from the patient.
D. HIPAA prohibits insurers from making treatment and/or payment for a patient's psychiatric condition contingent on whether psychotherapy notes are disclosed.

The correct response is option D: HIPAA prohibits insurers from making treatment and/or payment for a patient's psychiatric condition contingent on whether psychotherapy notes are disclosed.

HIPAA implementation banned insurance companies from making treatment and/or payment contingent on whether a patient's psychotherapy notes are disclosed (option D is correct). American case law created guidelines governing the scope of therapist–patient confidentiality before the implementation of HIPAA (option A is incorrect). HIPAA requires that psychotherapy notes be stored separately from the rest of a patient's medical records to qualify for the law's added privacy protections (option B is incorrect). Privacy protections afforded to psychotherapy notes under HIPAA do not preclude disclosure of a patient's symptoms, treatment plan, and prognosis (option C is incorrect). **Chapter 8 (pp. 206–207)**

8.5   Which of the following statements about determinations of competence is *true*?

A. A determination of competence or incompetence must be made by a judge sitting in a court of law.
B. Although determination of competence can be made by any physician, psychiatrists may be more capable of conducting competence evaluations in clinical contexts.
C. A determination of competence has no impact on whether a person can provide informed consent for treatment.
D. A determination of competence is based solely on a patient's underlying cognitive abilities.

The correct response is option A: A determination of competence or incompetence must be made by a judge sitting in a court of law.

Determinations of competence or incompetence are made by a judge (option A is correct).

Decisions related to a patient's *capacity*, not competence, are based on clinical appraisals that can be made by any physician concerning an individual's ability to function in regard to a specific demand or situation (option B is incorrect).

Only competent persons can provide informed consent for treatment. A patient who has been deemed incompetent in the eyes of the law requires a substitute decision maker to provide informed consent (option C is incorrect).

In the case of *In the Guardianship of John Roe* (1992), the Court ruled that a man with schizophrenia was incompetent to make decisions about his treatment not because of any cognitive limitations, but because of his persistent denial that he had an actual illness (option D is incorrect). **Chapter 8 (pp. 207–208)**

8.6   In which of the following situations would it be considered risky for a physician to proceed with treatment before obtaining informed consent?

A. A patient requires emergent treatment to save her life but is unconscious and therefore unable to communicate with the treatment provider.
B. A patient who is able to make his own medical decisions knowingly waives the right to informed consent, preferring to defer to his physician's judgment.
C. A psychiatrist believes that her patient may become so ill or emotionally distraught by the disclosure of certain information that it would complicate or hinder treatment.
D. A patient has been deemed unable to make his own medical decisions but has a readily available legal guardian who can provide informed consent on his behalf.

The correct response is option C: A psychiatrist believes that her patient may become so ill or emotionally distraught by the disclosure of certain information that it would complicate or hinder treatment.

The concept of therapeutic privilege is considered a particularly risky and rarely invoked exception to informed consent. In 2016, the American Medical Association Code of Medical Ethics delineated that "withholding pertinent medical information from patients in the belief that disclosure is medically contraindicated creates a conflict between the physician's obligations to promote patient welfare and to respect patient autonomy" (American Medical Association Council on Ethical and Judicial Affairs 2016, Opinion 2.1.3) (option C is correct).

Informed consent is not necessary when a patient requires emergency treatment to save his or her life or to prevent serious harm (option A is incorrect).

Competent patients can knowingly and voluntarily "waive" their right to informed consent and may defer to their physician's judgment regarding treatment decisions (option B is incorrect).

In general, patients who are deemed incompetent for the purposes of medical decision making are not able to provide informed consent; however, the incompetent patient's legal guardian (or designated health care proxy) may provide informed consent on his or her behalf (option D is incorrect). **Chapter 8 (pp. 209–211)**

8.7 A 55-year-old financial executive with a diagnosis of bipolar I disorder is scheduled to be discharged from an inpatient psychiatric unit where he has been treated with lithium and olanzapine for an acute manic episode. He plans to return to the home which he owns and where he lives with his wife and two young children. Two years ago, after being discharged from the psychiatric hospital under similar circumstances, the patient threw a glass vase at the wall while intoxicated. Six months ago, the patient's wife bought him a vintage baseball bat that he proudly displays in the living room. In the violence risk assessment conducted by the psychiatrist, which of the following features in this patient's profile would likely represent the most serious risk factor for violence?

A. The patient's planned return to live with his wife and two young children.
B. The patient's history of relapsing to alcohol use when he returns to the outpatient setting.
C. The patient's recent acquisition of a baseball bat that is readily accessible.
D. The fact that the patient is undergoing treatment with multiple psychiatric medications.

The correct response is option B: The patient's history of relapsing to alcohol use when he returns to the outpatient setting.

An important consideration in a clinical violence risk assessment is an understanding of the subtype of violence a patient is displaying and/or is prone to engage in. Additional considerations when performing violence risk assessments include dynamic and static risk factors. Dynamic risk factors are subject to change; examples include substance intoxication, access to firearms, medication noncompliance, and absence of a stable living situation. Static risk factors, on the other hand, are not subject to change and are largely demographic or historical in nature. A history of previous violence, male gender, and early childhood trauma history are all examples of static variables that can influence violence risk.

In this case example, substance intoxication (i.e., the patient's history of alcohol use and resulting violence when he is at home) is the main risk factor that must be taken into account when completing a competent violence risk assessment (option B is correct). The patient's home ownership and family support are indicative of a stable living situation, lowering his risk for violence (option A is incorrect). While access to firearms would be an essential consideration when performing a violence risk assessment, access to sports memorabilia would not pose the same degree of risk (option C is incorrect). In contrast to medication noncompliance, treatment with multiple medications for psychiatric illness is not viewed as a risk factor for violence (option D is incorrect). **Chapter 8 (pp. 216–218)**

8.8   Which of the following populations is protected in all 50 states by statutes mandating that psychiatrists report suspected maltreatment?

A. Children who might be experiencing abuse.
B. Patients who have been medically or psychiatrically hospitalized within the last year.
C. Physically disabled adults.
D. Middle-aged adult patients living alone.

The correct response is option A: Children who might be experiencing abuse.

All U.S. states have statutes pertaining to the mandatory reporting of suspected child abuse (option A is correct). In addition, most jurisdictions mandate the reporting of maltreatment involving other vulnerable populations, including the elderly and adults with developmental disabilities.

Patients who have been medically or psychiatrically hospitalized within the last year, adults with physical disabilities, and middle-aged adult patients living alone do not constitute populations frequently protected by state statutes requiring mandated reporting (options B, C, and D are incorrect). **Chapter 8 (pp. 203, 207)**

8.9   A psychiatrist is subpoenaed to testify as a fact witness in his patient's civil case after the patient is suspended from her teaching position following accusations of sexual misconduct with a student. The psychiatrist has been treating the patient with both psychotherapy and medication management for the past 10 years. During this time, the patient has revealed her sexual fantasies involving her male students, but has consistently insisted that she would never act upon them. Which of the following would be considered an appropriate action by the psychiatrist in this case?

A. Providing expert witness testimony in addition to serving as a fact witness on the patient's behalf.
B. Thoroughly reviewing the subpoena with a psychiatric colleague before deciding whether to respond.

C. Altering the patient's psychotherapy records to remove information told to him in confidence that he fears might prove damaging to the patient's husband and minor children if publicly revealed.

D. Explaining to the patient that patient–psychiatrist privilege does not extend to all psychotherapeutic communications and that the scope of confidentiality will be determined by the court.

The correct response is option D: Explaining to the patient that patient–psychiatrist privilege does not extend to all psychotherapeutic communications and that the scope of confidentiality will be determined by the court.

There are exceptions to both confidentiality and patient–psychiatrist privilege that may be determined by the court (option D is correct). Ethical guidelines strongly discourage psychiatrists from taking on the role of both treatment provider and court expert with the same patient (option A is incorrect). The first step a clinician should take after receiving a subpoena is to seek advice from his or her institutional or personal legal counsel, not a psychiatric colleague (option B is incorrect). Clinicians should never attempt to alter or destroy records after receiving a subpoena (option C is incorrect). **Chapter 8 (pp. 203–204)**

References

American Medical Association Council on Ethical and Judicial Affairs: AMA Code of Medical Ethics. Chicago, IL, American Medical Association, 2016

Cruzan v Director of Missouri Department of Health, 497 US 261, 110 S Ct 2841, 111 L Ed 2d 224 (1990)

Health Insurance Portability and Accountability Act of 1996, Pub. L. No. 104–191, 110 Stat 1936

In the Guardianship of John Roe, 411 Mass 666 (1992)

Jaffee v Redmond, 518 US 1 (1996)

Lipari v Sears, Roebuck and Company, 497 F Supp 185 (D Neb 1980)

M'Naghten's Case, 10 CL & F. 200, 8 Eng. Rep. 718 (1843)

Tarasoff v Regents of the University of California, 17 Cal 3d 425, 551 P 2d 334; 131 Cal Rptr 14 (1976)

CHAPTER 9

Neurodevelopmental Disorders

9.1   The mother of a 10-year-old boy reports that for the past 9 months, she has noticed her son making pouting movements with his mouth every day. He also frequently clears his throat and shrugs his shoulders. The boy's teachers have commented that they have noticed similar behavior. What is the most appropriate diagnosis for this child?

   A. Tourette's disorder.
   B. Persistent tic disorder.
   C. Provisional tic disorder.
   D. Unspecified tic disorder.

The correct response is option C: Provisional tic disorder.

The DSM-5 (American Psychiatric Association 2013) diagnostic criteria for *Tourette's disorder* require a history of multiple motor tics and at least one vocal tic, lasting for more than 1 year since first tic onset (which must have occurred before age 18 years); the symptoms must not be attributable to another medical condition or the physiological effects of a substance (option A is incorrect). The diagnostic criteria for *persistent motor or vocal tic disorder* are the same as those for Tourette's disorder, except that the tics must involve either the motor or the vocal domain (but not both) (option B is incorrect). *Provisional tic disorder* can involve symptoms consistent with either Tourette's disorder or persistent tic disorders; however, the diagnosis is reserved for cases in which the duration of symptoms since first tic onset is less than 1 year (option C is correct). In cases in which tics are present but do not meet full criteria for a defined disorder, a DSM-5 diagnosis of *other specified tic disorder* or *unspecified tic disorder* may be considered (option D is incorrect). **Chapter 9 (p. 248)**

9.2   A child whose development tracked closely with that of her peers during early childhood, but then diverged in later childhood, would best be described as having which kind of developmental trajectory?

A. Typical.
B. Regressing.
C. Remitting.
D. Persisting–delayed.

The correct response is option B: Regressing.

A *typical* developmental trajectory is steady, relatively linear, and rapid through-out childhood and adolescence, and to a lesser degree in adulthood (option A is incorrect). A *regressing* trajectory appears relatively typical in early stages, only to diverge or regress from the trajectory of chronological-age peers at a later stage (option B is correct). A *remitting* trajectory is characterized by a pattern of delayed maturation throughout childhood and adolescence that ultimately converges with the trajectory of chronological-age peers in adulthood (option C is incorrect). A *persisting–delayed* trajectory is steady but persistently slower over time (option D is incorrect). **Chapter 9 (p. 226 [Figure 9–1])**

9.3 Which of the following findings on evaluation would satisfy Criterion B for the DSM-5 diagnosis of intellectual disability?

A. Onset of difficulties during adolescent period.
B. Intelligence testing scores more than 2 standard deviations below average.
C. Impaired adaptive functioning in everyday life across multiple domains.
D. Deficits in intellectual functions on clinical assessment.

The correct response is option C: Impaired adaptive functioning in everyday life across multiple domains.

DSM-5 Criterion C requires establishment of onset of symptoms during the de-velopmental period (option A is incorrect). Assessment for deficits in intellectual functions (DSM-5 Criterion A) involves clinical assessment and standardized in-telligence testing (option D is incorrect). Intellectual disability for Criterion A is defined as scores approximately two standard deviations below the expected population mean (option B is incorrect). The potential limitations of intelligence testing in accurately classifying disability underscore the importance of DSM-5 Criterion B, which requires evidence for impaired adaptive functioning in every-day life across academic/intellectual, social, and practical domains (option C is correct). **Chapter 9 (p. 229)**

9.4 A persistent deficit in articulation of spoken language should prompt consider-ation of which of the following disorders?

A. Speech sound disorder.
B. Language disorder.
C. Childhood-onset fluency disorder.
D. Social communication disorder.

The correct response is option A: Speech sound disorder.

Speech sound disorder encompasses deficits in the articulation or phonology of spoken language, as evidenced by persistent misarticulation of sounds beyond developmental norms (option A is correct).

Language disorder represents a category of deficits in the acquisition and use of language; DSM-5 defines impairments in the capacity to effectively produce, receive, or comprehend language signals within this diagnostic category (option B is incorrect).

Childhood-onset fluency disorder, or *stuttering*, affects a specific aspect of speech—that of oral fluency, which pertains to the rate and continuity of speech production (option C is incorrect).

Social (pragmatic) communication disorder is characterized by impairments in communicating for social purposes, adjusting communication to match the context of the conversation, observing rules of typical conversation, and understanding implicit meanings (option D is incorrect). **Chapter 9 (pp. 231, 233, 234, 236)**

9.5   Which of the following is considered a first-line treatment for attention-deficit/hyperactivity disorder (ADHD)?

A. Bupropion.
B. Tricyclic agents.
C. Alpha-agonists.
D. Atomoxetine.

The correct response is option D: Atomoxetine.

In ADHD, pharmacological interventions are often provided as first-line treatment rather than psychosocial intervention. Pharmacological treatment approaches such as the Texas Children's Medication Algorithm Project outline empirically based practices (Pliszka et al. 2000), including first-line treatment with stimulants, encompassing the methylphenidate and mixed amphetamine salt classes as well as atomoxetine (option D is correct). Other evidence-based approaches include alpha-agonists (option C is incorrect), bupropion (option A is incorrect), and tricyclic agents (option B is incorrect). **Chapter 9 (pp. 243–244)**

9.6   Behaviors such as excessive motor activity or restlessness in inappropriate contexts, fidgeting, and talkativeness are examples of which of the following?

A. Inattention.
B. Hyperactivity.
C. Impulsivity.
D. Stereotypies.

The correct response is option B: Hyperactivity.

ADHD involves persistent impairments along core axes of inattention or hyperactivity–impulsivity. Clinical manifestations of *inattention* may be seen in behaviors such as frequent distraction, carelessness due to difficulty sustaining focus, and disorganization in management of materials or time (option A is incorrect). Behavioral aspects of *hyperactivity* are seen in excessive motor activity or restlessness in inappropriate contexts, fidgeting, or talkativeness (option B is correct). In the related domain of *impulsivity*, clinical features may be identified in social intrusiveness or action without accompanying self-monitoring (option C is incorrect).

Stereotypic movement disorder (SMD) is broadly characterized by involuntary, coordinated, repetitive, seemingly driven but apparently purposeless motor behaviors (i.e., *stereotypies*), such as hand flapping, opening and closing of hands, head banging, and self-biting that cannot be attributed to other medical conditions or psychiatric disorders. These stereotypies usually begin in early childhood (option D is incorrect). **Chapter 9 (pp. 240, 247)**

9.7   Which of the following disorders is defined by difficulties in the acquisition or application of specific core academic skills?

A. Language disorder.
B. Intellectual disability.
C. Attention deficit/hyperactivity disorder.
D. Specific learning disorder.

The correct response is option D: Specific learning disorder.

As the name implies, *language disorder* represents a category of deficits in the acquisition and use of language. Whereas previous DSM editions defined expressive and mixed receptive–expressive subtypes, DSM-5 more broadly defines impairments in the capacity to effectively produce, receive, or comprehend language signals within this diagnostic category, while still recognizing that deficits may be more pronounced in either the receptive or the expressive domain (option A is incorrect).

Specific learning disorder encompasses impairments in academic skills and learning. From a nosological perspective, specific learning disorder impairments are differentiated from communication disorders in that they represent difficulties in the acquisition or application not of language abilities, but rather of specific core academic skills (option D is correct).

Regarding *intellectual disability*, the current DSM-5 schema incorporates both intellectual abilities and level of adaptive functioning as determinants for diagnostic criteria, requiring evidence for impairments in well-established cognitive faculties: verbal comprehension, working memory, perceptual reasoning, quantitative reasoning, abstract thought, and cognitive efficacy (option B is incorrect).

Attention-deficit/hyperactivity disorder involves persistent impairments along core axes of inattention or hyperactivity–impulsivity (option C is incorrect). **Chapter 9 (pp. 226–227, 231, 240, 244)**

9.8   A young child has deficits in social–emotional reciprocity and in nonverbal communicative behaviors used for social interaction, stereotyped motor movements, and highly restricted interest of abnormal intensity. What additional deficit must be present to meet criteria for a DSM-5 diagnosis of autism spectrum disorder (ASD)?

A. Ritualized patterns of verbal or nonverbal behavior.
B. Unusual interest in sensory aspects of the environment.
C. Deficits in developing, maintaining, and understanding relationships.
D. Inaccuracy of performance of gross and/or fine motor skills.

The correct response is option C: Deficits in developing, maintaining, and understanding relationships.

Per DSM-5, the diagnosis of ASD requires the presence three social communication criteria and at least two of four additional criteria, with onset of symptoms in the early developmental period. The three social communication criteria are 1) deficits in social–emotional reciprocity, 2) deficits in nonverbal communicative behaviors used for social interaction, and 3) deficits in developing, maintaining, and understanding relationships (option C is correct).
    The four additional criteria for ASD are as follows: 1) stereotyped or repetitive motor movements; 2) cognitive inflexibility or ritualized patterns of verbal or nonverbal behavior (option A is incorrect); 3) highly restricted, fixated interests that are abnormal in intensity or focus; and 4) hyperreactivity or hyporeactivity to sensory input or unusual interest in sensory aspects of the environment (option B is incorrect).
    Developmental coordination disorder is characterized by delays in development of coordinated motor skills, often manifesting as clumsiness and slowness, as well as inaccuracy of performance of gross and/or fine motor skills (option D is incorrect). **Chapter 9 (pp. 236–237, 246)**

9.9   Which of the following interventions is widely used and effective for treating the core symptoms of autism spectrum disorder (ASD)?

A. Habit reversal training.
B. Early Intensive Behavioral Intervention.
C. Organizational skills planning.
D. Motor skills intervention.

The correct response is option B: Early Intensive Behavioral Intervention.

Habit reversal training is an intervention used in Tourette's disorder, not ASD (option A is incorrect). When combined with pharmacological treatment, this behavioral intervention (delivered alone or as part of a treatment package such as Comprehensive Behavioral Intervention for Tics) was found to be effective (Dutta and Cavanna 2013).

Behavioral interventions are the most effective and widely used treatments for core symptoms of ASD. Systematic reviews of early intensive interventions indicate that the Early Intensive Behavioral Intervention and the Early Start Denver Model have the strongest evidence for improving language and cognitive skills in children with ASD (Warren et al. 2011) (option B is correct).

Even though pharmacological treatments (rather than behavioral interventions) are typically used as the first-line treatment for attention-deficit/hyperactivity disorder (ADHD), a number of therapy modalities—including organizational skills training and cognitive-behavioral therapy—may positively influence outcomes in ADHD (option C is incorrect).

In children with developmental coordination disorder, motor skills interventions were found to be effective in improving short-term cognitive, emotional, and other psychological aspects of motor competence and performance (Yu et al. 2018) (option D is incorrect). **Chapter 9 (pp. 240, 244, 247, 250)**

9.10 Which of the following disorders is characterized by involuntary, coordinated, repetitive, seemingly driven but apparently purposeless motor behaviors?

A. Stereotypic movement disorder.
B. Developmental coordination disorder.
C. Autism spectrum disorder.
D. Unspecified tic disorder.

The correct response is option A: Stereotypic movement disorder.

Stereotypic movement disorder is broadly characterized by involuntary, coordinated, repetitive, seemingly driven but apparently purposeless motor behaviors, such as hand flapping, opening and closing of hands, head banging, and self-biting, that cannot be attributed to other medical conditions or psychiatric disorders (option A is correct).

Developmental coordination disorder is characterized by delays in development of coordinated motor skills, often manifesting as clumsiness and slowness, as well as inaccuracy of performance of gross and/or fine motor skills (option B is incorrect).

Autism spectrum disorder is a neurodevelopmental disorder characterized by impairments in social communication and social interaction, repetitive and stereotyped behaviors, and/or sensory aberrations (option C is incorrect).

A tic is a sudden, rapid, recurrent, nonrhythmic motor movement or vocalization. In cases in which tics are present but do not meet full criteria for a defined disorder, a DSM-5 diagnosis of *other specified tic disorder* or *unspecified tic disorder* may be considered (option D is incorrect). **Chapter 9 (pp. 236, 246, 247, 248)**

9.11 Which of the following features would preclude a diagnosis of social communication disorder?

A. Onset of symptoms at an early age.
B. Difficulty observing rules of typical conversation.
C. Difficulty understanding implicit meanings.
D. Presence of repetitive behaviors.

The correct response is option D: Presence of repetitive behaviors.

Social (pragmatic) communication disorder (SPCD) is a new category in DSM-5 that relates to deficits in the pragmatic aspects of language. The disorder is characterized by impairments in communicating for social purposes, adjusting communication to match the context of the conversation, observing rules of typical conversation (option B is incorrect), and understanding implicit meanings (option C is incorrect). Per DSM-5, symptoms must have their onset at an early age (option A is incorrect), and the symptoms must not be attributable to another psychiatric, neurological, or medical disorder. Unlike individuals with autism spectrum disorder, individuals with SPCD do not have restricted and repetitive behaviors (option D is correct). **Chapter 9 (p. 236)**

9.12   A 13-year-old boy is referred by a school nurse to a local clinic for evaluation of school difficulties due to forgetting to complete school assignments and poor exam scores. The boy's mother recalls that her son was slow to begin speaking as a toddler and used to throw tantrums when she dropped him off at daycare. Given this patient's history, which of the following characteristics, if found to be present, would be consistent with a diagnosis of intellectual disability?

A. He requires frequent reminders to wear a coat and closed-toed shoes when it is snowing outside.
B. His memory deficits appeared after a concussion at age 12 years.
C. He has an IQ one standard deviation below the expected population mean.
D. He has difficulty completing assignments when at school but is able to complete homework assignments at home without assistance.

The correct response is option A: He requires frequent reminders to wear a coat and closed-toed shoes when it is snowing outside.

The DSM-5 intellectual disabilities category encompasses conditions characterized by delayed development of general mental abilities, which is associated with significant deficits in daily adaptive functioning. Diagnoses in this group include intellectual disability, global developmental delay, and unspecified intellectual disability, depending on criteria met (option B is incorrect).
   Assessment for deficits in intellectual functions (DSM-5 Criterion A) involves clinical assessment and standardized intelligence testing. Intellectual disability for Criterion A is then defined as scores approximately two standard deviations below the expected population mean (option C is incorrect).

The potential limitations of intelligence testing in accurately classifying disability underscore the importance of DSM-5 Criterion B, which requires evidence for impaired adaptive functioning in everyday life across academic/intellectual, social, and practical domains (option D is incorrect).

While prior versions of DSM defined intellectual disability primarily by intelligence quotient (IQ) scores, the current DSM-5 schema incorporates both intellectual abilities and level of adaptive functioning as determinants for diagnostic criteria (American Psychiatric Association 2013). An important innovation in DSM-5 is the increased emphasis on adaptive functioning (as opposed to intellectual capacity alone) as a foundational criterion for the diagnosis. In accordance with this heightened emphasis, behavioral manifestations of the condition are required to include evidence for difficulties in meeting standards for personal independence and social responsibility within the appropriate sociocultural and developmental context (option A is correct). **Chapter 9 (pp. 225–229)**

9.13 Which of the following statements correctly describes a way in which autism spectrum disorder (ASD) differs from social (pragmatic) communication disorder (SPCD)?

A. Deficits in nonverbal communication are found in SPCD but not in ASD.
B. Restrictive and repetitive behaviors are found in ASD but not in SPCD.
C. Onset of symptoms occurs at an early age in ASD but not in SPCD.
D. Evidence-based treatments are available for SPCD but not for ASD.

The correct response is option B: Restrictive and repetitive behaviors are found in ASD but not in SPCD.

Unlike individuals with ASD, individuals with SPCD do not have restricted and repetitive behaviors (option B is correct). Deficits in nonverbal communicative behaviors used for social interaction are found in both ASD and SPCD (option A is incorrect).

In the DSM-5 diagnostic criteria for both ASD and SPCD, symptoms must have their onset at an early age (option C is incorrect).

No evidence-based treatments have been developed for SPCD to date. Systematic reviews indicate that the Early Intensive Behavioral Intervention and the Early Start Denver Model have the strongest evidence for improving language and cognitive skills in children with ASD (option D is incorrect). **Chapter 9 (pp. 236–240)**

9.14 A 40-year-old man is transferred to your care with a diagnosis of schizoid personality disorder. As a child, the patient was moved to multiple different schools due to behavioral dysregulation and was brought to the emergency room numerous times due to head banging. The patient is socially isolated due to difficulty engaging in conversation. Which of the following additional characteristics, if discovered about this patient, would lead you to suspect autism spectrum disorder (ASD) as the correct diagnosis rather than schizoid personality disorder?

A. He is uninterested in socializing.
B. He has a counting compulsion, which he finds distressing.
C. He exhibits stereotypic movements.
D. He has no activities that he enjoys.

The correct response is option C: He exhibits stereotypic movements.

Per DSM-5, the diagnosis of ASD requires the presence of three social communication criteria and at least two of four additional criteria, with onset of symptoms in the early developmental period. The three social communication criteria are 1) deficits in social–emotional reciprocity, 2) deficits in nonverbal communicative behaviors used for social interaction, and 3) deficits in developing, maintaining, and understanding relationships. The four additional criteria for ASD are as follows: 1) stereotyped or repetitive motor movements (option C is correct); 2) cognitive inflexibility or ritualized patterns of verbal or nonverbal behavior; 3) highly restricted, fixated interests that are abnormal in intensity or focus (option D is incorrect); and 4) hyperreactivity or hyporeactivity to sensory input or unusual interest in sensory aspects of the environment.

A critical part of the process of case formulation is differential diagnosis to determine whether presenting symptoms are due to ASD, an independent condition, or the presence of co-occurring disorders. Poor eye contact and low social initiative are common manifestations in children and adults with ASD, but these symptoms are also frequently found in children with depression or anxiety and in individuals with schizoid personality disorder or avoidant personality disorder (option A is incorrect). However, whereas individuals with ASD often have abnormal psychomotor function and inattention, these symptoms are typically absent in schizoid and avoidant personality disorders.

Whereas rituals and compulsions can be part of both ASD and obsessive-compulsive disorder (OCD) symptomatology, they tend to be ego-syntonic in ASD but ego-dystonic in OCD (option B is incorrect). **Chapter 9 (pp. 236–237, 239)**

9.15 A 35-year-old man comes to your office because he is concerned that he might have attention-deficit/hyperactivity disorder (ADHD). Which of the following details, if present or discovered about this patient, would strongly support an ADHD diagnosis?

A. He reports having experienced an improved ability to concentrate after taking his friend's ADHD medication.
B. He reports that he is more restless as an adult than he was as a child.
C. He is able to provide a history of symptoms from when he was less than 12 years old.
D. He is male.

The correct response is option C: He is able to provide a history of symptoms from when he was less than 12 years old.

As required by DSM-5 Criterion B, ADHD symptoms must be present by the early stages of development (age <12 years) (option C is correct).

Diagnoses will typically be based on a thorough clinical assessment, entailing history of deficits in both inattentive and hyperactive–impulsive domains. History taking will focus on determining the age at onset of symptom presentation and placing symptoms within the context of a developmental and sociocultural framework. Response to ADHD medication is not a defining criterion for the diagnosis (option A is incorrect).

A common feature in the developmental course is the finding that symptoms associated with the hyperactivity domain generally decrease over time in most individuals with the diagnosis (option B is incorrect).

While there appear to be sex differences in prevalence, ADHD occurs in both males and females, and female sex does not rule out the diagnosis (option D is incorrect). **Chapter 9 (pp. 240–243)**

9.16   A 14-year-old girl is brought to your office by her mother because of worsening social isolation at school. The girl's teacher reports that she frequently appears to be daydreaming during class. The teacher also reports that the girl is always having to borrow her classmates' books because she forgets to bring her own. The patient was recently seen by a neurologist to evaluate the possibility of absence seizures, and her electroencephalogram was normal. In conjunction with the patient's history, which of the following features would lead you to suspect attention-deficit/hyperactivity disorder (ADHD) as the primary diagnosis?

A. The onset of the patient's problem was 1 year ago.
B. The patient is having symptoms only at school.
C. The patient is female.
D. The patient has trouble completing tasks at home as well as at school.

The correct response is option D: The patient has trouble completing tasks at home as well as at school.

An important aspect of ADHD symptoms is that they are not context-dependent, but instead manifest in multiple settings (e.g., home and school). Having difficulty completing tasks at home in addition to disorganization at school is consistent with a diagnosis of ADHD (option D is correct; option B is incorrect).

As required by DSM-5 Criterion B, ADHD symptoms must be present by the early stages of development (age <12 years) (option A is incorrect).

There appear to be sex differences in prevalence, with male:female ratios ranging from 2:1 to 4:1 (option C is incorrect). **Chapter 9 (pp. 240–241)**

9.17   A 15-year-old girl with a provisional diagnosis of tic disorder presents for evaluation. She has been experiencing symptoms of finger flexing and nose twitching. These symptoms have been bothersome, leading to difficulty completing tasks at school. Workup for underlying medical causes of the patient's symptoms has been negative. Which of the following characteristics would lead you to suspect that Tourette's disorder is the correct diagnosis?

A. The patient's symptoms have been present for the past 6 months.
B. The patient also has a phonic tic (throat clearing).
C. The patient is female.
D. The patient's symptoms have been worsening since the start of adolescence.

The correct response is option B: The patient also has a phonic tic (throat clearing).

The DSM-5 diagnostic criteria for Tourette's disorder require a history of multiple motor tics and at least one vocal tic, lasting for more than 1 year (option A is incorrect) since first tic onset (which must have occurred before age 18 years). Examples of simple motor tics include eye blinking, shoulder shrugging, eye rolling, nose twitching, mouth pouting, head jerking, muscle tensing, and finger flexing; examples of simple phonic tics include throat clearing (option B is correct), coughing, gulping, snorting, sniffing, grunting, barking, belching, and hiccuping.

There is evidence of sex differences, with a male-to-female predominance of 4 to 1 (option C is incorrect).

Tics manifest similarly across the life span. In patients with Tourette's disorder, onset of tic symptoms is typically between the ages of 4 and 6 years. The severity of symptoms is often at its peak between the ages of 10 and 12 years, with a decline in severity during adolescence (option D is incorrect). **Chapter 9 (pp. 248–249)**

9.18 Which of the following statements about stereotypic movement disorder (SMD) is *true*?

A. It is idiopathic by definition.
B. It is associated with higher cognitive functioning.
C. It typically involves movements such as eye blinking or mouth pouting.
D. There are multiple evidence-based therapies for its treatment.

The correct response is option A: It is idiopathic by definition.

According to DSM-5, SMD can be diagnosed only if the repetitive motor behaviors are not attributable to neurological, neurodevelopmental, or mental disorders. Therefore, by definition, stereotypic movement disorder is always idiopathic (option A is correct).

Stereotypic behaviors are associated with lower cognitive functioning. The prevalence of SMD-like behaviors is higher (4%–16%) in individuals with intellectual disability (Arron et al. 2011; Harris 2010) (option B is incorrect).

SMD is broadly characterized by involuntary, coordinated, repetitive, seemingly driven but apparently purposeless motor behaviors, such as hand flapping, opening and closing of hands, head banging, and self-biting, that cannot be attributed to other medical conditions or psychiatric disorders. Movements such as eye blinking or mouth pouting are examples of simple motor tics (option C is incorrect).

Evidence-based treatments for SMD are lacking. Behavior modification techniques, including habit reversal and differential reinforcement of other behaviors, have been employed (option D is incorrect). **Chapter 9 (pp. 247–248)**

9.19   A 9-year old boy presents to your clinic for evaluation of speech. He frequently repeats sounds and syllables when he speaks. His mother notes that the symptoms are worse in certain situations, and he tends to say he is sick on days when he has to present a project in front of the class. The boy's symptoms have responded well to therapy by a speech and language pathologist. On the basis of this presentation, you suspect that the patient has childhood-onset fluency disorder. Which of the following statements about this disorder is *true*?

A. Childhood-onset fluency disorder cannot co-occur with other language-based disorders.
B. Childhood-onset fluency disorder symptoms are more severe in a relaxed and familiar setting.
C. Childhood-onset fluency disorder symptoms usually start after age 10.
D. Childhood-onset fluency disorder specifically affects the rate and continuity of speech production.

The correct response is option D: Childhood-onset fluency disorder specifically affects the rate and continuity of speech production.

Childhood-onset fluency disorder, or stuttering, affects a specific aspect of speech—that of oral fluency, which pertains to the rate and continuity of speech production. Clinical evidence of dysfluency may take the form of repetitions of sounds or syllables ("s-s-s-orry") or blocking and prolongations of sounds (option D is correct).

Childhood-onset fluency disorder may co-occur with other language-based disorders, tic or motor disorders, and attention-deficit/hyperactivity disorder (option A is incorrect).

Severity of symptoms may be dependent on context or perceived pressure in situations where speech occurs (option B is incorrect).

The vast majority of childhood-onset fluency issues will be evident prior to 5 years of age. Dysfluency that emerges after adolescence is identified as an adult-onset dysfluency and is typically associated with a specific neurological or medical condition (option C is incorrect). **Chapter 9 (pp. 234–235)**

9.20   Which of the following disorders is defined by deficits in the articulation or phonology of spoken language such as difficulty using phonemes to produce intelligible speech?

A. Speech sound disorder.
B. Social (pragmatic) communication disorder.
C. Childhood-onset fluency disorder.
D. Language disorder.

The correct response is option A: Speech sound disorder.

Speech sound disorder encompasses deficits in the articulation or phonology of spoken language. Individuals with this condition may have difficulty using phonemes, the basic units of spoken language, to produce intelligible speech (option A is correct).

Social (pragmatic) communication disorder is a new category in DSM-5 that relates to deficits in the pragmatic aspects of language. The disorder is characterized by impairments in communicating for social purposes, adjusting communication to match the context of the conversation, observing rules of typical conversation, and understanding implicit meanings (option B is incorrect).

Childhood-onset fluency disorder, or stuttering, affects a specific aspect of speech—that of oral fluency, which pertains to the rate and continuity of speech production (option C is incorrect).

Language disorder represents a category of deficits in the acquisition and use of language. Whereas previous DSM editions defined expressive and mixed receptive–expressive subtypes, DSM-5 more broadly defines impairments in the capacity to effectively produce, receive, or comprehend language signals within this diagnostic category, while still recognizing that deficits may be more pronounced in either the receptive or the expressive domain (option D is incorrect). **Chapter 9 (pp. 231–236)**

References

American Psychiatric Association: Diagnostic and Statistical Manual of Mental Disorders, 4th Edition. Washington, DC, American Psychiatric Association, 1994

American Psychiatric Association: Diagnostic and Statistical Manual of Mental Disorders, 5th Edition. Arlington, VA, American Psychiatric Association, 2013

Arron K, Oliver C, Moss J, et al: The prevalence and phenomenology of self-injurious and aggressive behaviour in genetic syndromes. J Intellect Disabil Res 55(2):109–120, 2011 20977515

Dutta N, Cavanna AE: The effectiveness of habit reversal therapy in the treatment of Tourette syndrome and other chronic tic disorders: a systematic review. Funct Neurol 28(1):7–12, 2013 23731910

Harris JC: Advances in understanding behavioral phenotypes in neurogenetic syndromes. Am J Med Genet C Semin Med Genet 154C(4):389–399, 2010 20981768

Pliszka SR, Greenhill LL, Crismon ML, et al: The Texas Children's Medication Algorithm Project: report of the Texas Consensus Conference Panel on Medication Treatment of Childhood Attention-Deficit/Hyperactivity Disorder, part I: attention-deficit/hyperactivity disorder. J Am Acad Child Adolesc Psychiatry 39(7):908–919, 2000 10892234

Warren Z, McPheeters ML, Sathe N, et al: A systematic review of early intensive intervention for autism spectrum disorders. Pediatrics 127(5):e1303–e1311, 2011 21464190

Yu JJ, Burnett AF, Sit CH: Motor skill interventions in children with developmental coordination disorder: a systematic review and meta-analysis. Arch Phys Med Rehabil 99(10):2076–2099, 2018 29329670

CHAPTER 10

Schizophrenia Spectrum and Other Psychotic Disorders

10.1 *Posturing* is classified as what type of psychotic symptom?

A. Positive.
B. Negative.
C. Disorganization.
D. Cognitive impairment.

The correct response is option C: Disorganization.

Positive symptoms can take many forms, including hallucinations, hyperactivity and hypervigilance, mood lability, grandiosity, suspiciousness, and hostility (option A is incorrect).

Lists of negative symptoms have varied over time, but the National Institute of Mental Health Measurement and Treatment Research to Improve Cognition in Schizophrenia (NIMH MATRICS) studies focused on affective flattening, alogia, avolition, asociality, and anhedonia as the central symptoms (Foussias et al. 2014) (option B is incorrect).

Disorganization encompasses conceptual disorganization, disorientation, posturing and mannerisms, bizarre behavior, stereotyped thinking, poor attention, and inappropriate affect (Ventura et al. 2010) (option C is correct).

Schizophrenia is associated with significant cognitive impairment. Cognitive deficits can include impairments in processing speed, working memory, verbal learning, executive function, and social cognition (option D is incorrect). **Chapter 10 (p. 258)**

10.2 A patient's psychosis was well controlled on clozapine 300 mg/day when he was discharged. from the hospital. Two weeks later, he experiences a reemergence of psychotic symptoms, although his dosage has not changed and he has been observed taking his medication daily. Which of the following is the most likely reason for this symptom reemergence?

A. The patient began drinking copious amounts of grapefruit juice after leaving the hospital.
B. The patient began smoking heavily after leaving the hospital.
C. The patient began taking cimetidine for gastritis after leaving the hospital.
D. The patient began taking diltiazem for atrial fibrillation after leaving the hospital.

The correct response is option B: The patient began smoking heavily after leaving the hospital.

Nicotine use is far more common among persons with schizophrenia than among the general population. Most patients with schizophrenia who smoke began smoking before illness onset, suggesting that smoking is not solely a response to schizophrenia symptoms or to antipsychotic medication. Tobacco smoke *induces* cytochrome P450 (CYP) enzymes, leading to increased metabolization and reduced blood levels of clozapine. Therefore, patients on clozapine who resume smoking after being discharged from the hospital can experience emergence of psychosis (option B is correct).

Grapefruit juice, cimetidine, and diltiazem *inhibit* CYP enzymes and therefore produce *increased* levels of clozapine, which in turn would lead to increased side effects (e.g., constipation, sialorrhea) of clozapine, not increased psychosis (options A, C, and D are incorrect). **Chapter 10 (pp. 259–260); see also Chapter 29 ("Psychopharmacology"; pp. 794, 822)**

10.3   Which of the following is *not* a standard part of the workup for first-episode psychosis?

A. Thyroid-stimulating hormone (TSH).
B. HIV and syphilis testing.
C. Computed tomography (CT) scan of the head.
D. Urine toxicology.

The correct response is option C: Computed tomography (CT) scan of the head.

Routine laboratory testing, especially for newly diagnosed patients, should include a complete blood count, serum electrolytes (including calcium), blood urea nitrogen and creatinine, liver function tests, thyroid function tests (including TSH level), vitamin B_{12} level, HIV and syphilis tests, and drug screening (options A, B, and D are incorrect). Other diagnostic tests, including neuroimaging, electroencephalography, and genotypic and serological assessments, are not usually performed for patients presenting with a first episode of psychosis unless there is suspicion of an underlying medical condition such as a neurodegenerative disease or substance-induced psychosis (option C is correct). **Chapter 10 (p. 263)**

10.4   Temporal lobe seizures are often associated with which of the following types of psychotic symptoms?

A. Visual hallucinations.

B. Olfactory hallucinations.

C. Bizarre behavior.

D. Echolalia.

The correct response is option B: Olfactory hallucinations.

Visual hallucinations are most commonly seen in psychosis related to primary neurocognitive disorders such as Lewy body dementia (option A is incorrect). *Olfactory hallucinations* can result from temporal lobe seizures (option B is correct). *Bizarre behavior* is a component of *disorganization*, a core feature of schizophrenia that also encompasses conceptual disorganization, disorientation, posturing and mannerisms, stereotyped thinking, poor attention, and inappropriate affect (option C is incorrect). *Echolalia* is a phenomenon seen in catatonia and tic disorders (option D is incorrect). **Chapter 10 (pp. 258, 259, 264 [Table 10–2]); see also Chapter 9 ("Neurodevelopmental Disorders"; p. 248) and Chapter 25 ("Neurocognitive Disorders"; p. 681, 698)**

10.5 A patient presents with subacute-onset psychotic symptoms, changes in behavior, seizures, and memory loss. Which of the following is the most likely cause of these symptoms?

A. Mitochondrial disease.

B. HIV-associated central nervous system (CNS) infection.

C. Cocaine intoxication.

D. Limbic encephalitis.

The correct response is option D: Limbic encephalitis.

Mitochondrial diseases involve organs in different systems, and a patient with a mitochondrial disease would likely have multiple system involvement as opposed to just neuropsychiatric symptoms (option A is incorrect). HIV-associated CNS infection is more likely to be acute than subacute and also often includes delusions (option B is incorrect). Cocaine intoxication is an acute rather than subacute cause of psychosis and is unlikely to manifest in memory loss (option C is incorrect). Limbic encephalitis has a subacute onset and can include memory loss and seizures (option D is correct). **Chapter 10 (p. 264 [Table 10–2])**

10.6 Which of the following stages of schizophrenia is associated with the highest risk of suicide as well as neuroimaging evidence of cortical thinning?

A. Premorbid stage.

B. Prodromal stage.

C. Progressive stage.

D. Chronic–residual stage.

The correct response is option C: Progressive stage.

The natural history of schizophrenia involves four stages of illness: premorbid, prodromal, progressive, and chronic–residual. In the *premorbid stage* of illness, individuals who will eventually develop schizophrenia do not yet exhibit significant signs or symptoms of the illness. A number of studies have identified subtle differences between individuals who later develop schizophrenia and those who do not, including physical abnormalities, motor abnormalities, and deficits in intellectual and social functioning. The *prodromal stage* is characterized by signs and symptoms that suggest impending psychosis. These may include attenuated psychotic symptoms (e.g., exaggerated thoughts with partially preserved insight), transient psychotic symptoms (e.g., brief in duration, spontaneously remitting), or a significant decrease in functioning. The *progressive stage* of schizophrenia begins when overt psychotic symptoms appear (positive symptoms, negative symptoms, or disorganization) and cause significant social and occupational dysfunction. Clinical deterioration is common during cycles of relapses and remissions. Notably, the progressive phase of illness is the period of highest suicide risk. Furthermore, structural brain changes have been observed during the progressive phase, including thinning of the cortex, particularly the frontal, temporal, and parietal cortex (option C is correct; options A, B, and D are incorrect). The *chronic–residual stage* is characterized by persistent residual symptoms and disability that may remain stable and without progression. Outcomes are highly variable. Chronic illness and poor functioning are extremely common, but a minority of patients show near-remission or full remission between exacerbations. **Chapter 10 (pp. 266–267)**

10.7 A patient develops a temperature of 102°F, rigidity, confusion, and hypotension after a rapid increase in his fluphenazine dosage. Which of the following is the most likely diagnosis?

A. Serotonin syndrome.
B. Neuroleptic malignant syndrome.
C. Drug reaction with eosinophilia and systemic symptoms.
D. Central nervous system (CNS) infection.

The correct response is option B: Neuroleptic malignant syndrome.

Although serotonin syndrome can present with confusion, fevers, and rigidity, it is unlikely to result from dopamine D_2 receptor blockade of a first-generation antipsychotic (option A is incorrect).

With high dosages of a high-potency antipsychotic, patients can develop neuroleptic malignant syndrome (NMS), characterized by delirium, autonomic instability, rigidity, dystonia, fever, and lab abnormalities including elevated creatine kinase and elevated hepatic enzymes (option B is correct).

Most phenothiazines are associated with increased photosensitivity and risk of sunburn. Additionally, skin pigmentation changes to a grayish color have been observed with chlorpromazine. The U.S. Food and Drug Administration issued a warning regarding risk of serious skin reactions, including drug reaction with eosinophilia and systemic symptoms (DRESS), for olanzapine and ziprasidone. DRESS is characterized by a severe rash and systemic symptoms including fever (38°C to 40°C [100.4°F to 104°F]), malaise, lymphadenopathy, and symptoms related to visceral involvement (option C is incorrect).

CNS infection can present with fever and confusion but would be unlikely to result from uptitration of a medication (option D is incorrect). **Chapter 10 (pp. 265, 270); see also Chapter 25 ("Neurocognitive Disorders"; p. 690) and Chapter 29 ("Psychopharmacology"; pp. 810, 813, 831–832)**

10.8   There are low levels of this neurotransmitter in patients with schizophrenia in comparison with healthy control subjects. Moreover, psychotic symptoms result from administration of agents that are antagonists for the receptors that mediate this neurotransmitter. Based on these findings, which of the following neurotransmitters *not targeted by current medications* has been hypothesized to play an important role in schizophrenia?

A. Glutamate.
B. Dopamine.
C. Serotonin.
D. GABA.

The correct response is option A: Glutamate.

Glutamate has been hypothesized to play a role in schizophrenia (option A is correct). Glutamate is the most abundant neurotransmitter in the brain. It is mediated by *N*-methyl-D-aspartate (NMDA) receptors, and its pathways involve the cortex, limbic system, and thalamus—regions that are implicated in schizophrenia. Glutamate levels have been found to be lower in the cerebrospinal fluid of patients with schizophrenia. NMDA receptor antagonists such as phencyclidine and ketamine can trigger psychotic symptoms. Anti-NMDA receptor encephalitis can result in psychotic symptoms that resemble schizophrenia (Yang and Tsai 2017).

The dopamine hypothesis posits that patients with schizophrenia have increased dopaminergic activity, especially in the mesolimbic dopamine pathway. Consistent with this hypothesis, positron emission tomography studies have shown that patients with schizophrenia have increased dopamine activity in the striatum and midbrain origins of neurons. Antipsychotics cause varying degrees of blockade at the dopamine D_2 receptor in the mesolimbic pathway, which effectively treats the positive symptoms of schizophrenia (option B is incorrect).

A role for serotonin has been suggested by the observation that lysergic acid diethylamide (LSD) causes hallucinations. However, there is currently no direct evidence for serotonergic dysfunction in the pathogenesis of schizophrenia (Yang and Tsai 2017) (option C is incorrect).

Alterations in the GABA (γ-aminobutyric acid) neurotransmitter system have been reported in clinical and basic neuroscience schizophrenia studies and in animal models. GABA is the primary inhibitory neurotransmitter in the central nervous system. GABA abnormalities may contribute to problems with neural synchrony, γ oscillations, and working memory impairments (synchrony of neural oscillations is important for memory, perception, and consciousness) (Yang and Tsai 2017). Although GABA dysfunction may lead to cognitive problems, and people with schizophrenia show differences in GABA circuitry in comparison with control populations, psychotic symptoms generally do not arise from GABA antagonists such as flumazenil (option D is incorrect). **Chapter 10 (pp. 271, 274–275)**

References

Foussias G, Agid O, Fervaha G, et al: Negative symptoms of schizophrenia: clinical features, relevance to real world functioning and specificity versus other CNS disorders. Eur Neuropsychopharmacol 24(5):693–709, 2014 24275699

Ventura J, Thames AD, Wood RC, et al: Disorganization and reality distortion in schizophrenia: a meta-analysis of the relationship between positive symptoms and neurocognitive deficits. Schizophr Res 121(1–3):1–14, 2010 20579855

Yang AC, Tsai SJ: New targets for schizophrenia treatment beyond the dopamine hypothesis. Int J Mol Sci 18(8):1689, 2017 28771182

CHAPTER 11

Bipolar and Related Disorders

11.1   A 35-year-old woman with a history of bipolar disorder is brought to the emergency department by her husband for suicidal ideation. He reports that his wife abruptly quit her job as a computer programmer 10 days ago to start working on a book about climate change. He notes that this behavior is very atypical for her, and she has been staying up day and night filling notebooks with senseless writing. She apparently never gets tired. Over the past week, she has been increasingly irritable and moody, cries frequently, and has been talking about death. On interview, the patient states that she needs to be discharged immediately so that she can get back to writing an "extremely important" book about the global climate crisis. She reports strong feelings of guilt regarding her own role in the "destruction of the environment." The mental status exam is notable for rapid and pressured speech, "depressed" mood, labile affect, tangential thought processes, and suicidal ideation. Which of the following diagnoses best describes this patient's current mood episode?

A. Manic episode with anxious distress.
B. Hypomanic episode with mixed features.
C. Major depressive episode with mixed features.
D. Manic episode with mixed features.

The correct response is option D: Manic episode with mixed features.

Manic episodes are distinguished from hypomanic episodes by their *minimum duration* (7 days [fewer if hospitalization is necessary] for manic vs. 4 days for hypomanic) and *severity* (manic requires that psychosis, psychiatric hospitalization, and/or severe functional impairment be present during the episode, whereas hypomanic requires that none of these be present). This patient is demonstrating increased goal-directed activity, irritable and labile mood, decreased need for sleep, increased talkativeness, racing thoughts, and impulsivity. Collateral information suggests that these symptoms have been present for at least 10 days (option B is incorrect). On the basis of these symptoms, the patient meets full DSM-5 (American Psychiatric Association 2013) criteria for a manic episode. However, the patient also reports depressed mood, excessive guilt, and thoughts of suicide, which are typically associated with depressive episodes. The DSM-5 "with mixed features" episode specifier can be applied when full criteria are met for a manic episode, concurrent with at least three (out of a total of six) nonoverlapping symptoms of depression. Thus, this patient, who meets full criteria for mania in addition to demonstrating three symptoms of depression, would receive a diagnosis of *manic episode with mixed features* (option D is correct).

The DSM-5 "with anxious distress" specifier can be applied when at least two (out of a total of five) anxiety symptoms are present during the mood episode. This patient is not demonstrating any of the anxiety symptoms required for the "with anxious distress" specifier (option A is incorrect).

This patient does not meet full criteria for a major depressive episode (option C is incorrect). **Chapter 11 (pp. 280–283)**

11.2   Which of the following statements accurately describes how suicide rates among patients with bipolar disorder differ from rates in the general population?

A. Compared with individuals in the general population, patients with bipolar disorder have increased rates of both attempted and completed suicide.
B. Compared with individuals in the general population, patients with bipolar disorder have increased rates of attempted suicide but not of completed suicide.
C. Compared with individuals in the general population, patients with bipolar disorder have increased rates of completed suicide but not of attempted suicide.
D. The rates of attempted and completed suicide among patients with bipolar disorder are about the same as those in the general population.

The correct response is option A: Compared with individuals in the general population, patients with bipolar disorder have increased rates of both attempted and completed suicide.

The estimated annual rates of attempted and completed suicide among bipolar disorder patients are 3.9% and 1.4%, respectively, which are considerably higher than the corresponding rates among the general population (0.5% and 0.02%, respectively) (option A is correct; options B, C, and D are incorrect). Moreover, patients with bipolar disorder are more likely than individuals in the general population to complete suicide attempts, as demonstrated by the higher ratio of completed to attempted suicide in individuals with bipolar disorder (approximately 1:3) compared with that in the general population (1:20 to 1:40) (Baldessarini et al. 2006). **Chapter 11 (pp. 286–287)**

11.3   You are treating a 25-year-old man with bipolar I disorder who was admitted 5 days ago to an inpatient psychiatric unit for treatment of acute mania with mixed features. On admission, he received a loading dose of divalproex 20 mg/kg and was started on divalproex 750 mg/day, which 2 days ago was increased to 1,000 mg/day. The patient continues to be euphoric with an irritable edge, is intrusive, and is sleeping only 3 hours a night. You order a 12-hour serum divalproex trough level and find it to be 75 µg/mL. Which of the following would be the most appropriate next step in managing this patient's mood stabilizer?

A. Decrease divalproex to 750 mg/day.
B. Increase divalproex to 1,250 mg/day.
C. Switch to lithium 300 mg bid.
D. Switch to lamotrigine 25 mg bid daily.

The correct response is option B: Increase divalproex to 1,250 mg/day.

Divalproex is U.S. Food and Drug Administration (FDA) approved for monotherapy treatment of acute mania and can be started at 750 mg/day with or without a loading dose of 20 mg/kg; thus, this initial regimen is a reasonable choice for a young man admitted for treatment of acute mania. Therapeutic divalproex levels are considered to be 50–125 µg/mL; however, there appears to be a greater clinical benefit for acute mania in the 85–125 µg/mL range. Therefore, in this case, where clinically the patient still appears manic and the serum divalproex level is only 75 µg/mL, the patient's divalproex dosage should be increased (option B is correct; option A is incorrect) and his serum divalproex level rechecked.

Lithium is a less appropriate choice for this patient, given that he is experiencing acute mania with mixed features, which (together with rapid cycling) may be predictive of lower response to lithium (Bobo 2017) (option C is incorrect). Lamotrigine is not FDA approved for the treatment of acute mania (option D is incorrect). **Chapter 11 (pp. 290–292)**

11.4 A 38-year-old woman with a history of bipolar I disorder presents to her outpatient psychiatrist reporting 3 weeks of a symptom constellation consistent with an episode of acute bipolar depression. What U.S. Food and Drug Administration (FDA)–approved medications are currently available to treat this patient?

A. Olanzapine-fluoxetine (combination), sertraline, and quetiapine.
B. Olanzapine-fluoxetine (combination), quetiapine, and lurasidone.
C. Lithium, lurasidone, and quetiapine.
D. Divalproex, lurasidone, and quetiapine.

The correct response is option B: Olanzapine-fluoxetine (combination), quetiapine, and lurasidone.

As of fall 2018, only three medications were FDA approved for the treatment of acute bipolar depression: olanzapine–fluoxetine combination therapy, quetiapine, and lurasidone (option B is correct). Lithium is FDA approved for the long-term maintenance treatment of bipolar disorder but not for the treatment of acute bipolar depression (option C is incorrect). Divalproex is not FDA approved for either acute bipolar depression or longer-term maintenance treatment (option D is incorrect). Antidepressant monotherapy is not recommended in patients with bipolar I disorder (option A is incorrect). **Chapter 11 (pp. 291 [Table 11–4], 295–296, 300)**

11.5   The patient described in question 11.4 is started on quetiapine, and the dosage is increased to 300 mg/day (taken nightly). She continues on this medication for 4 weeks and experiences improvement in her sleep quality, but her low mood, poor concentration, poor appetite, decreased interest, and feelings of guilt persist. She denies any concurrent manic symptoms and does not have a history of rapid cycling. She reports that a number of years ago, her depression was effectively treated with escitalopram, and she asks her psychiatrist whether it might be possible/appropriate for her to receive this medication again. How should the psychiatrist respond?

A. "No, patients with a diagnosis of bipolar I disorder should never be treated with antidepressants because of the risk of inducing mania."
B. "No, patients with a diagnosis of bipolar I disorder should never be treated with antidepressants because they are ineffective."
C. "Yes, we can taper off and discontinue the quetiapine, and then start escitalopram."
D. "Yes, you could start taking escitalopram in addition to quetiapine."

The correct response is option D: "Yes, you could start taking escitalopram in addition to quetiapine."

The use of antidepressants in individuals with bipolar and related disorders is a topic of considerable controversy. Despite the fact that no antidepressants are U.S. Food and Drug Administration approved for the treatment of bipolar disorder, antidepressants are among the most widely used pharmacotherapies for individuals with bipolar disorder, being prescribed in as many as 50% of patients (Baldessarini et al. 2007), likely in part because of the scarcity of adequately tolerated alternative agents for bipolar depression. In 2013, the International Society for Bipolar Disorders Task Force issued a consensus statement providing clinical recommendations for antidepressant use in bipolar disorder (Pacchiarotti et al. 2013). One of the primary recommendations stated that "Adjunctive antidepressants may be used for acutely depressed bipolar I or II disorder patients who previously had a positive response to antidepressants" (option D is correct; options A and B are incorrect).

    The Task Force further recommended that adjunctive antidepressants be avoided in acutely depressed bipolar disorder patients experiencing two or more concurrent core manic symptoms in the presence of rapid cycling, and finally, that antidepressant monotherapy be avoided in patients with bipolar I disorder (option C is incorrect). **Chapter 11 (pp. 299–300)**

11.6   A 31-year-old man is admitted to an inpatient unit for treatment of acute mania. His psychiatrist is pondering whether to initiate treatment with lithium or divalproex. Which of the following features, if present in the patient's current presentation or history, might support use of divalproex rather than lithium?

A. A history of rapid cycling (i.e., four or more mood episodes within 1 year).
B. A family history of bipolar disorder in the patient's mother, who has been stable on lithium for many years.
C. A current presentation consistent with euphoric mania.
D. No prior history of manic episodes.

The correct response is option A: A history of rapid cycling (i.e., four or more mood episodes within 1 year).

Both lithium and divalproex are U.S. Food and Drug Administration approved for the treatment of acute mania; however, certain clinical features—such as mixed states or rapid cycling—may predict a lower likelihood of response to lithium (Bobo 2017) (option A is correct). In contrast, individuals presenting with classic euphoric mania, fewer prior episodes, and a family history of lithium response may be more likely to respond to lithium (options B, C, and D are incorrect). **Chapter 11 (pp. 290–292)**

11.7   Which of the following statements regarding the use of psychotherapy in treatment of patients with bipolar disorder is *true*?

A. Psychotherapy is most effective in treatment of acute manic episodes.
B. Psychotherapy is most effective in treatment of acute depressive episodes.
C. Psychotherapy has demonstrated benefit in preventing mood episode recurrence in euthymic patients.
D. Psychotherapy alone (without medications) is the first-line treatment for patients with bipolar disorder.

The correct response is option C: Psychotherapy has demonstrated benefit in preventing mood episode recurrence in euthymic patients.

Although pharmacological treatment is the mainstay of bipolar disorder management, adjunctive psychotherapy is an important component of a comprehensive treatment plan. Psychosocial interventions, when added to medications, can improve outcomes for bipolar patients by alleviating subsyndromal mood symptoms, enabling early detection of emerging mood episodes, increasing medication adherence, enhancing interpersonal functioning, and potentially targeting comorbid conditions such as anxiety and personality disorders (option D is incorrect).
    Four evidence-based psychotherapeutic interventions for bipolar disorder have been evaluated in randomized controlled trials: group psychoeducation, family-focused therapy, cognitive-behavioral therapy, and interpersonal and social rhythm therapy (Reiser et al. 2017). The controlled studies for these varied psychotherapeutic interventions have primarily demonstrated their benefit in preventing mood episode recurrence in euthymic patients (option C is correct), whereas their efficacy in treating acute mood episodes may prove less robust (options A and B are incorrect). **Chapter 11 (p. 301)**

11.8   A 46-year-old man with a history of hypertension and bipolar I disorder is brought to the emergency department by his wife because he has been acting sleepy and "confused" for the last few hours. She explains that both of them have recently had a stomach virus, with several days of vomiting and diarrhea. She is now recovered, but her husband continues to have vomiting and diarrhea. This morning, she was concerned that he seemed to be sleepier than usual and forgot where to get a water glass in their kitchen. On exam, the patient is lethargic, is not fully oriented, and shows a coarse tremor and an ataxic gait. He does not have any rigidity or myoclonus. Among medications routinely prescribed for maintenance treatment of bipolar disorder, which of the following would be most likely to account for the patient's presentation?

A. Lamotrigine.
B. Olanzapine.
C. Lithium.
D. Divalproex.

The correct response is option C: Lithium.

This patient, who has a history of bipolar disorder, is likely receiving long-term maintenance treatment. Medications approved by the FDA for monotherapy maintenance treatment of bipolar I disorder include lithium, lamotrigine, olanzapine, aripiprazole, and risperidone (long-acting formulation). Given the patient's reported history of a recent gastrointestinal illness with significant fluid loss due to vomiting and diarrhea, he may have transiently decreased renal function. Lithium serum levels are sensitive to fluctuations in hydration status and can reach toxic levels when there is decreased renal function. Early signs of lithium toxicity include nausea, vomiting, and diarrhea, while later signs include neurological symptoms such as confusion and ataxia (option C is correct; options A, B, and D are incorrect).

Lamotrigine and olanzapine are metabolized by the liver, and serum levels are unlikely to be affected by renal function. Divalproex can cause gastrointestinal side effects, including nausea, diarrhea, and dyspepsia, and at toxic levels can lead to neurological symptoms, including confusion and ataxia, but not coarse tremor. Divalproex is also metabolized in the liver, and serum levels are unlikely to be impacted by decreased renal function. **Chapter 11 (pp. 290–292, 297–298)**

11.9   An 18-year-old woman presents to the emergency room because of suicidal ideation. She reports a month of low mood, anhedonia, poor sleep, daytime fatigue, and feelings of worthlessness in addition to the recent onset of suicidal thoughts. She has not previously experienced a depressive episode. Which of the following aspects of this patient's presentation might lead the evaluating psychiatrist to consider bipolar disorder (in addition to unipolar depression) in the differential diagnosis?

A. Presence of suicidal ideation.
B. The patient's age.

C. Presence of insomnia.

D. The patient's gender.

The correct response is option B: The patient's age.

About half of patients with bipolar disorder will experience depression as their first mood episode, leading to challenges making an initial bipolar diagnosis, which in turn can lead to delays in appropriate treatment. Key risk factors that may lead a clinician to suspect a possible bipolar diagnosis in a patient initially presenting with depression include early age at onset (i.e., younger than 25 years) of the first major depressive episode (option B is correct), a first-degree family history of bipolar disorder, and the presence of psychotic features associated with depression (Bobo 2017).

Both suicidal ideation and insomnia are symptoms of a major depressive episode and are not necessarily suggestive of bipolar disorder (options A and C are incorrect).

Although some data suggest that among individuals with bipolar disorder, women are more likely than men to experience rapid cycling and mixed states, the overall prevalence of bipolar disorder is roughly equal in women and men (option D is incorrect). **Chapter 11 (pp. 280, 286–287, 288–289)**

11.10 A 31-year-old man with a history of bipolar disorder consults his psychiatrist about changing his maintenance medication regimen. He is tired of taking pills every day and asks if he could be treated with a long-acting injectable medication. Which of the following medications is U.S. Food and Drug Administration (FDA) approved for the maintenance treatment of bipolar disorder and is available in a long-acting injectable formulation?

A. Ziprasidone.

B. Haloperidol.

C. Fluphenazine.

D. Aripiprazole.

The correct response is option D: Aripiprazole.

Five second-generation antipsychotics have been FDA approved for the longer-term maintenance treatment of bipolar disorder: olanzapine, risperidone, quetiapine, ziprasidone, and aripiprazole. Of those, only risperidone and aripiprazole are available in a long-acting injectable formulation (option D is correct; option A is incorrect).

Fluphenazine and haloperidol are first-generation antipsychotics that are available in decanoate form and are FDA approved for the maintenance treatment of schizophrenia; however, they lack an indication for the maintenance treatment of bipolar disorder (options B and C are incorrect). **Chapter 11 (pp. 291, 298–299); see also Chapter 29 ("Psychopharmacology"; pp. 801–802 [Table 29–2])**

References

American Psychiatric Association: Diagnostic and Statistical Manual of Mental Disorders, 5th Edition. Arlington, VA, American Psychiatric Association, 2013

Baldessarini RJ, Pompili M, Tondo L: Suicide in bipolar disorder: risks and management. CNS Spectr 11(6):465–471, 2006 16816785

Baldessarini RJ, Leahy L, Arcona S, et al: Patterns of psychotropic drug prescription for U.S. patients with diagnoses of bipolar disorders. Psychiatr Serv 58(1):85–91, 2007 17215417

Bobo WV: The diagnosis and management of bipolar I and II disorders: clinical practice update. Mayo Clin Proc 92(10):1532–1551, 2017 28888714

Pacchiarotti I, Bond DJ, Baldessarini RJ, et al: The International Society for Bipolar Disorders (ISBD) task force report on antidepressant use in bipolar disorders. Am J Psychiatry 170(11):1249–1262, 2013 24030475

Reiser RP, Thompson LW, Johnson SL, et al: Bipolar Disorder. Boston, MA, Hogrefe, 2017

CHAPTER 12

Depressive Disorders

12.1 An 8-year-old boy is brought to clinic by his parents, who report that for the past year, their son has had severe behavioral outbursts, including punching and kicking his parents. He appears very irritable throughout the day, and his parents state that over the past year, he has screamed and lashed out multiple times each week, including at home, school, and soccer practice. His parents say he is almost never calm and happy. Which of the following interventions should be considered for this child?

A. Sertraline.
B. Lithium.
C. Insight-oriented psychotherapy.
D. Play therapy.

The correct response is option A: Sertraline.

This boy's behavior indicates he has disruptive mood dysregulation disorder (DMDD). The core phenomenology of DMDD is characterized by frequent and severe verbal and/or behavioral outbursts (in response to common stressors) that are pervasive, are outside the developmental stage, and occur in the background of a chronic negative mood. The onset is between ages 6 and 10 years. The current approach to management is symptomatic and problem focused. Optimal treatment for individuals with DMDD is not clear, and several individual and combined treatments are under consideration; however, there is no currently validated treatment for this disorder. Irritability has been shown to be responsive to selective serotonin reuptake inhibitors (SSRIs) in the context of a nonbipolar illness (option A is correct).

A small placebo-controlled study of lithium treatment of DMDD was negative (option B is incorrect), whereas results of trials of divalproex and risperidone have provided some support for use of these agents in management of the irritability (Leibenluft 2011). Although no formal psychotherapy trials have been reported, anecdotal reports indicate that irritability and aggression have improved with behavioral management strategies (options C and D are incorrect). **Chapter 12 (pp. 308–309, 311–312)**

12.2   Which of the following is a key feature of disruptive mood dysregulation disorder (DMDD) that can help distinguish it from other disorders that also cause behavioral problems?

A. Boredom and poor concentration.
B. Chronic irritability punctuated by periodic outbursts.
C. Periods of irritability combined with increased energy.
D. Normal mood punctuated by periodic outbursts.

The correct response is option B: Chronic irritability punctuated by periodic outbursts.

The key phenomenological feature of DMDD is irritability that is both acutely reactive and persistently chronic (option B is correct).

Individuals with pediatric bipolar disorder exhibit discrete episodes of mood disturbance with sustained volitional and cognitive changes. Distinct periods of euphoria, grandiosity, racing thoughts, and lack of need for sleep in a sustained energized state characterize bipolar disorder rather than DMDD (option C is incorrect). In contrast, DMDD is a disorder with acute temperamental outbursts on a background of chronic irritability. An explosive, chronically cranky, sensitive, and unhappy child will more likely have DMDD.

Attention-deficit/hyperactivity disorder (ADHD) may frequently coexist with DMDD, and the diagnosis is made according to the criteria of ADHD. The chronic irritability of DMDD may contribute to the appearance of boredom and difficulty maintaining focus that are part of ADHD (option A is incorrect). The impulsivity of ADHD is unlikely to be confused with the profound outbursts of temper in DMDD.

Intermittent explosive disorder is an exclusion diagnostic category for a child with frequent outbursts of temper (similar to a child with DMDD) but with no evidence of persistent mood disruption between outbursts. A child with chronic and persistent annoyed, sensitive, and irritable mood with temper outbursts would receive a diagnosis of DMDD; a child with "normal" mood between temper outbursts would receive a diagnosis of intermittent explosive disorder (option D is incorrect). **Chapter 12 (pp. 309–311)**

12.3   A 66-year-old man presents to your clinic at the urging of his wife, for "not being himself" for the past 6 months. He complains of poor sleep, poor appetite, slowed movements, and low energy; however, he denies depressed mood, saying he feels "fine." Which of the following additional symptoms would be required to meet criteria for a diagnosis of major depressive disorder (MDD)?

A. Anhedonia.
B. Insomnia.
C. Change in weight.
D. Feelings of worthlessness.

The correct response is option A: Anhedonia.

Criterion A in the DSM-5 (American Psychiatric Association 2013) diagnostic criteria for MDD requires the individual to have experienced at least five of nine listed symptoms simultaneously during a 2-week period and to have undergone a change from previous functioning. Either depressed mood or anhedonia (loss of interest or pleasure) must be one of the symptoms (option A is correct). Anhedonia is the second anchor criterion of depression. Its insidious onset in the absence of depressed mood may be associated with diminished capacity to recognize the presence of a depressive episode. Key to the assessment is the qualitative change and reference points that include timelines and activities. People who know the patient well (e.g., family members) may be immeasurably helpful in providing necessary clinical data to establish these criteria.

Appetite change and unintended weight loss reflect the physical and metabolic symptoms related to depression; the desire to eat, the pleasure of a favorite food, and the volitional drive of self-care are diminished (option C is incorrect).

Patterns of sleep disturbances within a depressive episode vary across individuals, and an individual may experience episode variability and evolution of the depressive sleep pattern over time. Characteristically, the individual feels that he or she is not getting enough sleep and experiences fatigue or exhaustion during waking hours (option B is incorrect).

An individual with MDD may have feelings of unworthiness or excessive or inappropriate guilt that are delusional (e.g., unfounded blaming of self for a major catastrophe) (option D is incorrect). **Chapter 12 (pp. 312–313)**

12.4   Which of the following symptoms, if present only during a major depressive episode, would *not* be suggestive of a separate diagnosis?

A. Bizarre delusions.
B. Weight loss.
C. Hypersomnia.
D. Panic attacks.

The correct response is option D: Panic attacks.

Anxiety and substance use disorders may be considered comorbid to depression—and commonly are—or may, in fact, be the primary disorder. An axiom by some is that for individuals with co-occurring depressive symptoms, anxiety, and panic, all should be treated concomitantly, with less regard for which was the primary presenting problem. The rationale is that anxiety is routinely a symptom itself and is extremely common during a depressive episode, and panic attacks occurring only during a depressive episode do not merit a separate diagnosis of panic disorder (option D is correct).

A thorough psychiatric examination will consider and weigh the evidence for psychotic illness, such as schizophrenia, although there may be mood-congruent or mood-incongruent psychotic features within major depressive disorder that manifest with expressions of guilt. The more systematized and bizarre the psychotic features are, the greater the likelihood that a schizophrenia-phenotypic-spectrum illness is present (option A is incorrect).

Some of the criterion signs and symptoms of a major depressive episode are identical to those of general medical conditions (e.g., weight loss with untreated diabetes, fatigue with cancer, hypersomnia early in pregnancy, insomnia later in pregnancy or during the postpartum period) (options B and C are incorrect). A newly diagnosed patient with depression clearly warrants a comprehensive medical examination that includes standard hematological and biochemistry screens as well as other screens indicated by the physical examination. **Chapter 12 (p. 318)**

12.5   A 45-year-old man with major depressive disorder presents to your clinic 1 week after starting an antidepressant. The patient had an abusive childhood and is recently divorced. He reports that work colleagues have commented that he "seems more motivated," but he still feels depressed and anxious and continues to experience some suicidal thoughts and feelings of despondency. Which of the following features in this patient's history portends a good initial response to antidepressant medication?

A. Stressor immediately prior to current episode.
B. The patient's adverse childhood experiences.
C. Prominent anxious features.
D. Increased motivation and energy.

The correct response is option D: Increased motivation and energy.

The course of symptoms throughout an episode varies according to the success of targeted treatment of symptoms. Because volition and energy may pick up early in treatment relative to mood and emotional symptoms, a patient may feel distressed that others comment that he or she appears somewhat better even though he or she still feels emotionally lousy, sad, and overwhelmed. The improvement in volition and energy is generally a good sign of initial response to treatment (option D is correct); however, the lag in improvement in mood relative to improvement in volition may result in despondency and suicidal behavior.

Adverse childhood experiences, particularly when there are multiple experiences of diverse types, comprise a set of potent risk factors for major depressive disorder and are often associated with poor response to treatment (option B is incorrect).

Stressful life events are well recognized as precipitants of major depressive episodes, but the presence or absence of adverse life events near the onset of episodes does not appear to provide a useful guide to prognosis or treatment selection (option A is incorrect).

Features associated with lower recovery rates, other than current episode duration, include psychosis, prominent anxiety (option C is incorrect), personality disorders, and severe symptomatology. **Chapter 12 (p. 315)**

12.6   A 76-year-old man with major depressive disorder (MDD) and chronic kidney disease returns to clinic for follow-up. He started escitalopram 8 weeks ago at 20 mg/day, with a dosage increase to 30 mg/day 4 weeks ago. He reports mild improvement, and his Patient Health Questionnaire–9 score has improved by 50%. He has experienced mild side effects, which he states are tolerable, but he does not want to increase the dosage. What is the next best step in management?

A. Augment with lithium.
B. Augment with aripiprazole.
C. Switch to another selective serotonin reuptake inhibitor.
D. Recommend electroconvulsive therapy (ECT).

The correct response is option B: Augment with aripiprazole.

If response is poor after 8 weeks of antidepressant monotherapy at appropriate dosages, then it would be strongly recommended to conduct a pharmacogenomic assessment and, depending on results, either change the antidepressant, add an adjunctive medication to the antidepressant, or add psychotherapy if that has not been used. Adjunctive medication should be considered when the initial antidepressant is well tolerated and is showing a greater than 25% response in terms of improvement on a depression rating scale (option C is incorrect).

First-line choices for adjunctive therapy to an antidepressant in the situation of partial response include low dosages of aripiprazole, quetiapine, or risperidone (option B is correct).

Additional adjunctive medication choices that are second line but that may be particularly familiar or well tolerated include brexpiprazole, lamotrigine, lithium, bupropion, and the thyroid hormone triiodothyronine (T_3) (option A is incorrect).

In addition to psychotherapy and medication, brain stimulation techniques, including ECT and repetitive transcranial magnetic stimulation, have first-line evidence for efficacy in adult MDD. In general, ECT will be reserved for severe depression or for situations of extreme clinical need, such as a highly suicidal patient, a patient with prominent psychotic symptoms, or a medically vulnerable patient with other health concerns, including pregnancy or medical conditions that interfere with use of antidepressant medications (option D is incorrect). **Chapter 12 (pp. 321–322)**

12.7   A 62-year-old woman with a history of major depressive disorder (MDD) is brought in by her son for evaluation and treatment. She reports having depression off and on for many years, dating back to her adolescence. She is reluctant to start treatment due to a dislike of doctors. Which of the following elements in this patient's profile and history most strongly suggest that she will experience more severe recurrences in the future?

A. She is an older adult.
B. She is female.
C. She had previous untreated episodes of depression.
D. She was brought to treatment by her son.

The correct response is option C: She had previous untreated episodes of depression.

Despite consistent differences between genders in prevalence rates for depressive disorders and in suicide rates, there appear to be no clear differences by gender in phenomenology, course, or treatment response (option B is incorrect).

Similarly, there are no clear effects of current age on the course or treatment response of MDD (option A is incorrect). Some symptom differences exist, however, such that reverse vegetative symptoms are more likely in younger individuals, and melancholic symptoms, particularly psychomotor slowing, are more common in older individuals.

There are inadequate data about specific effects of aging on long-term course of untreated MDD, but available data consistently suggest that individuals with untreated or inadequately treated MDD appear to experience more recurrences as years pass (option C is correct). Additionally, with each episode, they experience longer episodes that occur closer together, and these episodes appear to become more difficult to treat with each ensuing episode (Greden 2003; Greden et al. 2011; Kupfer et al. 1992).

The prognosis for MDD is influenced by vulnerability factors (untoward life events and stressful environmental influences) and protective factors (supportive relationships and nurturing environment) (option D is incorrect). The prognosis is positively influenced by a long-term strategy for medical and psychological management that focuses on the patient as well as his or her family and environment and maximizes the protective factors and minimizes the vulnerabilities. **Chapter 12 (pp. 316–317, 323)**

12.8 Which of the following is a major clinical feature that differentiates persistent depressive disorder (dysthymia) from major depressive disorder (MDD)?

A. Concomitant presence of anxious features.
B. Lack of changes in appetite and sleep.
C. Chronic subthreshold low mood.
D. Greater response to psychotherapy.

The correct response is option C: Chronic subthreshold low mood.

The core phenomenological feature of persistent depressive disorder is a long-standing subthreshold depression with vicissitudes of mood and temperament (option C is correct).

Symptoms may change daily or weekly. The individual often has a sullen disposition, with low energy and drive, preoccupation with guilt and failure, and a tendency to ruminate. Complaints and symptoms tend to outweigh the physical signs. Common subjective symptoms include sadness, diminished concentration or indecisiveness, a pervasive sense of hopelessness, and low self-worth or self-esteem and a generally "unhappy" aura; objective clinical signs include appetite and sleep disturbances (increased or decreased) and notable changes in energy levels (option B is incorrect).

The care and psychiatric management of a patient with persistent depressive disorder may be challenging because of chronicity and paucity of controlled trials. A meta-analytic review of 16 randomized trials (Cuijpers et al. 2010) concluded that psychotherapy had a small but significant effect but that it was less effective than pharmacotherapy in direct comparisons, especially selective serotonin reuptake inhibitors (SSRIs), and that combined pharmacotherapy and psychotherapy treatment was more effective than either alone (option D is incorrect). This pattern is comparable to that found with MDD.

In clinical practice, concomitant anxiety occurs frequently and tends to result in many patients being treated concomitantly with SSRIs and an anxiolytic, usually a benzodiazepine (option A is incorrect). **Chapter 12 (pp. 323, 325)**

12.9   A 37-year-old woman with a history of premenstrual dysphoric disorder (PMDD) presents to your clinic for treatment. You initiate treatment with a selective serotonin reuptake inhibitor (SSRI) and she quickly reports a benefit; however, she complains of sexual dysfunction and asks for some way to reduce this side effect. Which of the following is the best strategy to do so while maintaining a good therapeutic effect?

A. Continue the SSRI unchanged.
B. Increase her caffeine intake.
C. Take the SSRI only in the days prior to the onset of menses.
D. Decrease physical activity.

The correct response is option C: Take the SSRI only in the days prior to the onset of menses.

The management of PMDD includes a discussion of environmental and medical interventions. Lifestyle modifications that are encouraged and recommended include reductions in use of caffeine, salt, alcohol, and tobacco (option B is incorrect).

In addition, regular physical activity, relaxation, and psychotherapy are integrated (Zukov et al. 2010) (option D is incorrect).

An impressive pharmacological observation is the rapid response of PMDD to SSRIs. An SSRI antidepressant may be used in the 7–10 days prior to the onset of menses (option C is correct) or be taken on a regular basis. The relief of symptoms is usually immediate (within 24 hours).

Patients who respond to SSRIs may develop their own approach to determining when to start and stop the medication during their menstrual cycles (option A is incorrect). Systematic evaluation of therapeutic interventions with self-ratings of symptoms and response will guide the clinician and patient to an effective treatment strategy. **Chapter 12 (pp. 327–328)**

12.10 A 45-year-old man with a long history of alcohol use disorder presents to your clinic. He states that he has been sober for the past 6 months. He remains very depressed and despondent, and his wife confirms his history. Which of the following is the most likely diagnosis?

A. Alcohol withdrawal syndrome.
B. Demoralization.
C. Substance/medication-induced depressive disorder (SMIDD).
D. Major depressive disorder (MDD).

The correct response is option D: Major depressive disorder (MDD).

SMIDD is a broad category, and the causal substance driving the depressive episode is less critical than the observation of an association between the substance and the depression. DSM-5 stipulates that the substance must be known to be capable of producing a depressive disorder. An empirical test would be a month of abstinence from the suspected substance, and if the depression resolves, it is likely to have been caused by or associated with SMIDD (option C is incorrect). The depression is considered to be independent of the substance abuse if depression clearly occurred prior to the onset of abuse or continues once abstinence is reliably achieved for at least 1 month (option D is correct).

An alcohol-dependent person who becomes demoralized and overwhelmed by the effects of drinking may meet criteria for MDD for a significant portion of a 2-week period and might therefore be considered to have SMIDD (option B is incorrect). However if the alcohol-dependent person is successfully withdrawn from alcohol and maintains sobriety for more than 1 month but continues to have signs and symptoms of depression, the diagnosis would be MDD and not SMIDD (option A is incorrect). **Chapter 12 (pp. 328–330)**

References

American Psychiatric Association: Diagnostic and Statistical Manual of Mental Disorders, 5th Edition. Arlington, VA, American Psychiatric Association, 2013
Cuijpers P, van Straten A, Schuurmans J, et al: Psychotherapy for chronic major depression and dysthymia: a meta-analysis. Clin Psychol Rev 30(1):51–62, 2010 19781837
Greden JF: Physical symptoms of depression: unmet needs. J Clin Psychiatry 64 (suppl 7):5–11, 2003 12755646
Greden JF, Riba MB, McInnis MG: Treatment Resistant Depression: A Roadmap for Effective Care. Washington, DC, American Psychiatric Publishing, 2011
Kupfer DJ, Frank E, Perel JM, et al: Five-year outcome for maintenance therapies in recurrent depression. Arch Gen Psychiatry 49(10):769–773, 1992 1417428
Leibenluft E: Severe mood dysregulation, irritability, and the diagnostic boundaries of bipolar disorder in youths. Am J Psychiatry 168(2):129–142, 2011 21123313
Zukov I, Ptácek R, Raboch J, et al: Premenstrual dysphoric disorder—review of actual findings about mental disorders related to menstrual cycle and possibilities of their therapy. Prague Med Rep 111(1):12–24, 2010 20359434

CHAPTER 13

Anxiety Disorders

13.1   Which of the following factors increases the likelihood of having an anxiety disorder?

A. Male sex.
B. Married marital status.
C. White race.
D. High socioeconomic status.

The correct response is option C: White race.

Studies have shown a constellation of risk factors that, for the most part, are common to all of the anxiety disorders (Kessler et al. 2010). Female sex, younger age, single or divorced marital status, low socioeconomic status, poor social supports, and low education are associated with an increased likelihood of anxiety disorders (options A, B, and D are incorrect). White individuals are more likely than individuals from ethnic minority groups to have anxiety disorders (option C is correct). **Chapter 13 (p. 342)**

13.2   Which of the following anxiety disorders carries the highest lifetime prevalence in the United States?

A. Specific phobia.
B. Panic disorder.
C. Generalized anxiety disorder.
D. Agoraphobia.

The correct response is option A: Specific phobia.

Among anxiety disorders, phobias, particularly specific phobia and social anxiety disorder, are the most common conditions, with lifetime prevalence rates greater than 10% (Kessler et al. 2012) (option A is correct).

Panic disorder, generalized anxiety disorder, agoraphobia, and separation anxiety disorder have lifetime prevalence rates between 2% and 7% (Kessler et al. 2012) (options B, C, and D are incorrect). **Chapter 13 (p. 342)**

13.3 What is the most likely comorbid diagnosis in patients with generalized anxiety disorder?

A. Major depressive disorder.
B. Another anxiety disorder.
C. Alcohol use disorder.
D. Borderline personality disorder.

The correct response is option B: Another anxiety disorder.

Comorbidity of anxiety disorders with other conditions often leads to poorer outcomes and affects treatment. The most common comorbidity is the presence of another anxiety disorder (option B is correct; options A, C, and D are incorrect). Mood and substance use (including nicotine and alcohol) disorders also commonly co-occur with anxiety disorders. Because anxiety disorders often precede the onset of mood disorders and substance use, early interventions to treat anxiety disorders may prevent mood and substance use disorders. Anxiety disorders are also commonly comorbid with personality disorders, such as borderline, antisocial, and avoidant personality disorders (El-Gabalawy et al. 2013). **Chapter 13 (p. 342)**

13.4 A 30-year-old woman comes to your office for evaluation. She reports several visits to the emergency room in the past 2 months for evaluation of new-onset episodes of paroxysmal chest pain and shortness of breath, often accompanied by diaphoresis and intense fears of dying. Despite negative findings from a thorough medical workup, the patient remains convinced she has a heart condition that will kill her and spends a significant amount of time worrying that her symptoms will return. She has been avoiding strenuous physical activity, although she is still unsure about what triggered her previous episodes. What is the most likely diagnosis for this patient?

A. Panic disorder.
B. Generalized anxiety disorder.
C. Illness anxiety disorder.
D. Specific phobia.

The correct response is option A: Panic disorder.

Panic attacks are sudden, sometimes unexpected episodes of severe anxiety (although they may become more context specific and less unexpected over time), accompanied by an array of physical (e.g., cardiorespiratory, otoneurological, gastrointestinal, and/or autonomic) symptoms. These attacks are extremely frightening, particularly because they seem to occur out of the blue and without explanation (option A is correct).

Panic attacks can occur in individuals with specific phobias when exposed to the feared object (common examples are heights, snakes, and spiders), which this patient does not describe (option D is incorrect).

Persons with panic disorder commonly believe that their intense somatic symptoms are indicative of a serious physical illness (e.g., cardiac, neurological). In illness anxiety disorder, however, there is the belief that an illness is present without the experience of strong somatic symptoms (option C is incorrect).

Whereas nervousness, physical symptoms, and focal worries are indeed seen in virtually all of the anxiety disorders, what distinguishes generalized anxiety disorder from the others is the multifocal and pervasive nature of the worries, which this patient also does not describe (option B is incorrect). **Chapter 13 (pp. 351–352)**

13.5 A patient comes to the emergency room reporting symptoms consistent with a panic attack. Which of the following, if found in the patient's medical history, would most likely be the direct cause of the patient's panic attacks?

A. Mitral valve prolapse.
B. Sleep apnea.
C. Asthma.
D. Hyperthyroidism.

The correct response is option D: Hyperthyroidism.

Comorbid medical problems—such as mitral valve prolapse, asthma, Meniere's disease, migraine, and sleep apnea—can accentuate panic symptoms or be accentuated by them, but these co-occurring conditions would rarely, if ever, be considered the cause of an individual's panic attacks (Craske and Stein 2016) (options A, B, and C are incorrect).

In contrast, panic attacks (and, when recurrent, panic disorder) can occur as a direct result of common conditions such as hyperthyroidism and caffeine and other stimulant (e.g., cocaine, methamphetamine) use/abuse and, more rarely, with disorders such as pheochromocytoma or complex partial seizures (option D is correct). **Chapter 13 (p. 353)**

13.6 The medical history and emergency department workup of the patient described in question 13.5 reveal no significant abnormalities, and he appears calmer after administration of oral lorazepam 1 mg. However, the patient continues to appear distressed and tearful. When you evaluate him, he tells you "This is the third time this month that I've come to the emergency room and they can't find anything wrong with me and tell me that it's all in my head. I'm going to walk out of here still feeling terrible." What is the next best course of action to take?

A. Offer another dose of lorazepam 0.5 mg.
B. Provide reassurance and empathic listening.
C. Refer the patient for Holter monitor and cardiac consultation.
D. Ask about symptoms of depression and suicidal ideation.

The correct response is option D: Ask about symptoms of depression and suicidal ideation.

In most instances, a thorough medical history, physical examination, routine electrocardiogram, thyroid-stimulating hormone blood level, and urine or blood drug screening are sufficient as a first-pass "rule out" for such conditions. Yet, when dictated by the patient's history, additional tests may be indicated (e.g., frequent palpitations indicating the need for a Holter monitor, echocardiogram, and/or cardiology consultation). Given that this patient has no abnormalities in basic workup and medical history, no further workup is needed at this time (option C is incorrect).

Clinicians should also be aware that patients with panic disorder may be at heightened risk of suicide. Panic attacks are now so well recognized in certain medical settings, such as the emergency department, that it is common practice to identify them appropriately as such, provide reassurance, and send the patient home (option B is incorrect).

The first dose of benzodiazepine helped with the anxiety, and there is no indication that a second dose is needed at this time (option A is incorrect).

It is incumbent on clinicians in these settings to inquire about comorbid depression in general, and about suicidal ideation and plans in particular (option D is correct). **Chapter 13 (pp. 353–354)**

13.7   A 55-year-old man comes to your office for an evaluation. He describes an intense fear of traveling on the subway since he had a panic attack 10 years ago on a very crowded car. Now he refuses to travel on the subway and avoids many social situations with friends because of similar fears of "being trapped somewhere." What is the most likely diagnosis for this patient?

A. Social anxiety disorder.
B. Posttraumatic stress disorder.
C. Agoraphobia.
D. Specific phobia.

The correct response is option C: Agoraphobia.

Criterion A of the DSM-5 (American Psychiatric Association 2013) diagnostic criteria for agoraphobia refers to marked fear or anxiety regarding two or more of the following five situations: 1) using public transportation, 2) being in open spaces, 3) being in enclosed places, 4) standing in line or being in a crowd, or 5) being outside of the home alone (option C is correct).

Individually, each of the situations within the typical agoraphobic clusters could be considered a specific phobia if it were truly specific (i.e., isolated to that particular situation). What ties these situations together under agoraphobia is the fact that the individual will have several fears from these clusters of situations, accompanied by the aforementioned prototypical fears of being incapacitated, unable to escape, or unable to obtain help if symptoms emerge (option D is incorrect).

Another disorder that may be difficult to differentiate from agoraphobia is posttraumatic stress disorder (PTSD), in which an individual may have multiple feared situations from the agoraphobia clusters, including leaving home; however, in PTSD, the fears and avoidance are tied to memories of specific traumatic experiences, which are typically absent in agoraphobia (option B is incorrect).

Social anxiety disorder and agoraphobia can both be associated with fear and avoidance of similar types of situations (e.g., crowds), but the nature of the cognitions differs. Individuals with social anxiety disorder will report that they avoid situations because of fear of embarrassment or humiliation, whereas individuals with agoraphobia will report that they avoid situations because of fear of incapacitation or difficulty in escaping should help not be available (option A is incorrect). **Chapter 13 (pp. 357–358)**

13.8   A 40-year-old man with a history of a specific phobia of needles comes to your office seeking treatment. He is due for routine but required blood work in 6 weeks, and he describes significant anticipatory anxiety surrounding the appointment. Which of the following pharmacological options would be most appropriate for this patient?

A. Escitalopram.
B. Lorazepam.
C. Duloxetine.
D. Buspirone.

The correct response is option B: Lorazepam.

The algorithm for treatment of specific phobia includes consideration of cognitive-behavioral therapy first, and using benzodiazepines as needed (options A and C are incorrect).

Benzodiazepines are the best-established pharmacotherapy for treating anxiety that is predictable and limited to particular situations (e.g., specific phobia such as flying phobia or needle phobia), for which they can be prescribed on an as-needed basis (option B is correct).

Buspirone is a nonbenzodiazepine anxiolytic with efficacy limited to the treatment of generalized anxiety disorder (Stein and Sareen 2015) (option D is incorrect). **Chapter 13 (pp. 362 [Figure 13–3], 367)**

13.9   A 7-year-old boy is brought to your office for an evaluation prompted by recent disruptive behavior in school. His teachers report frequent tantrums and yelling, daily stomachaches with trips to the nurse's office, and excessive crying that interferes with his ability to focus in class. In your office, he continually fidgets with his mother's skirt, does not direct his attention toward you, and cries when his mother steps out of the office. What is the most likely diagnosis for this patient?

A. Panic disorder.
B. Social anxiety disorder.
C. Generalized anxiety disorder.
D. Separation anxiety disorder.

The correct response is option D: Separation anxiety disorder.

Separation anxiety disorder should be diagnosed when there is evidence of developmentally inappropriate and excessive anxiety occurring on separation (or threat of separation) from significant attachment figures. In children, this extreme anxiety is usually manifested by excessive crying, tantrums, physical complaints, and other manifestations of fear and avoidance of separation (option D is correct).

Social anxiety disorder is characterized by a marked fear of social and performance situations that often results in avoidance. Many patients with social anxiety disorder have extensive social fears spanning multiple social situations, unlike this child, whose symptoms as described here center on separation from his mother (option B is incorrect).

Similarly, *generalized anxiety disorder* is also characterized by fears that span various domains, which are not evident in this case (option C is incorrect).

Panic disorder will also enter the differential diagnosis, and in fact, patients with separation anxiety may have panic attacks when faced with an unwanted separation from a significant attachment figure. What distinguishes panic disorder from separation anxiety disorder is the unexpected nature of the panic attacks, unlike in this patient, where symptoms are clearly linked to separation (option A is incorrect). **Chapter 13 (pp. 344, 349)**

13.10 A 25-year-old graduate student who is in ongoing psychotherapy with a clinical social worker is referred to you by his therapist for a pharmacological consultation. He gives a history of severe anxiety that is interfering with his ability to complete his thesis. On questioning, the young man admits to using alcohol to help control his symptoms, stating that drinking 3–4 beers is the only thing that reduces his anxiety. He is ambivalent about decreasing his current intake of alcohol because he experiences overwhelming anxiety when he does not drink. His symptoms are consistent with severe generalized anxiety, and he informs you that he was diagnosed with generalized anxiety disorder as a teenager. Which of the following medications would you recommend at this time?

A. Naltrexone.
B. Gabapentin.
C. Sertraline.
D. Lorazepam.

The correct response is option C: Sertraline.

The presence of current comorbidity with other medical disorders such as mood, substance use, and personality disorders also affects the management of anxiety disorders. Alcohol and other substance use disorders are frequently comorbid with anxiety disorders, and self-medication with alcohol and drugs to reduce tension and anxiety is common among people with anxiety disorders. Understanding the vicious cycle of anxiety symptoms, in which self-medication with alcohol and drugs leads to a rebound of anxiety, is important for both the patient and the clinician. Whereas in the past, recommendations specified that clinicians should insist on abstinence before treating comorbid anxiety and substance use disorders, current thinking favors concurrent treatment of both disorders whenever feasible. In this case, the patient is in consistent psychotherapy but is ambivalent about seeking substance use–specific treatment at this time (option A is incorrect).

Treating his comorbid anxiety with a selective serotonin reuptake inhibitor, which is the first-line psychopharmacological treatment for generalized anxiety disorder, would be the most appropriate intervention (option C is correct; options B and D are incorrect). **Chapter 13 (pp. 361, 362 [Figure 13–3])**

References

American Psychiatric Association: Diagnostic and Statistical Manual of Mental Disorders, 5th Edition. Arlington, VA, American Psychiatric Association, 2013

Craske MG, Stein MB: Anxiety. Lancet 388(10063):3048–3059, 2016 27349358

El-Gabalawy R, Tsai J, Harpaz-Rotem I, et al: Predominant typologies of psychopathology in the United States: a latent class analysis. J Psychiatr Res 47(11):1649–1657, 2013 23978394

Kessler RC, Ruscio AM, Shear K, et al: Epidemiology of anxiety disorders. Curr Top Behav Neurosci 2:21–35, 2010 21309104

Kessler RC, Petukhova M, Sampson NA, et al: Twelve-month and lifetime prevalence and lifetime morbid risk of anxiety and mood disorders in the United States. Int J Methods Psychiatr Res 21(3):169–184, 2012 22865617

Stein MB, Sareen J: CLINICAL PRACTICE. Generalized anxiety disorder. N Engl J Med 373(21):2059–2068, 2015 26580998

CHAPTER 14

Obsessive-Compulsive and Related Disorders

14.1 Which of the following psychiatric disorders has the highest rate of comorbidity with obsessive-compulsive disorder (OCD) and should be screened for when making that diagnosis?

A. Autism spectrum disorder.
B. Tourette's disorder.
C. Major depressive disorder.
D. Stereotypic movement disorder.

The correct response is option C: Major depressive disorder.

An Epidemiologic Catchment Area study found that two-thirds of patients with OCD met criteria for at least one other psychiatric illness during their lifetime (Karno et al. 1988). The most common comorbid psychiatric diagnosis is major depressive disorder (option C is correct). Approximately one-third of individuals with OCD are currently experiencing a major depressive episode, and two-thirds will experience a major depressive episode during their lifetime.

Conversely, OCD is one of the most common comorbidities in patients diagnosed with autism spectrum disorder, Tourette's disorder, or stereotypic movement disorder (options A, B, and D are incorrect). **Chapter 14 (pp. 372–373); see also Chapter 9 ("Neurodevelopmental Disorders"; pp. 239, 248, 250)**

14.2 A 23-year-old patient with obsessive-compulsive disorder (OCD) has tried sertraline, fluoxetine, and fluvoxamine at full therapeutic dosages for 2 months each without improvement. Which of the following pharmacological augmentation strategies would be the most appropriate in this situation?

A. Continue fluvoxamine and add bupropion.
B. Continue fluvoxamine and add aripiprazole.
C. Continue fluvoxamine and add imipramine.
D. Discontinue fluvoxamine and start citalopram.

The correct response is option B: Continue fluvoxamine and add aripiprazole.

Meta-analyses have generally found that 40%–60% of patients with OCD achieve response (defined as at least a 25%–35% decrease in OCD symptoms) when treated with serotonin reuptake inhibitors (SRIs) (Greist et al. 1995). These meta-analyses, as well as a small number of head-to-head studies, have failed to demonstrate superior efficacy of any SRI over the others (option D is incorrect).

There is no evidence supporting the use of dopaminergic antidepressants (e.g., bupropion) in the treatment of OCD, and there is strong evidence from clinical trials that tricyclic antidepressants other than clomipramine are not effective in the treatment of OCD (options A and C are incorrect).

There have long been data supporting the use of dopaminergic antagonists (antipsychotics) to augment the effects of SRIs in the treatment of OCD. The atypical antipsychotics are most often used for this indication; however, because of these agents' side-effect burden, clinicians should use them with caution and an understanding of the risks and benefits. At this juncture, strong evidence exists only for risperidone and aripiprazole, although other atypical antipsychotics are commonly used as well (Veale et al. 2014) (option B is correct). Dosages are usually in the low to moderate range (e.g., risperidone 1–4 mg/day), and response after augmentation is typically seen within 1–4 weeks. **Chapter 14 (p. 375)**

14.3 A 42-year-old divorced woman (BMI: 22 kg/m^2) presents to her psychiatrist because of overwhelming anxiety and distress about her "fat" stomach. She frequently scrutinizes her appearance in the mirror and compares herself with other women. She now wears loose-fitting clothing to hide her abdomen, and she has stopped dating because of her conviction that potential partners would be "disgusted" by this defect. Which of the following would be the most appropriate diagnosis for this patient?

A. Body dysmorphic disorder.
B. Bulimia nervosa.
C. Anorexia nervosa.
D. Social anxiety disorder.

The correct response is option A: Body dysmorphic disorder.

There are several different causes of social avoidance. In *body dysmorphic disorder* (BDD), the patient's avoidance of social situations is based on a concern that others will negatively evaluate a perceived defect or flaw in the individual's physical appearance (in this case, the patient's abdomen) (option A is correct). Conversely, in *social anxiety disorder*, the concern is that others will negatively evaluate the individual's internal self (e.g., personality, intelligence) (option D is incorrect).

This difference between the two disorders can be difficult to elicit, and almost 40% of those diagnosed with BDD have comorbid social anxiety disorder at some point. Finally, weight concerns occurring in the context of an eating disorder preclude the diagnosis of BDD; however, this patient does not report restrictive eating habits (options B and C are incorrect). **Chapter 14 (pp. 376–377); see also Chapter 13 ("Anxiety Disorders"; p. 350)**

14.4 Which of the following represents the first-line intervention for a newly diagnosed patient with obsessive-compulsive disorder (OCD)?

A. Selective serotonin reuptake inhibitors (SSRIs).
B. Clomipramine.
C. Cognitive therapy.
D. Exposure and response prevention (ERP) therapy.

The correct response is option D: Exposure and response prevention (ERP) therapy.

Although all of the options above are considered acceptable treatments for OCD, ERP is a highly effective treatment for OCD and is considered to be the first-line intervention for the disorder (option D is correct). A study by Foa and Kozak (1996), defining "response" as a 30% or greater improvement in OCD symptoms, found that the response rate across more than a dozen studies of ERP was 76%–83%. In contrast, meta-analyses have generally found that 40%–60% of patients with OCD achieve response (defined as at least a 25%–35% decrease in OCD symptoms) when treated with serotonin reuptake inhibitors (SRIs) (Greist et al. 1995). Moreover, it is noteworthy that the few studies that have compared ERP with pharmacotherapy (e.g., Foa et al. 2005) have found that ERP was superior (options A and B are incorrect).

In terms of pharmacotherapy, the SRIs—which include all of the selective serotonin reuptake inhibitors (SSRIs) as well as clomipramine—represent the first-line pharmacotherapy intervention for OCD (Bandelow et al. 2008). When SRIs are used for treating OCD, it is important that high dosages be used, because response rates are higher with high-dosage treatment compared with low-dosage treatment. Of note, some studies have suggested that combining ERP with pharmacotherapy results in lower relapse rates in patients with OCD when they discontinue pharmacotherapy.

Cognitive therapy is a form of psychotherapy that seeks to identify and modify maladaptive beliefs (Wilhelm et al. 2009). Meta-analyses of psychotherapies in OCD (Öst et al. 2015; Rosa-Alcázar et al. 2008) found similar effect size estimates for cognitive therapy and ERP (option C is incorrect). **Chapter 14 (pp. 374–375)**

14.5 Which of the following statements accurately describes a way in which hoarding disorder differs from obsessive-compulsive disorder (OCD)?

A. Unlike OCD symptoms, hoarding disorder symptoms are typically chronic and unchanging over time.
B. Whereas clinically significant distress or impairment in important areas of functioning is required for a DSM-5 diagnosis of OCD, such distress or impairment is not required for a diagnosis of hoarding disorder.

C. Behavioral therapy is typically the first-line therapy for hoarding disorder, but not for OCD.

D. OCD has a strong heritable component, but hoarding disorder does not.

The correct response is option A: Unlike OCD symptoms, hoarding disorder symptoms are typically chronic and unchanging over time.

Hoarding had been considered a subtype of OCD, but when different OCD symptom factors were examined, hoarding was found to be clearly distinct from the others (Bloch et al. 2008; Mataix-Cols et al. 2010). Unlike symptoms of OCD, hoarding symptoms, while chronic, are rarely associated with a waxing and waning course, and instead show relatively little change over time (Tolin et al. 2010) (option A is correct).

The DSM-5 (American Psychiatric Association 2013) diagnostic criteria for hoarding disorder require that the hoarding behaviors cause "clinically significant distress or impairment in social, occupational, or other important areas of functioning (including maintaining a safe environment for self and others)" (option B is incorrect).

For both OCD and hoarding disorder, behavioral therapy is considered the first-line treatment (option C is incorrect). In hoarding disorder, the behavioral therapy focuses on removing hoarded items from the environment (increasing outflow) and providing skills to decrease future hoarding (decreasing inflow) (Frost and Tolin 2008).

Twin studies have shown that there is a strong heritable component to OCD, with concordance rates of between 80% and 87% in monozygotic twins and between 47% and 50% in dizygotic twins (van Grootheest et al. 2005). There also appears to be a genetic component in hoarding disorder. Approximately 50% of hoarders report a first-degree relative who hoards, and twin studies suggest that approximately 50% of the variability in hoarding is attributable to genetic factors (Iervolino et al. 2009). **Chapter 14 (pp. 372, 373, 375, 379–380)**

14.6   Which of the following neurostimulation therapies have been approved by the U.S. Food and Drug Administration (FDA) for use in the treatment of patients with intractable obsessive-compulsive disorder (OCD)?

A. Deep brain stimulation and repetitive transcranial magnetic stimulation.
B. Electroconvulsive therapy and deep brain stimulation.
C. Vagus nerve stimulation and deep brain stimulation.
D. Electroconvulsive therapy and repetitive transcranial magnetic stimulation.

The correct response is option A: Deep brain stimulation and repetitive transcranial magnetic stimulation.

In 2009, the FDA approved the use of deep brain stimulation (DBS) targeted at the ventral capsule/ventral striatum for treatment-refractory OCD (Keen et al. 2017).

In 2018, repetitive transcranial magnetic stimulation (rTMS) received FDA approval for the treatment of OCD (option A is correct).

Electroconvulsive therapy is the oldest and most rapidly acting and the most effective treatment for depression and catatonia; however, it has not shown benefit for OCD (options B and D are incorrect).

Vagus nerve stimulation is an FDA-approved treatment for epilepsy as well as for treatment-resistant unipolar and bipolar depression, but not for OCD (option C is incorrect). **Chapter 14 (pp. 375–376); see also Chapter 30 ("Brain Stimulation Therapies"; pp. 867, 871, 881, 893)**

14.7 A 13-year-old girl who regularly abuses marijuana and ecstasy told her mother that she believes her hair is "being contaminated from an external force" that is "infecting her brain," and she hears an external voice commanding her to "remove the hair," because otherwise she will "die of infection." Her mother has found large amounts of hair in her daughter's shower drain. The girl is missing eyelashes and patches of hair from her head. What is the appropriate DSM-5 diagnosis?

A. Trichotillomania (hair-pulling disorder).
B. Psychotic disorder.
C. Obsessive-compulsive disorder (OCD).
D. Body dysmorphic disorder (BDD).

The correct response is option B: Psychotic disorder.

Individuals with psychotic disorders may remove hair as a result of a delusion or hallucination (option B is correct). The DSM-5 (American Psychiatric Association 2013) diagnosis of hair-pulling disorder would not apply in this case (option A is incorrect).

It is of paramount importance to avoid misattributing hair loss caused by a medical condition to hair pulling. It is also possible that OCD or BDD may manifest symptoms consistent with hair-pulling disorder. For example, patients may pull their hair because they feel it is contaminated (OCD) or because they perceive it as a physical defect (BDD) (options C and D are incorrect). **Chapter 14 (pp. 381–382)**

14.8 Which of the following treatments for excoriation disorder was found to be *ineffective* in clinical trials?

A. Lamotrigine.
B. Fluoxetine.
C. *N*-acetylcysteine.
D. Habit-reversal therapy.

The correct response is option A: Lamotrigine.

Behavioral treatment of excoriation disorder is identical to that of hair-pulling disorder (i.e., based on habit-reversal therapy). The only randomized trial of habit-reversal therapy for skin picking found it to be superior to a wait-list control condition (Teng et al. 2006) (option D is incorrect).

To date, four double-blind, placebo-controlled trials of pharmacotherapy treatment of skin picking have been published. In one placebo-controlled trial with fluoxetine, 80% of patients assigned to fluoxetine were classified as responders (as measured with the Clinical Global Impression–Improvement scale) versus only 27.3% of those treated with placebo (Simeon et al. 1997) (option B is incorrect).

Another trial demonstrated efficacy for N-acetylcysteine (Grant et al. 2016) (option C is incorrect).

Two other trials were unable to demonstrate efficacy for citalopram (Arbabi et al. 2008) or lamotrigine (Grant et al. 2010) (option A is correct). **Chapter 14 (pp. 384–385)**

References

American Psychiatric Association: Diagnostic and Statistical Manual of Mental Disorders, 5th Edition. Arlington, VA, American Psychiatric Association, 2013

Arbabi M, Farnia V, Balighi K, et al: Efficacy of citalopram in treatment of pathological skin picking, a randomized double blind placebo controlled trial. Acta Medica Iranica 46(5):367–372, 2008

Bandelow B, Zohar J, Hollander E, et al: World Federation of Societies of Biological Psychiatry (WFSBP) guidelines for the pharmacological treatment of anxiety, obsessive-compulsive and post-traumatic stress disorders—first revision. World J Biol Psychiatry 9(4):248–312, 2008 18949648

Bloch MH, Landeros-Weisenberger A, Rosario MC, et al: Meta-analysis of the symptom structure of obsessive-compulsive disorder. Am J Psychiatry 165(12):1532–1542, 2008 18923068

Foa EB, Kozak MJ: Psychological treatment for obsessive-compulsive disorder, in Long-Term Treatments for Anxiety Disorders. Edited by Mavissakalian MR, Prien RF. Washington, DC, American Psychiatric Press, 1996, pp 285–309

Foa EB, Liebowitz MR, Kozak MJ, et al: Randomized, placebo-controlled trial of exposure and ritual prevention, clomipramine, and their combination in the treatment of obsessive-compulsive disorder. Am J Psychiatry 162(1):151–161, 2005 15625214

Frost RO, Tolin DF: Compulsive hoarding, in Clinical Handbook of Obsessive-Compulsive Disorder and Related Problems. Edited by Abramowitz JS, Taylor S, McKay D. Baltimore, MD, Johns Hopkins University Press, 2008, pp 76–94

Grant JE, Odlaug BL, Chamberlain SR, et al: A double-blind, placebo-controlled trial of lamotrigine for pathological skin picking: treatment efficacy and neurocognitive predictors of response. J Clin Psychopharmacol 30(4):396–403, 2010 20531220

Grant JE, Chamberlain SR, Redden SA, et al: N-acetylcysteine in the treatment of excoriation disorder: a randomized clinical trial. JAMA Psychiatry 73(5):490–496, 2016 27007062

Greist JH, Jefferson JW, Kobak KA, et al: Efficacy and tolerability of serotonin transport inhibitors in obsessive-compulsive disorder. A meta-analysis. Arch Gen Psychiatry 52(1):53–60, 1995 7811162

Iervolino AC, Perroud N, Fullana MA, et al: Prevalence and heritability of compulsive hoarding: a twin study. Am J Psychiatry 166(10):1156–1161, 2009 19687130

Karno M, Golding JM, Sorenson SB, et al: The epidemiology of obsessive-compulsive disorder in five US communities. Arch Gen Psychiatry 45(12):1094–1099, 1988 3264144

Keen EC, Widge AS, Dougherty DD: Functional neurosurgery in severe and treatment-refractory OCD, in Obsessive-Compulsive Disorder: Phenomenology, Pathophysiology, and Treatment. Edited by Pittenger C. New York, Oxford University Press, 2017, pp 507–516

Mataix-Cols D, Frost RO, Pertusa A, et al: Hoarding disorder: a new diagnosis for DSM-V? Depress Anxiety 27(6):556–572, 2010 20336805

Öst LG, Havnen A, Hansen B, et al: Cognitive behavioral treatments of obsessive-compulsive disorder. A systematic review and meta-analysis of studies published 1993–2014. Clin Psychol Rev 40:156–169, 2015 26117062

Rosa-Alcázar AI, Sánchez-Meca J, Gómez-Conesa A, et al: Psychological treatment of obsessive-compulsive disorder: a meta-analysis. Clin Psychol Rev 28(8):1310–1325, 2008 18701199

Simeon D, Stein DJ, Gross S, et al: A double-blind trial of fluoxetine in pathological skin picking. J Clin Psychiatry 58(8):341–347, 1997 9515971

Teng EJ, Woods DW, Twohig MP: Habit reversal as a treatment for chronic skin picking: a pilot investigation. Behav Modif 30(4):411–422, 2006 16723422

Tolin DF, Meunier SA, Frost RO, et al: Course of compulsive hoarding and its relationship to life events. Depress Anxiety 27(9):829–838, 2010 20336803

van Grootheest DS, Cath DC, Beekman AT, et al: Twin studies on obsessive-compulsive disorder: a review. Twin Res Hum Genet 8(5):450–458, 2005 16212834

Veale D, Anson M, Miles S, et al: Efficacy of cognitive behaviour therapy versus anxiety management for body dysmorphic disorder: a randomised controlled trial. Psychother Psychosom 83(6):341–353, 2014 25323062

Wilhelm S, Steketee G, Fama JM, et al: Modular cognitive therapy for obsessive-compulsive disorder: a wait-list controlled trial. J Cogn Psychother 23(4):294–305, 2009 21072138

CHAPTER 15

Trauma- and Stressor-Related Disorders

15.1   An *increase* in which of the following physiological parameters is typically observed following the traumatic event in patients with posttraumatic stress disorder (PTSD)?

A. Serum cortisol levels.
B. Activity of the amygdala.
C. Activity of the ventromedial prefrontal cortex.
D. Heart rate variability.

The correct response is option B: Activity of the amygdala.

The general change following the traumatic event is the induction of a persistent state of alarm, hyperalertness, and sensitivity to threat, characterized by hyper(re)activity of the amygdala (Hughes and Shin 2011) (option B is correct).

Brain structures that have been found to inhibit the expression of conditioned fear, in part by facilitating extinction, including the ventromedial prefrontal cortex (vmPFC), are hypo(re)active (option C is incorrect). The amygdala and the vmPFC have an inverse relationship—the more active the vmPFC is, the less active the amygdala is, and vice versa.

Paralleling the heightened sympathetic nervous system (re)activity in PTSD is hypoactivity of the parasympathetic nervous system, manifested in decreased heart rate variability (option D is incorrect), which has been found to predict mortality.

The most surprising finding in biological research of PTSD has been that cortisol is not elevated, as might be expected according to a classical stress model (option A is incorrect); if anything, cortisol is reduced (Yehuda 2002). **Chapter 15 (pp. 396–397)**

15.2 Besides the requirement that the child has experienced extremes of social neglect or insufficient care that are presumed to have led to the child's disturbed behavior, what other diagnostic criterion is shared between the DSM-5 diagnoses of reactive attachment disorder (RAD) and disinhibited social engagement disorder (DSED)?

A. Attachment of the child to putative caregivers must be absent or grossly underdeveloped.
B. The diagnosis may not be made in children with autism spectrum disorder.
C. The disturbance in the child's behavior must be evident before 5 years of age.
D. The child must have a developmental age of at least 9 months.

The correct response is option D: The child must have a developmental age of at least 9 months.

DSM-5 (American Psychiatric Association 2013) describes the essential feature of RAD as absent or grossly underdeveloped attachment between the child and putative caregiving adults. DSED, in contrast, can occur in children who lack attachments, who have established attachments, or who have secure attachments (option A is incorrect), with some studies showing none and others identifying secure attachment (Zeanah and Gleason 2015).

Whereas the DSM-5 diagnosis for RAD requires that criteria not be met for autism spectrum disorder and that the disturbance be evident before 5 years of age, the DSED diagnosis does not include these requirements (options B and C are incorrect).

In both RAD and DSED, the child must be cognitively at least 9 months old (option D is correct), given that these diagnoses should not be made in children who are developmentally unable to form selective attachments. **Chapter 15 (pp. 402–404)**

15.3 Which of the following options best reflects the first-line treatment approach recommended by the 2010 American Academy of Child and Adolescent Psychiatry (AACAP) *Practice Parameter for the Assessment and Treatment of Children and Adolescents With Posttraumatic Stress Disorder (PTSD)*?

A. Start trauma-focused cognitive-behavioral therapy (CBT).
B. Start fluoxetine 10 mg/day.
C. Start lorazepam 0.5 mg at bedtime.
D. Start clonidine 0.05 mg at bedtime.

The correct response is option A: Start trauma-focused cognitive-behavioral therapy (CBT).

The AACAP practice parameter (Cohen et al. 2010) cautioned that because of possible hyperarousal with irritability, poor sleep, or inattention, selective serotonin reuptake inhibitor (SSRI) monotherapy may not be an optimal treatment for children with PTSD (Robb et al. 2010). Therefore, the AACAP advised beginning with an evidence-based targeted psychotherapy such as trauma-focused CBT (first-line choice) and adding an SSRI (second-line choice) if severity of symptoms indicates a need for more interventions (option A is correct; option B is incorrect).

Other than SSRIs, there are no other medications for consideration, and there is no updated AACAP guideline or U.S. Food and Drug Administration approval for a medication treatment of PTSD or other trauma- and stressor-related disorders in children. Despite wide clinical use of benzodiazepines or clonidine for treatment of PTSD, no evidence-based study has established their benefit for this indication (options C and D are incorrect). **Chapter 15 (p. 419)**

15.4 One week after presenting to the emergency department immediately following a reported sexual assault by a stranger, an 18-year-old woman is referred for follow-up with a health care provider. She reports multiple symptoms consistent with psychological trauma and screens positive on a brief instrument for acute stress disorder. Which of the following early posttrauma psychotherapeutic interventions has been shown to be *unhelpful* and *possibly harmful*?

A. Psychoeducation about typical trauma responses.
B. Psychological debriefing.
C. Brief trauma-focused supportive psychotherapy.
D. Multisession cognitive-behavioral therapy (CBT).

The correct response is option B: Psychological debriefing.

In a meta-analysis and systematic review of acute stress disorder, brief trauma-focused supportive therapy was found to be the most effective therapy for reducing posttraumatic stress disorder (PTSD) symptom severity (Roberts et al. 2009, 2010) (option C is incorrect). Multisession CBT has been recommended for trauma survivors with acute trauma symptoms consistent with acute stress disorder, and there is evidence that it may provide some benefit to those with subthreshold symptoms (option D is incorrect). Psychoeducation about typical trauma responses also may be helpful (option A is incorrect). Although once believed to be effective, psychological debriefing has been shown not to reduce PTSD incidence or symptom severity; for some, it may even be harmful, in that it may disrupt naturally occurring coping mechanisms (Rose et al. 2002; van Emmerik et al. 2002) (option B is correct). **Chapter 15 (pp. 413–414)**

15.5 Along with prolonged exposure therapy, which of the following psychotherapy approaches possesses the best evidence for treating posttraumatic stress disorder (PTSD) symptoms?

A. Present-centered therapy.
B. Stress inoculation training.
C. Cognitive processing therapy.
D. Group cognitive-behavioral therapy.

The correct response is option C: Cognitive processing therapy.

Prolonged exposure therapy and cognitive processing therapy are the evidence-based therapies with the greatest amount of empirical support for treating PTSD (option C is correct). Non-trauma-focused therapies, including stress inoculation training and present-centered therapy, have some but weaker support in treating PTSD (options A and B are incorrect). Group therapies have been found to be less effective than individual therapies in reducing PTSD symptoms (option D is incorrect), despite being comparably effective for reducing depression and suicidal ideation (Resick et al. 2017). **Chapter 15 (pp. 415, 416)**

15.6   A 28–year old man starts seeing a therapist several months after his father died suddenly of a heart attack at age 50 years. Since the days immediately following his father's death, the patient has suffered from profound distress over the loss, experiencing daily low mood, poor concentration, and fatigue, with a feeling of "heaviness" throughout his body. His performance at work suffers, and he ultimately quits his job. He dwells on memories of his father and has had frequent thoughts of death, wishing that he and his father could be reunited, although he denies active self-harm ideation or behaviors. These symptoms persist for a year; however, there is no evident increase in irritability or anger, hypervigilance, exaggerated startle, sleep disturbance, or avoidance behavior. What is the most appropriate DSM-5 diagnosis?

A. Acute stress disorder.
B. Posttraumatic stress disorder.
C. Adjustment disorder with depressed mood.
D. Other specified trauma- and stressor-related disorder.

The correct response is option D: Other specified trauma- and stressor-related disorder.

In DSM-5's formulation of *acute stress disorder*, the disturbance has a duration of no more than 30 days, starting immediately after the trauma (option A is incorrect). Likewise, for *adjustment disorder*, the symptoms do not persist longer than an additional 6 months after the stressor has terminated (option C is incorrect). The diagnosis of *posttraumatic stress disorder* requires at least one intrusion symptom, one avoidance symptom, two negative cognition or mood symptoms, and two altered arousal and reactivity symptoms or behaviors; in this case, the avoidance criterion is noted to be entirely absent (option B is incorrect). DSM-5 lists five examples of presentations for which an "other specified" designation might be appropriate, including the presentations of *adjustment-like disorders with prolonged duration of more than 6 months without prolonged duration of stressor* and *persistent complex bereavement disorder* (listed in "Conditions for Further Study" in Section III of DSM-5), either of which could fit the symptom profile in this vignette (option D is correct). **Chapter 15 (p. 426; Table 15–3 [p. 406], Table 15–5 [p. 421], Table 15–6 [p. 423])**

15.7 Which of the following is a diagnostic criterion for DSM-5 acute stress disorder (ASD)?

A. At least three dissociative symptoms must be present.
B. Nine or more symptoms from any of five categories are required.
C. Symptoms must persist for at least 2 days after the trauma.
D. Symptoms may persist for up to 2 months after the trauma.

The correct response is option B: Nine or more symptoms from any of five categories are required.

In DSM-IV-TR (American Psychiatric Association 2000), the diagnostic criteria for ASD required the presence of at least three of five dissociative symptoms. In DSM-5, the diagnosis of ASD still includes, but no longer requires, dissociative symptoms (option A is incorrect). Instead, the DSM-5 ASD diagnosis requires the presence of at least 9 of 14 symptoms in any of five categories—intrusion symptoms, negative mood, dissociative symptoms, avoidance symptoms, and arousal symptoms—beginning or worsening after the traumatic event and persisting for 3 days (instead of the 2 days required in DSM-IV [American Psychiatric Association 1994]) to 1 month after the trauma (option B is correct; options C and D are incorrect). The new DSM-5 threshold of 9 of 14 symptoms is based on an analysis of data from Israel, the United Kingdom, and Australia (Bryant et al. 2011). **Chapter 15 (pp. 420–421)**

15.8 Which of the following specific cognitive-behavioral therapies (CBTs) for post-traumatic stress disorder (PTSD) recommended in the 2017 VA/DoD *Clinical Practice Guideline for Management of Post-Traumatic Stress* has been shown to be comparable in efficacy to prolonged exposure therapy?

A. Brief eclectic psychotherapy.
B. Narrative exposure therapy.
C. Written narrative exposure therapy.
D. Eye movement desensitization and reprocessing.

The correct response is option D: Eye movement desensitization and reprocessing.

The 2017 VA/DoD guidelines (U.S. Department of Veterans Affairs and U.S. Department of Defense 2017) suggested that various specific CBTs for PTSD, including brief eclectic psychotherapy, narrative exposure therapy, written narrative exposure, and eye movement desensitization and reprocessing (EMDR), can all be beneficial as a PTSD treatment, with EMDR having the most supporting data of these and efficacy similar to that of prolonged exposure therapy (option D is correct; options A, B, and C are incorrect). EMDR involves trauma recall, emotional processing, and cognitive reappraisal strategies accompanied by eye movement tracking or other forms of bilateral stimulation. **Chapter 15 (pp. 415–416)**

References

American Psychiatric Association: Diagnostic and Statistical Manual of Mental Disorders, 4th Edition. Washington, DC, American Psychiatric Association, 1994

American Psychiatric Association: Diagnostic and Statistical Manual of Mental Disorders, 4th Edition, Text Revision. Washington, DC, American Psychiatric Association, 2000

American Psychiatric Association: Diagnostic and Statistical Manual of Mental Disorders, 5th Edition. Arlington, VA, American Psychiatric Association, 2013

Bryant RA, Friedman MJ, Spiegel D, et al: A review of acute stress disorder in DSM-5. Depress Anxiety 28(9):802–817, 2011 21910186

Cohen JA, Bukstein O, Walter H, et al: Practice parameter for the assessment and treatment of children and adolescents with posttraumatic stress disorder. J Am Acad Child Adolesc Psychiatry 49(4):414–430, 2010 20410735

Hughes KC, Shin LM: Functional neuroimaging studies of post-traumatic stress disorder. Expert Rev Neurother 11(2):275–285, 2011 21306214

Resick PA, Wachen JS, Dondanville KA, et al: Effect of group vs individual cognitive processing therapy in active-duty military seeking treatment for posttraumatic stress disorder: a randomized clinical trial. JAMA Psychiatry 74(1):28–36, 2017 27893032

Robb AS, Cueva JE, Sporn J, et al: Sertraline treatment of children and adolescents with posttraumatic stress disorder: a double-blind, placebo-controlled trial. J Child Adolesc Psychopharmacol 20(6):463–471, 2010 21186964

Roberts NP, Kitchiner NJ, Kenardy J, Bisson JI: Systematic review and meta-analysis of multiple-session early interventions following traumatic events. Am J Psychiatry 166(3):293–301, 2009 19188285

Roberts NP, Kitchiner NJ, Kenardy J, Bisson JI: Early psychological interventions to treat acute traumatic stress symptoms. Cochrane Database Syst Rev (3):CD007944, 2010 20238359

Rose S, Bisson J, Churchill R, Wessely S: Psychological debriefing for preventing post traumatic stress disorder (PTSD). Cochrane Database Syst Rev (2):CD000560, 2002 12076399

U.S. Department of Veterans Affairs, U.S. Department of Defense: VA/DoD Clinical Practice Guideline for Management of Post-Traumatic Stress (Publ No 10Q-CPG/PTSD-04). Washington, DC, Veterans Health Administration, Department of Veterans Affairs and Health Affairs, Department of Defense, Office of Quality and Performance, 2017

van Emmerik AA, Kamphuis JH, Hulsbosch AM, Emmelkamp PM: Single session debriefing after psychological trauma: a meta-analysis. Lancet 360(9335):766–771, 2002 12241834

Yehuda R: Post-traumatic stress disorder. N Engl J Med 346(2):108–114, 2002 11784878

Zeanah CH, Gleason MM: Annual research review: Attachment disorders in early childhood—clinical presentation, causes, correlates, and treatment. J Child Psychol Psychiatry 56(3):207–222, 2015 25359236

C H A P T E R 1 6

Dissociative Disorders

16.1   Which of the following is an effective treatment option for dissociative identity disorder (DID)?

A. Antidepressants.
B. Benzodiazepines.
C. Antipsychotics.
D. Psychotherapy.

The correct response is option D: Psychotherapy.

Psychotherapy can help patients with DID gain control over the dissociative process underlying their symptoms. The fundamental psychotherapeutic stance should involve meeting patients halfway, in the sense of acknowledging that they experience themselves as fragmented, yet the reality is that the fundamental problem is a failure of integration of conflicting memories and aspects of the self. The ultimate goal of psychotherapy for patients with DID is integration of the disparate states. Hypnosis can be helpful in therapy as well as in diagnosis. It can be helpful in facilitating access to dissociated personalities. The tactical-integration model for the treatment of dissociative disorders consists of structured cognitive-behavioral–based treatments that foster symptom relief, followed by integration of the personalities and/or ego states into one mainstream of consciousness. In addition, both cognitive analytic therapy (CAT) (Kellett 2005; Ryle and Fawkes 2007) and dialectical behavior therapy (DBT) (Braakmann et al. 2007) have been found to be helpful as adjunctive or primary treatment of patients with DID (option D is correct).

To date, no good evidence shows that medication of any type has a direct therapeutic effect on the dissociative process manifested by patients with DID. Thus, pharmacological treatment has been limited to the control of signs and symptoms afflicting patients with DID or comorbid conditions rather than the treatment of dissociation per se. The use of antidepressants should be limited to the treatment of DID patients who experience symptoms of major depressive disorder (Barkin and Kluft 1986) (option A is incorrect).

Benzodiazepines have at times been used to facilitate recall through controlling secondary anxiety associated with retrieval of traumatic memories. However, these effects may be nonspecific at best (option B is incorrect).

Antipsychotics are rarely useful in reducing dissociative symptoms (option C is incorrect). **Chapter 16 (pp. 452–453, 456–460)**

16.2   In addition to psychotherapy, which of the following has shown some efficacy in the reduction of depersonalization symptoms?

A. Antidepressants.
B. Psychostimulants.
C. Naltrexone.
D. Benzodiazepines.

The correct response is option C: Naltrexone.

There is no known pharmacotherapy for the treatment of depersonalization/derealization disorder. Virtually all types of psychotropic medications, including psychostimulants, antidepressants, antipsychotics, anticonvulsants, and benzodiazepines, have been tried with modest success in individuals with depersonalization or derealization symptoms (options A, B, and D are incorrect).

In an open trial of naltrexone (dosage ranged between 100 and 250 mg/day), the authors reported an average 30% reduction of symptoms of depersonalization as measured by three validated dissociation scales (Simeon et al. 2005) (option C is correct). **Chapter 16 (p. 466)**

16.3   Which of the following is the underlying disturbance in all dissociative disorders?

A. Poor reality testing.
B. Disturbance in the integration of mental contents.
C. Deficit in memory encoding and storage.
D. Disturbance in identity formation.

The correct response is option B: Disturbance in the integration of mental contents.

The dissociative disorders involve a disturbance in the integrated organization of consciousness, memory, identity, emotion, perception, body representation, motor control, and behavior. The problem is the failure of integration or the decontextualization of information, rather than the contents of the fragments (option B is correct).

Depersonalization/derealization disorder is primarily a disturbance in the integration of perceptual experience. Different from those with delusional disorders and other psychotic processes, those with depersonalization/derealization disorder have intact reality testing. Patients are aware of some distortion in their perceptual experience and therefore are not delusional (option A is incorrect).

Dissociative amnesia is the classical functional disorder of memory and involves difficulty in retrieving discrete components of autobiographical–episodic memory (Kritchevsky et al. 2004; Spiegel et al. 2011). It does not, however, involve a difficulty in memory storage, as in Wernicke-Korsakoff syndrome (option C is incorrect).

Fragmentation of identity results in dissociative identity disorder (option D is incorrect). **Chapter 16 (pp. 437, 460, 464)**

16.4   What is the hallmark characteristic of dissociative identity disorder (DID)?

A. Disordered perception.
B. Poor memory integration.
C. Fragmentation of identity.
D. Multiple personalities.

The correct response is option C: Fragmentation of identity.

The dissociative disorders involve a disturbance in the integrated organization of consciousness, memory, identity, emotion, perception, body representation, motor control, and behavior. *Fragmentation of identity* results in DID (option C is correct). As specified in the DSM-5 (American Psychiatric Association 2013) diagnostic criteria, the hallmark of DID is "disruption of identity characterized by [the presence of] two or more distinct personality states, which may be described in some cultures as an experience of possession" (p. 292).

Disordered perception yields depersonalization/derealization disorder (option A is incorrect).

The identity temporarily lost during dissociative states or the aspects of the self that are fragmented in DID are two-dimensional aspects of an overall personality structure. In this sense, it has been said that patients with DID do not have *more than* one personality but rather have *less than* one personality (option D is incorrect).

When *memories are poorly integrated*, the resulting disorder is dissociative amnesia (option B is incorrect). **Chapter 16 (pp. 437, 446)**

16.5   Which of the following is the most common dissociative disorder?

A. Dissociative identity disorder.
B. Dissociative amnesia.
C. Depersonalization/derealization.
D. Dissociative fugue.

The correct response is option B: Dissociative amnesia.

Dissociative amnesia is considered the most common of the dissociative disorders (option B is correct; options A and C are incorrect). Amnesia is a symptom commonly found in several other dissociative and anxiety disorders, including somatic symptom disorder, DID, acute stress disorder, and posttraumatic stress disorder. A higher incidence of dissociative amnesia has been described in the context of war and natural and other disasters (Maldonado et al. 2002). There appears to be a direct relationship between the severity of the exposure to trauma and the incidence of amnesia. Dissociative amnesia is the classical functional disorder of memory and involves difficulty in retrieving discrete components of autobiographical–episodic memory (Kritchevsky et al. 2004; Spiegel et al. 2011).

In DSM-5, *dissociative fugue* was removed as a separate diagnostic entity, and fugue is now a subtype of dissociative amnesia designated by use of the specifier "with dissociative fugue" when dissociative amnesia also involves purposeful travel or bewildered wandering (option D is incorrect). **Chapter 16 (pp. 437, 448 [Table 16–2], 460)**

16.6   Which of the following disorders is characterized by an inability to recall important personal information, usually of a traumatic or stressful nature, that cannot be explained by ordinary forgetfulness in the absence of overt brain pathology or substance use?

A. Dissociative identity disorder.
B. Acute stress disorder.
C. Dissociative amnesia.
D. Depersonalization/derealization.

The correct response is option C: Dissociative amnesia.

As specified in the DSM-5 diagnostic criteria, the hallmark of *dissociative amnesia* is the inability to recall important personal information, usually of a traumatic or stressful nature, that cannot be explained by ordinary forgetfulness in the absence of overt brain pathology or substance use (option C is correct).

The hallmark of *dissociative identity disorder* is "disruption of identity characterized by [the presence of] two or more distinct personality states, which may be described in some cultures as an experience of possession" (American Psychiatric Association 2013, p. 292) (option A is incorrect).

Acute stress disorder (see Chapter 15, "Trauma- and Stressor-Related Disorders") is characterized by exposure to actual or threatened death, serious injury, or sexual violation and presence of nine (or more) posttrauma symptoms from any of the five categories of intrusion, negative mood, dissociation, avoidance, and arousal. The disturbance has a duration of 3–30 days, starting immediately after the trauma, and causes clinically significant distress or impairment (option B is incorrect).

The essential feature of depersonalization/derealization disorder is the presence of *depersonalization* (i.e., persistent feelings of unreality, detachment, or estrangement from oneself or one's body, usually with the feeling that one is an outside observer of one's own mental processes), *derealization* (i.e., experiences of unreality or detachment with respect to surroundings), or both (option D is incorrect). **Chapter 16 (pp. 421, 446, 460, 464); see also Chapter 15 ("Trauma- and Stressor-Related Disorders"; p. 421)**

16.7   Which of the following types of memory is most affected in dissociative amnesia?

A. Episodic memory.
B. Short-term memory.
C. Implicit memory.
D. Procedural memory.

The correct response is option A: Episodic memory.

Patients with "psychogenic" or dissociative amnesia typically differ from patients with the neurological amnestic syndrome in that memory for their personal life histories is much more severely affected than is their ability to learn and retain new information; that is, they have isolated retrograde amnesia (Brandt and Van Gorp 2006) (option B is incorrect).

Dissociative amnesia has three primary characteristics:

1. The memory loss is episodic. Explicit (or episodic) memory involves recall of personal experiences identified with the self (e.g., "I was at the ball game last week") (option A is correct). The first-person recollection of certain events is lost, rather than knowledge of procedures (option D is incorrect).
2. The memory loss is for a discrete period of time. It is not vagueness or the inefficient retrieval of memories, but rather a dense unavailability of memories that had been clearly accessible. Unlike the amnestic disorders, such as from damage to the medial temporal lobe in surgery, or in Wernicke-Korsakoff syndrome, there is usually no difficulty in learning new episodic information. However, a dissociative syndrome of continuous difficulty in incorporating new information may mimic organic amnestic syndromes.
3. The memory loss is generally for events of a traumatic or stressful nature. Implicit (or semantic) memory involves the execution of routine operations, such as riding a bicycle or typing (option C is incorrect).

Chapter 16 (pp. 440, 460–461)

16.8   A 33-year-old male veteran with a history of posttraumatic stress disorder presents with memory difficulties. Two weeks ago, the patient showed up to work and found out that he had quit his job the day before, despite having no recollection of it. The patient has also found new purchases in his home that he does not recall making. He has no history of traumatic brain injury, overt brain pathology, or substance use. What is the most likely diagnosis?

A. Dissociative identity disorder.
B. Depersonalization/derealization.
C. Dissociative amnesia.
D. Dissociative fugue.

The correct response is option C: Dissociative amnesia.

As specified in the DSM-5 diagnostic criteria, the hallmark of *dissociative amnesia* is the inability to recall important personal information, usually of a traumatic or stressful nature, that cannot be explained by ordinary forgetfulness in the absence of overt brain pathology or substance use. Such individuals initially may not be aware of the memory loss; however, they may find, for example, new purchases in their homes but have no memory of having obtained them. They report being told that they have done or said things that they cannot remember (option C is correct).

Individuals with *dissociative amnesia* generally do not have disturbances of identity, except to the extent that their identity is influenced by the warded-off memory (option A is incorrect).

However, those with the *fugue subtype of dissociative amnesia* may have more pervasive amnesia for personal identity, sometimes coupled with aimless wandering or purposeful travel (option D is incorrect).

The essential feature of *depersonalization/derealization disorder* is the presence of depersonalization (i.e., persistent feelings of unreality, detachment, or estrangement from oneself or one's body, usually with the feeling that one is an outside observer of one's own mental processes), derealization (i.e., experiences of unreality or detachment with respect to surroundings), or both (option B is incorrect). **Chapter 16 (pp. 460–462, 464)**

16.9   Which of the following statements regarding the *dissociative subtype of posttraumatic stress disorder* (PTSD+DS) is accurate?

   A. Functional magnetic resonance imaging (fMRI) research has shown lesser amygdala connectivity to regions involved in consciousness, awareness, and proprioception in PTSD+DS patients.
   B. fMRI research has shown frontal hyperactivity and limbic hypoactivity in patients with PTSD+DS during exposure to trauma-related imagery.
   C. fMRI research has shown frontal hypoactivity and limbic hyperactivity in patients with PTSD+DS during exposure to trauma-related imagery.
   D. fMRI research has shown lesser amygdala functional connectivity to prefrontal regions involved in emotional regulation in PTSD+DS patients.

The correct response is option B: fMRI research has shown frontal hyperactivity and limbic hypoactivity in patients with PTSD+DS during exposure to trauma-related imagery.

DSM-5 includes a dissociative subtype of PTSD (i.e., PTSD+DS). A systematic literature review of latent class and profile analytic studies of PTSD lent support to the PTSD dissociative subtype (PTSD+DS), primarily characterized by depersonalization and derealization (Hansen et al. 2017). fMRI research has identified a dissociative subtype of PTSD that is notably different from the more common hyperarousal pattern (Lanius et al. 2010; Nicholson et al. 2017). The *dissociative sub-*

type involves frontal hyperactivity coupled with limbic hypoactivity (option B is correct), consistent with cognitive suppression of emotional response, whereas the more common *hyperarousal subtype* of PTSD is associated with the opposite pattern: limbic hyperactivity and hypofrontality (Brand et al. 2012) (option C is incorrect).

More recent research has shown that among patients with PTSD, the PTSD+DS group exhibited *greater* amygdala functional connectivity to prefrontal regions involved in emotion regulation (bilateral basolateral amygdala [BLA] and left centromedial amygdala [CMA] to the middle frontal gyrus and bilateral CMA to the medial frontal gyrus) than the PTSD non-DS group (Nicholson et al. 2015) (option D is incorrect).

Also, the PTSD+DS group showed *greater* amygdala connectivity to regions involved in consciousness, awareness, and proprioception implicated in depersonalization and derealization (left BLA to superior parietal lobe and cerebellar culmen, and left CMA to dorsal posterior cingulate and precuneus) (option A is incorrect). **Chapter 16 (pp. 439, 444–446)**

16.10 Which of the following statements accurately describes a way in which *dissociation* and *repression* differ?

A. The organizational structure of mental contents is horizontal in dissociation and vertical in repression.
B. In dissociation, the barrier preventing access to mental contents is dynamic conflict; in repression, the barrier is amnesia.
C. Retrieval of dissociated information often can be accomplished through interpretation, whereas retrieval of repressed information usually requires hypnosis.
D. Dissociation is a response to unwanted wishes and fears, whereas repression is often elicited as a defense against trauma.

The correct response is option A: The organizational structure of mental contents is horizontal in dissociation and vertical in repression.

As a general model for keeping information out of conscious awareness, *repression* differs from *dissociation* in several important ways (Table 16–1). The organizational structure of mental contents in dissociation is considered to be horizontal, with subunits of information divided from one another but equally available to consciousness (Hilgard 1977). Repressed information, on the other hand, is presumed to be stored in an archaeological manner, at various depths, and therefore, different components are not equally accessible (Freud 1923/1961) (option A is correct).

Subunits of information are presumed to be divided by amnesic barriers in dissociation, whereas dynamic conflict, or motivated forgetting, is the mechanism underlying repression (option B is incorrect).

Dissociation is often elicited as a defense, especially after episodes of physical trauma, whereas repression is a response to warded-off fears and wishes or a response to other dynamic conflicts (option D is incorrect).

TABLE 16–1. Differences between dissociation and repression

	Dissociation	Repression
Organizational structure[a]	Horizontal	Vertical
Barriers[b]	Amnesia	Dynamic conflict
Etiology[c]	Trauma	Developmental conflict over unacceptable wishes
Contents[d]	Untransformed: traumatic memories	Disguised, primary process: dreams, slips
Means of access[e]	Hypnosis	Interpretation
Psychotherapy[f]	Access, control, and working through of traumatic memories	Interpretation, transference

[a]The organizational structure of mental contents in dissociation is considered to be horizontal, with subunits of information divided from one another but equally available to consciousness (Hilgard 1977). Repressed information, on the other hand, is presumed to be stored in an archaeological manner, at various depths, and therefore, different components are not equally accessible (Freud 1923/1961).

[b]Subunits of information are presumed to be divided by amnesic barriers in dissociation, whereas dynamic conflict, or motivated forgetting, is the mechanism underlying repression.

[c]The information kept out of awareness in dissociation often involves a discrete and sharply delimited period, usually a traumatic experience, whereas repressed information may involve a variety of experiences, fears, or wishes scattered across time. Dissociation is often elicited as a defense, especially after episodes of physical trauma, whereas repression is a response to warded-off fears and wishes or a response to other dynamic conflicts.

[d]Dissociated information is stored in a discrete and untransformed manner, whereas repressed information is usually disguised and fragmented. Even when repressed information becomes available to consciousness, its meaning is hidden (e.g., in dreams, slips of the tongue).

[e]Retrieval of dissociated information often can be direct. Techniques such as hypnosis can be used to access warded-off memories. In contrast, uncovering repressed information often requires repeated recall trials through intense questioning, psychotherapy, or psychoanalysis with subsequent interpretation (i.e., of dreams).

[f]The focus of psychotherapy for dissociation is integration via control of access to dissociated states and working through of traumatic memories. The classical psychotherapy for repression involves interpretation, including working through the transference.

Retrieval of dissociated information often can be direct. Techniques such as hypnosis can be used to access warded-off memories. In contrast, uncovering repressed information often requires repeated recall trials through intense questioning, psychotherapy, or psychoanalysis with subsequent interpretation (i.e., of dreams) (option C is incorrect). **Chapter 16 (Table 16–1 [p. 440])**

References

American Psychiatric Association: Diagnostic and Statistical Manual of Mental Disorders, 5th Edition. Arlington, VA, American Psychiatric Association, 2013

Barkin RBB, Kluft RP: The dilemma of drug therapy for multiple personality disorder, in Treatment of Multiple Personality Disorder. Edited by Braun B. Washington, DC, American Psychiatric Press, 1986, pp 107–132

Braakmann D, Ludewig S, Milde J, et al: Dissociative symptoms during treatment of borderline personality disorder [in German]. Psychother Psychosom Med Psychol 57(3–4):154–160, 2007 17523235

Brand BL, Lanius R, Vermetten E, et al: Where are we going? An update on assessment, treatment, and neurobiological research in dissociative disorders as we move toward the DSM 5. J Trauma Dissociation 13(1):9–31, 2012 22211439

Brandt J, Van Gorp WG: Functional ("psychogenic") amnesia. Semin Neurol 26(3):331–340, 2006 16791779

Freud S: The ego and the id (1923), in Standard Edition of the Complete Psychological Works of Sigmund Freud, Volume 19: The Ego and the Id and Other Works (1923–1925). Translated by Strachey J. Edited by Freud A. London, Hogarth, 1961, pp 1–66

Hansen M, Ross J, Armour C: Evidence of the dissociative PTSD subtype: a systematic literature review of latent class and profile analytic studies of PTSD. J Affect Disord 213:59–69, 2017 28192736

Hilgard ER: The problem of divided consciousness: a neodissociation interpretation. Ann NY Acad Sci 296:48–59, 1977 279254

Kellett S: The treatment of dissociative identity disorder with cognitive analytic therapy: experimental evidence of sudden gains. J Trauma Dissociation 6(3):55–81, 2005 16172082

Kritchevsky M, Chang J, Squire LR: Functional amnesia: clinical description and neuropsychological profile of 10 cases. Learn Mem 11(2):213–226, 2004 15054137

Lanius RA, Vermetten E, Loewenstein RJ, et al: Emotion modulation in PTSD: clinical and neurobiological evidence for a dissociative subtype. Am J Psychiatry 167(6):640–647, 2010 20360318

Lanius RA, Brand B, Vermetten E, et al: The dissociative subtype of posttraumatic stress disorder: rationale, clinical and neurobiological evidence, and implications. Depress Anxiety 29(8):701–708, 2012 22431063

Maldonado J, Butler L, Spiegel D: Treatment for dissociative disorders, in A Guide to Treatments That Work, 2nd Edition. Edited by Nathan PE, Gorman JM. New York, Oxford University Press, 2002, pp 463–496

Nicholson AA, Densmore M, Frewen PA, et al: The dissociative subtype of posttraumatic stress disorder: unique resting-state functional connectivity of basolateral and centromedial amygdala complexes. Neuropsychopharmacology 40(10):2317–2326, 2015 25790021

Nicholson AA, Friston KJ, Zeidman P, et al: Dynamic causal modeling in PTSD and its dissociative subtype: bottom-up versus top-down processing within fear and emotion regulation circuitry. Hum Brain Mapp 38(11):5551–5561, 2017 28836726

Ryle A, Fawkes L: Multiplicity of selves and others: cognitive analytic therapy. J Clin Psychol 63(2):165–174, 2007 17173319

Simeon D, Greenberg J, Nelson D, et al: Dissociation and posttraumatic stress 1 year after the World Trade Center disaster: follow-up of a longitudinal survey. J Clin Psychiatry 66(2):231–237, 2005 15705010

Spiegel D, Loewenstein RJ, Lewis-Fernández R, et al: Dissociative disorders in DSM-5. Depress Anxiety 28(12):E17–E45, 2011 22134959

CHAPTER 17

Somatic Symptom and Related Disorders

17.1 A 36-year-old man with a history of major depressive disorder, cerebral palsy, seizures, and multiple musculoskeletal injuries is psychiatrically hospitalized following a self-aborted high-lethality suicide attempt. His depressive symptoms and suicidality occur in the setting of chronic pain and excessive worry related to his muscle injuries. His intense fear of future reinjury has led him to alternately engage in prolonged sedentary periods and periods of obsessive adherence to physical therapy exercise regimens, which often result in increased pain. In addition to major depressive disorder, which psychiatric diagnosis best explains this patient's symptoms?

A. Chronic pain secondary to cerebral palsy.
B. Somatic symptom disorder.
C. Obsessive-compulsive disorder.
D. Illness anxiety disorder.

The correct response is option B: Somatic symptom disorder.

Although this patient suffers from cerebral palsy and has incurred numerous musculoskeletal injuries resulting in chronic pain, the DSM-5 (American Psychiatric Association 2013) criteria for somatic symptom disorder do not require that the symptoms be medically unexplained (option A is incorrect), nor are specific numbers or types of symptoms needed to meet the diagnosis.

Rather, the additional core feature of this diagnosis is the presence of abnormal thoughts, feelings, and behaviors associated with symptoms. This patient's excessive worry and behaviors, such as prolonged sedentary periods and excessive exercise, are characteristic of the distress and maladaptive thoughts, feelings, and behaviors associated with somatic symptoms disorder (option B is correct).

Obsessive-compulsive disorder could result in excessive time and energy being devoted to health concerns or somatic symptoms; however, obsessions would be accompanied by compulsions focused on reducing anxiety (option C is incorrect).

Illness anxiety disorder may be characterized by maladaptive thoughts and behaviors similar to those seen in somatic symptom disorder but would not include the presence of significant somatic symptoms (option D is incorrect). **Chapter 17 (pp. 476–479)**

17.2   A 43-year-old woman with a history of anxiety and panic attacks has long-standing symptoms of anxiety and a 2-year history of postprandial abdominal pain and dyspepsia. She thinks about these gastroenterological symptoms constantly. Consequently, she avoids eating, leading to a 50-pound weight loss. She has undergone significant medical workup, including endoscopy, barium esophagram, esophageal manometry, and computed tomography of the abdomen and pelvis, as well as a small bacterial overgrowth study, all of which yielded normal findings. Which of the following would be the best initial step in this patient's treatment?

A. Start sertraline 25 mg/day with plans to titrate to the maximum effective dosage.
B. Order a colonoscopy and further gastroenterological workup.
C. Confront the patient about her negative workup.
D. Start amitriptyline 10 mg/day and initiate a course of cognitive-behavioral therapy.

The correct response is option D: Start amitriptyline 10 mg/day and initiate a course of cognitive-behavioral therapy.

Somatic symptom disorder is difficult to treat, and there appears to be no single superior treatment approach. Physicians should be cautious about ordering repetitive, unnecessary, and invasive medical/surgical workups, which can cause iatrogenic illness (option B is incorrect).

Primary care physicians generally can manage patients with somatic symptom disorder adequately, but the expertise of a consulting psychiatrist has been shown to be useful. In short, patients require an empathic, supportive, and functional approach to address their suffering (option C is incorrect). Cloninger (1994) provided three important general principles for treatment management for these patients: 1) establish a firm therapeutic alliance with the patient, 2) educate the patient about the manifestations of somatic symptom disorder, and 3) provide consistent reassurance. Implementation of these suggestions may greatly facilitate clinical management of somatic symptom disorder and prevent potentially serious complications, including the effects of unnecessary diagnostic and therapeutic procedures (iatrogenic illness) (Kurlansik and Maffei 2016).

In 2001, the National Institute of Mental Health funded a single-blind, active control, parallel-assignment interventional study of cognitive-behavioral therapy (CBT) for somatization disorder in the primary care setting (Allen et al. 2006). This study found that CBT with psychiatric consultation was more effective in improving symptoms and functioning than psychiatric consultation alone (option D is correct). Other studies have found that "health anxious" patients experienced sustained symptomatic benefit from CBT over 2 years, with no significant effect on total health costs (Kurlansik and Maffei 2016).

With regard to psychopharmacology, systematic reviews have shown that antidepressants can provide substantial benefits in somatic symptom disorder. Tricyclic antidepressants (TCAs) had a greater likelihood of effectiveness in comparison with selective serotonin reuptake inhibitors (SSRIs) (Kurlansik and Maffei 2016) (option A is incorrect). Amitriptyline, the most studied TCA, and fluoxetine, in the SSRI class, both showed benefits in the domains of pain, functional status, global well-being, sleep, morning stiffness, and tender points (Kurlansik and Maffei 2016) (option D is correct). **Chapter 17 (pp. 480–481, 487–488)**

17.3 A 31-year-old woman with a history of generalized anxiety disorder that has been well managed on escitalopram presents to your office with significant concerns about having breast cancer. She has a family history of breast cancer in her mother. The patient reports that as a child, she had the traumatic experience of watching her mother go through chemotherapy and ultimately die. She is preoccupied with the thought that she could have breast cancer, examines her breasts daily, and makes frequent visits to her primary care physician. This preoccupation has affected her ability to fully attend to the needs of her child. Which of the following diagnoses best explains this patient's presentation?

A. Adjustment disorder.
B. Obsessive-compulsive disorder.
C. Illness anxiety disorder.
D. Somatic symptom disorder.

The correct response is option C: Illness anxiety disorder.

Illness anxiety disorder is characterized by a preoccupation with having or acquiring a serious illness (Table 17–1). A key feature of the disorder is the absence of significant somatic symptoms; the patient's distress derives not from any specific physical complaints but rather from anxiety surrounding the possibility of having a dreaded illness (option C is correct).

Adjustment disorder should be considered in patients whose symptoms have not met the duration or severity criteria for illness anxiety disorder and are clearly in response to a specific event. This consideration may be particularly relevant when the event leading to the adjustment disorder is health related (option A is incorrect).

Preoccupations in *obsessive-compulsive disorder* would be expected to focus on a fear of getting the disease in the future, as opposed to a focus on current symptoms, and would also generally involve additional obsessions or compulsions (option B is incorrect).

The diagnosis of *somatic symptom disorder* requires the presence of at least one significant bodily symptom (option D is incorrect). **Chapter 17 (pp. 481–482; Table 17–1 [p. 477])**

TABLE 17–1. Somatic symptom and related disorders: principal DSM-5 diagnostic criteria

	Somatic symptom disorder	Illness anxiety disorder	Conversion disorder	Psychological factors affecting other medical conditions	Factitious disorder (imposed on self or another)
Core symptom	Presence of one or more somatic symptoms that are distressing or result in significant disruption to daily life	Preoccupation with having or acquiring a serious illness (no symptom need be present)	Presence of one or more symptoms of altered voluntary motor or sensory function	Presence of a medical symptom or condition	Falsification of physical or psychological signs or symptoms (or induction of injury or disease) associated with identified deception
Essential feature(s)	Individual manifests excessive thoughts, feelings, or behaviors related to the somatic symptoms or associated health concerns.	A high level of anxiety about health is present. Individual manifests excessive health-related behaviors or maladaptive avoidance.	Clinical findings provide evidence that symptoms are incompatible with recognized neurological or medical conditions.	Psychological or behavioral factors adversely affect the medical condition.	Individual presents self (or another) as being ill. Deceptive intent is evident even in the absence of obvious external rewards.
Symptom duration	Symptomatic state (as opposed to any one symptom) is persistent (typically lasting more than 6 months).	Preoccupation has been present for at least 6 months.	None specified	None specified	None specified

Note. For the complete DSM-5 diagnostic criteria, please refer to pp. 309–327 in DSM-5 (American Psychiatric Association 2013).

17.4   A 24-year-old woman who has a history of one major depressive episode that responded well to fluoxetine (which was subsequently discontinued) and who is
currently in a long-term relationship with a boyfriend presents to her primary
care physician with overwhelming concerns about having human papillomavirus
(HPV). Despite having a negative Pap smear and no other symptoms consistent
with infection with the virus (e.g., condylomas, evidence of cervical cancer), the
patient continually worries about the prospect of having HPV. These worries
have interfered with her ability to concentrate at work and to function appropriately in her social life. Which of the following would be the best treatment option
for this patient?

A. Have the primary care physician restart fluoxetine and continue with regular
Pap smear screening at the recommended intervals.
B. Provide reassurance that the patient shows no evidence of HPV and encour-
age her to make a follow-up appointment if she develops new symptoms.
C. Refer the patient for cognitive-behavioral therapy without pharmacothera-
peutic intervention.
D. Make a psychiatric referral for cognitive-behavioral therapy, schedule regular
office visits to provide support, and restart fluoxetine.

**The correct response is option D: Make a psychiatric referral for cognitive-
behavioral therapy, schedule regular office visits to provide support, and restart fluoxetine.**

Treatment of DSM-5 illness anxiety disorder has not yet been thoroughly studied,
but research on and clinical experience with hypochondriasis remain relevant. Patients referred early for psychiatric evaluation and treatment of hypochondriasis
appear to have a better prognosis than those receiving only medical evaluations
and treatments (option A is incorrect).

As with other somatic symptom and related disorders, psychiatric referrals
should be made with sensitivity and awareness of stigma related to mental illness.
Patients may feel dissatisfied by reassurance that their symptoms are "not serious"
and may avoid psychiatric referral due to anger over being told that their symptoms are "all in their head" (option B is incorrect). Therefore, the referring physician should emphasize that the patient's distress is serious and that psychiatric
evaluation will be a supplement to, not a replacement for, continued medical care.

In patients with hypochondriasis, research has suggested that selective serotonin reuptake inhibitor treatment is useful for both acute and long-term treatment, with significant portions of patients achieving remission (Schweitzer et al.
2011). Stoudemire (1988) suggested an approach featuring consistent treatment,
generally by the same physician, with supportive, regularly scheduled office visits not focused on the evaluation of symptoms. Psychotherapeutic approaches
may be greatly enhanced by effective pharmacotherapy. Cognitive-behavioral
therapy (CBT) was found to be most effective, with one study reporting that 57%
of CBT-treated patients showed a reduction in hypochondriacal beliefs at 12-
month follow-up (Barsky and Ahern 2004) (option D is correct).

A combined approach of medication and psychotherapy is believed to have synergistic effects (option C is incorrect). **Chapter 17 (pp. 482–483)**

17.5   A 29-year-old woman with a medical history of partial complex seizures who is currently taking phenytoin (100 mg tid) presents to the emergency room 30 minutes after an episode of loss of consciousness and generalized limb shaking. Her boyfriend, who is accompanying her, states that this episode is similar to previous seizures and occurred immediately following a heated argument between the two of them. The patient, now awake and not experiencing residual symptoms but clearly in distress, states that she remembers falling on the floor with her eyes closed and her arms moving from side to side uncontrollably. Findings from her neurological examination and computed tomography (head without intravenous contrast) are within normal limits. Which of the following would be the best initial step in this patient's treatment?

A. Increase phenytoin to 100 mg qid, as her documented history of a seizure disorder indicates that she must be having epileptiform events.
B. Obtain a neurological consultation and order video electroencephalographic (vEEG) monitoring to capture a typical seizure event.
C. Obtain a psychiatric consultation, given the likely diagnosis of conversion disorder.
D. Confront the patient with the fact that her symptoms are inconsistent with the neurological examination findings and with known physiological presentations of seizures.

The correct response is option B: Obtain a neurological consultation and order video electroencephalographic (vEEG) monitoring to capture a typical seizure event.

The essential feature of conversion disorder is the presence of symptoms of altered motor or sensory function that (as evidenced by clinical findings) are incompatible with any recognized neurological or medical condition and are not better explained by another medical or mental disorder (see Table 17–1). There may be episodes of abnormal generalized limb shaking with apparent impairment or loss of consciousness that resemble epileptic seizures (also called *psychogenic* or *nonepileptic seizures*). The DSM-5 criteria for conversion disorder explicitly require neurological examination findings that are inconsistent with any known neurological disease; such findings include seizures involving long duration, fluctuating course, asynchronous movements, pelvic thrusting, side-to-side head or body movement, closed eyes during the episode, ictal crying, and memory recall. Complicating diagnosis is the fact that physical illness and conversion disorder are not mutually exclusive. Patients with documented neurological illness also may have "pseudosymptoms"; for example, patients with epilepsy may also have psychogenic nonepileptic seizures (PNES), previously described as "pseudoseizures" (option A is incorrect).

PNES have been researched extensively, and a multitude of terms have been used to describe these events. A conversion disorder diagnosis may be appropriate for certain patients experiencing such episodes who meet the full criteria. Diagnosis of PNES is currently most reliably established by ruling out epilepsy by using vEEG monitoring to capture a typical seizure event without an electrographic ictal pattern (option B is correct).

One major problem with conversion symptoms is the risk of applying a conversion disorder diagnosis when a true illness is present. Physicians should consider the risks of misdiagnosis when making a diagnosis of conversion disorder (option C is incorrect).

Generally, the initial aim in treating conversion disorder is the removal of the symptom. In any situation, direct confrontation is not recommended. Such a communication may cause a patient to feel even more isolated (option D is incorrect). **Chapter 17 (pp. 483–485, 487; Table 17–1 [p. 477])**

17.6 A 34-year-old woman with no significant medical history develops unilateral vision loss that becomes progressively worse over the course of 6 weeks, followed by difficulty walking due to right-sided weakness of the lower extremity. After these symptoms have persisted for several months, the woman presents to the emergency department at the urging of her family members. She is admitted to the neurological service with concerns for multiple sclerosis. Extensive workup, including a brain magnetic resonance imaging scan, yields unremarkable findings. In the absence of any neurophysiological explanation or findings, a diagnosis of conversion disorder is made by the consulting psychiatrist. Following a brief psychotherapeutic intervention, the patient's symptoms rapidly improve. When discharged, she has returned to her usual state of health. Which of the following features of this patient's profile may indicate a good prognosis?

A. Prompt resolution of the conversion symptoms.
B. Slow onset of symptoms.
C. Absence of clearly identifiable stress at the time of onset.
D. Long interval between onset of symptoms and institution of treatment.

The correct response is option A: Prompt resolution of the conversion symptoms.

The onset of conversion disorder is generally acute, but it may be characterized by gradually increasing symptomatology. The typical course of individual conversion symptoms is generally short; half to nearly all patients show disappearance of symptoms by the time of hospital discharge. Factors typically associated with good prognosis include acute onset (option B is incorrect), presence of clearly identifiable stress at the time of onset (option C is incorrect), and short interval between onset and institution of treatment (option D is incorrect). It does appear that prompt resolution of conversion symptoms is important in that a longer duration of conversion symptoms is associated with greater risk of recurrence and chronic disability (option A is correct). **Chapter 17 (pp. 486–487)**

17.7   A 42-year-old homeless man presents to the hospital complaining of fever and chills. He is febrile, hypotensive, and found to have *E. Coli* bacteremia. He is promptly started on intravenous (IV) antibiotics for treatment of sepsis. After initially demonstrating significant improvement, on day 3, the patient spikes a fever and decompensates. Shortly afterward, nursing staff discover numerous syringes filled with feces in the patient's backpack, leading the clinical staff to suspect that he has been injecting himself with them. Which of the following would be the best next step in the treatment of this patient?

A. Conduct regular room searches of all patient's belongings.
B. Confront the patient so that he can admit to his deception.
C. Continue with IV antibiotics and do not inform the patient of any change in treatment plan.
D. Involve the hospital administration and schedule regular treatment team meetings.

The correct response is option D: Involve the hospital administration and schedule regular treatment team meetings.

Treatment of factitious disorder can be divided into acute and long-term methods. Initially the diagnosis must be confirmed. Previously used methods of confirming the diagnosis, such as searching patients' belongings for paraphernalia used in producing symptoms, may continue to be tempting for clinicians, but such methods violate ethical and most likely legal boundaries (option A is incorrect). For this reason and because of the potentially strong countertransference reactions engendered by the patients, some authors have recommended early involvement of hospital administration when a diagnosis of factitious disorder is suspected. Treatment team meetings are recommended to help coordinate efforts between providers and to allow for the management of negative emotions toward patients (option D is correct).

Once the contribution of a general medical illness has been factored out, the patient must be informed of a change in the treatment plan, and an attempt must be made to enlist the patient in that plan (option C is incorrect). The literature generally refers to this process as containing an element of "confrontation." There is now general agreement that treatment begins at this point, and that it is best done indirectly, with minimal expectation that the patient "confess" or acknowledge the deception (option B is incorrect). **Chapter 17 (p. 492)**

17.8   A 29-year old man with a history of type 1 diabetes mellitus is bought to the emergency room unconscious and is found to have a blood glucose level of 36 mg/dL. He is quickly stabilized with dextrose infusions, and after recovery, states that he "must not have eaten enough today." Soon afterward, the man's girlfriend arrives and discloses to the attending physician that the patient has been intentionally self-administering too much insulin, resulting in multiple recent hypoglycemic episodes requiring hospitalization. Exasperated, the girlfriend says she cannot understand why he would be doing such a thing. Which of the following diagnoses would be most appropriate for this patient?

A. Borderline personality disorder.
B. Somatic symptom disorder.
C. Factitious disorder.
D. Malingering.

The correct response is option C: Factitious disorder.

The essential feature in factitious disorder is falsification of physical or psychological signs or symptoms, or induction of injury or disease, with evidence of deceptive intent (see Table 17–1) (option C is correct).

Given the inherent duplicity in the presentation of factitious disorder, establishing a diagnosis and differentiating from other conditions may be difficult. *Malingering* can be distinguished from factitious disorder by the presence of personal gain resulting from the symptoms (option D is incorrect).

Although self-harm behaviors such as the cutting common in *borderline personality disorder* might appear similar to the deliberate induction of injury in factitious disorder, such self-injurious behaviors would not possess the required association with identified deception (option A is incorrect).

Similarly, *somatic symptom disorder* lacks evidence of feigned symptoms, instead being defined by maladaptive thoughts, behaviors, and feelings associated with a symptom (option B is incorrect). **Chapter 17 (pp. 489–490; Table 17–1 [p. 477])**

17.9 A 27-year-old homeless man with an extensive history of high-risk sexual behavior and drug use is seen by a primary care physician for flu-like symptoms. The patients tests positive for HIV. He is referred to an HIV clinic and started on appropriate antiretroviral therapy. The patient, in denial of his diagnosis, continues to engage in regular unprotected sex, is nonadherent to his medications, and escalates his use of crystal methamphetamine. Several months later, the patient self-presents to the emergency room with paranoia and evidence of methamphetamine intoxication. His laboratory testing reveals a rapidly declining CD4 count and a high HIV viral load. Which of the following diagnoses best explains this patient's presentation?

A. Illness anxiety disorder.
B. Other specified mental disorder due to another medical condition.
C. Somatic symptom disorder.
D. Psychological factors affecting other medical conditions.

The correct response is option D: Psychological factors affecting other medical conditions.

The relationship between psychological factors and medical illness is familiar to many clinicians and often to their patients as well. Many of the treatment challenges faced by primary care and hospital-based physicians are further complicated by patient factors such as poor adherence to treatment plans, maladaptive coping styles, and persistent high-risk behavior. Although these factors (defined loosely) are present in many patients, the DSM-5 *psychological factors affecting other medical conditions* (PFAOMC) diagnosis is reserved for cases in which patient psychological factors are judged to have clinically significant impact on a medical condition (see Table 17–1). In this vignette, the patient's maladaptive coping strategy (escalation of crystal methamphetamine use), continuing disregard for the dangers of unprotected sex, and nonadherence to lifesaving antiretroviral therapy have led to a precipitous decline in his health (option D is correct).

Several other somatic symptom and related disorders must be differentiated from PFAOMC. *Somatic symptom disorder* may include the same psychological distress or maladaptive behaviors that would help to meet criteria for the PFAOMC diagnosis. However, the core of the latter diagnosis is the presence of a medical condition, the course of which has been adversely altered by psychological factors. By contrast, a diagnosable medical condition need not be present in somatic symptoms disorder; instead, the focus is on the maladaptive thoughts, behaviors, and feelings associated with a symptom (option C is incorrect).

Illness anxiety disorder shares with PFAOMC a relationship between a psychological symptom and health concerns, but in that diagnosis, no serious medical illness is present (option A is incorrect).

DSM-5 includes the diagnosis *other specified mental disorder due to another medical condition* (in the chapter "Other Mental Disorders") to capture presentations in which a medical condition is judged to be causing symptoms of a mental disorder through direct physiological means. However, the salient problem of the patient in this vignette is not mental disorder symptoms caused by HIV; rather, it is worsening of his HIV disease caused by maladaptive coping styles and health-related behaviors—most significantly, the patient's failure to take the medication he needs to stay alive (option B is incorrect). **Chapter 17 (pp. 488–489; Table 17–1 [p. 477])**

17.10 A 31-year-old woman, 16 weeks pregnant, has worried constantly about congenital illness and fetal malformations ever since she first learned she was pregnant. She has undergone all routine screening, including ultrasonography at appropriate intervals, but has not felt reassured by the lack of any abnormal findings. More recently, she has begun scheduling numerous urgent appointments to see her OB/GYN even though she is not experiencing any new physical symptoms. This anxiety has also begun to interfere with her sleep and has become a source of conflict between her and her partner. Which of the following diagnoses best explains this patient's symptoms?

A. Brief somatic symptom disorder.
B. Illness anxiety disorder without excessive health-related behaviors.
C. Brief illness anxiety disorder.
D. Pseudocyesis.

The correct response is option C: Brief illness anxiety disorder.

Two additional somatic symptom and related disorder diagnostic categories are provided in DSM-5. The categories of *other specified somatic symptom and related disorder* and *unspecified somatic symptom and related disorder* may be applied to presentations that are characteristic of a somatic symptom and related disorder and that cause clinically significant impairment but do not meet full criteria for any of the disorders in this diagnostic class. For an "other specified" diagnosis, the clinician records the specific reason that full criteria are not met; for an "unspecified" diagnosis, no reason need be given. Use of the latter category should be reserved for exceptionally uncommon situations in which there is insufficient information to make a more specific diagnosis.

DSM-5 provides four examples of presentations for which the other specified somatic symptom and related disorder designation might be appropriate:

1. Brief somatic symptom disorder—Duration of symptoms is less than 6 months (option A is incorrect).
2. Brief illness anxiety disorder—Duration of symptoms is less than 6 months (option C is correct).
3. Illness anxiety disorder without excessive health-related behaviors—Criterion D for illness anxiety disorder is not met (option B is incorrect).
4. Pseudocyesis—A false belief of being pregnant that is associated with objective signs and reported symptoms of pregnancy (option D is incorrect).

Chapter 17 (p. 493)

References

Allen LA, Woolfolk RL, Escobar JI, et al: Cognitive-behavioral therapy for somatization disorder: a randomized controlled trial. Arch Intern Med 166(14):1512–1518, 2006 16864762

American Psychiatric Association: Diagnostic and Statistical Manual of Mental Disorders, 5th Edition. Arlington, VA, American Psychiatric Association, 2013

Barsky AJ, Ahern DK: Cognitive behavior therapy for hypochondriasis. JAMA 291(12):1464–1470, 2004 15039413

Cloninger CR: Somatoform and dissociative disorders, in The Medical Basis of Psychiatry, 2nd Edition. Edited by Winokur G, Clayton P. Philadelphia, PA, WB Saunders, 1994, pp 169–192

Kurlansik SL, Maffei MS: Somatic symptom disorder. Am Fam Physician 93(1):49–54, 2016 26760840

Schweitzer PJ, Zafar U, Pavlicova M, et al: Long-term follow-up of hypochondriasis after selective serotonin reuptake inhibitor treatment. J Clin Psychopharmacol 31(3):365–368, 2011 21508861

Stoudemire GA: Somatoform disorders, factitious disorders, and malingering, in The American Psychiatric Press Textbook of Psychiatry. Edited by Talbott JA, Hales RE, Yudofsky SC. Washington, DC, American Psychiatric Press, 1988, pp 533–556

CHAPTER 18

Eating and Feeding Disorders

18.1 A 28-year-old woman (BMI: 16.8 kg/m^2) presents to a medical clinic at her family's insistence. When asked, she states that she does not feel there is any problem with her weight, although she admits to symptoms of disordered eating since she was a teenager. Her initial complaint is only of feeling anxious and depressed. She is highly preoccupied with her body shape, which she has always perceived to be "too fat" (causing persistent low self-esteem), and she diets and exercises excessively in order to counterbalance episodes of overeating during which she feels "out of control." What is the most appropriate diagnosis for this patient?

A. Bulimia nervosa.
B. Anorexia nervosa.
C. Major depressive episode.
D. Avoidant/restrictive food intake disorder.

The correct response is option B: Anorexia nervosa.

This patient possesses all of the essential features of anorexia nervosa: An imbalance of energy intake to expenditure is present, leading to clinically significant weight loss for age, height, and gender (i.e., low BMI). The patient experiences severe anxiety or fear about gaining weight and/or engages in ongoing behaviors such as overexercise, dietary restriction, or purging that interfere with weight gain. The patient has the perception that her body weight is not low despite significant weight loss, or denies that the weight loss is medically serious. The patient's self-worth is highly dependent on weight or body shape. Although restrictive eating based on fear of weight gain is the primary presentation of anorexia nervosa, binge eating and purging follow in about half of cases (option B is correct).

In order to have bulimia nervosa, the patient must not have anorexia nervosa, nor have clinically significant low weight (option A is incorrect).

Patients with anorexia nervosa often appear withdrawn, depressed, and anxious; however, the major theme of this presentation is better characterized by an eating disorder, and this patient does not fulfill criteria for a major depressive episode (option C is incorrect).

With avoidant/restrictive food intake disorder, the eating problems do not involve weight or shape concerns and are not specifically associated with anorexia nervosa or bulimia nervosa (option D is incorrect). **Chapter 18 (pp. 498–499, 502, 510)**

18.2   A 24-year-old woman (BMI: 19.8 kg/m^2) comes in for help with her eating habits. She reports that over the past year, she has had repeated, uncontrollable overeating episodes at least twice weekly. She desperately fears "getting too heavy," and thus has begun inducing vomiting regularly after every such episode. You inform her that while all of the following medications have some data for efficacy in treating her condition, only one is U.S. Food and Drug Administration (FDA) approved for this purpose. What is this medication?

A. Nortriptyline.
B. Topiramate.
C. Selegiline.
D. Fluoxetine.

The correct response is option D: Fluoxetine.

The first controlled studies of the use of medication to treat bulimia nervosa were of the tricyclic antidepressants and monoamine oxidase inhibitors, demonstrating the superiority of both to placebo in reducing binge eating and purging. These studies were eventually followed by studies demonstrating that fluoxetine (60 mg/day) was superior to placebo in treating bulimia nervosa, as are most of the serotonin reuptake inhibitors. Fluoxetine is currently the only medication approved by the FDA for the treatment of bulimia nervosa (option D is correct; options A, B, and C are incorrect). Antiepileptics (e.g., topiramate) have shown some promise in treating bulimia nervosa, although dropout rates in controlled studies have been higher than dropout rates with antidepressants, largely because of side effects. **Chapter 18 (pp. 505–506)**

18.3   A 26-year-old woman (BMI: 34.2 kg/m^2) presents for evaluation for bariatric surgery. She reports episodes of rapid, excessive eating multiple times a week over the past 6 months, after which she feels overly full, and ashamed about the amount she has eaten. She denies overexercising, inducing vomiting, using diuretics, or engaging in any other compensatory weight-loss behavior, but she talks at length about how closely her self-esteem depends on her body image. She is worried that she may have bulimia nervosa. You tell her that you suspect she has binge-eating disorder (BED). What is the reason for your distinction?

A. She does not have anorexia nervosa.
B. Her binge-eating episodes do not occur every day.
C. She is not engaging in inappropriate behaviors to prevent weight gain.
D. She bases her self-esteem heavily on her body image.

The correct response is option C: She is not engaging in inappropriate behaviors to prevent weight gain.

Criteria for both bulimia nervosa and BED include that the patient does not have anorexia, and also allow for the patient to have less-than-daily binge-eating episodes (options A and B are incorrect).

Self-worth highly dependent on weight or body shape is an essential feature of both bulimia nervosa and BED (option D is incorrect).

Unlike bulimia nervosa, BED does not involve compensatory behaviors such as self-induced vomiting, excessive exercise, or laxative and diuretic abuse (option C is correct). Bulimia nervosa usually occurs in individuals who are of normal weight or who are slightly overweight; BED more often occurs in individuals who are overweight or obese (note this patient's elevated BMI). In bulimia nervosa, binge eating is considered to be a response to restriction of food intake (not seen in this patient), whereas in BED, binge eating occurs in the context of overall chaotic and unregulated eating patterns. **Chapter 18 (pp. 502, 506–507)**

18.4   The parents of a 12-year-old boy (weight: <5th percentile for age) report that since his early years, their son has had a rather anxious temperament and has been an exceptionally picky eater. He tends to rigidly stick to a handful of bland food options, rejecting all others because they "taste bad" or "feel weird when I eat them." The boy understands that his weight is low, but his efforts to gain weight have been stymied by significant anxiety around eating. Which of the following diagnoses best explains this patient's eating habits and struggles with low weight?

A. Anxiety disorder.
B. Avoidant-restrictive food intake disorder.
C. Normal childhood development.
D. Autism spectrum disorder.

The correct response is option B: Avoidant-restrictive food intake disorder.

DSM-5 (American Psychiatric Association 2013) diagnostic criteria for avoidant-restrictive food intake disorder (ARFID) include food restriction or avoidance without shape or weight concerns or intentional efforts to lose weight that results in significant weight loss and nutritional deficiencies. Some patients present with highly selective eating; neophobia (the fear of new things) related to food types; or hypersensitivity to food texture, appearance, and taste. Patients are aware that they are low weight and may express a wish to eat more and gain weight, but their anxiety and fear prevent them from consuming enough to do so (option B is correct; option C is incorrect).

Patients with autism spectrum disorder (ASD) frequently display selective eating patterns, so it is not surprising that ARFID is sometimes confused with ASD and other neurodevelopmental disorders; however, there is no evidence in this case for other feeding-unrelated symptoms (option D is incorrect).

Anxiety disorders and anxious traits as well as depressive symptoms often predate the development of ARFID, but this description of food avoidance with significant weight loss and anxiety associated only with food is more consistent with ARFID (option A is incorrect). **Chapter 18 (p. 509)**

18.5   A 13-year-old girl (weight: <5th percentile for age) is brought in to your clinic by her parents, who are concerned about her weight and recently decreased appetite. The patient denies any concerns about weight or body image, insisting that she is simply not hungry and has never had much interest in food. She appears generally downcast, although she does speak excitedly about upping her swim schedule to twice-daily practices in order to make the varsity team at her school. You speak to her parents alone, who convey that their daughter has seemed depressed over the past few months, and who tearfully report that they recently found extensively highlighted dieting magazines under her bed, along with myriad journal entries expressing her fears of "becoming heavy" and "looking too big." What diagnosis most likely explains this patient's new habits and weight loss?

A. Bulimia nervosa.
B. Anorexia nervosa.
C. Avoidant-restrictive food intake disorder.
D. Major depressive episode.

The correct response is option B: Anorexia nervosa.

There is evidence that anorexia nervosa symptoms may be expressed differently in childhood and adolescence compared with adulthood. Children and adolescents are often incapable of verbalizing abstract thoughts; therefore, behaviors such as food refusal that lead to malnutrition may manifest as nonverbal representations of emotional experiences. For this reason, parental reports about the child's behavior are critical, given that self-report is often unreliable due to of lack of insight, minimization, and denial by the child or adolescent. Some young patients deny body image or weight concerns at assessment and insist they just are not hungry or complain of abdominal discomfort. While self-starvation persists, academic and athletic pursuits usually continue and sometimes become more compulsive and driven (option B is correct).

Patients with anorexia nervosa often appear withdrawn, depressed, and anxious; however, severe anxiety or fear about gaining weight and/or ongoing behaviors such as overexercise, dietary restriction, or purging that interfere with weight gain, is an essential feature of anorexia nervosa and is evident in this patient (option D is incorrect).

Bulimia nervosa usually occurs in patients who are of normal weight or who are slightly overweight (option A is incorrect).

Avoidant-restrictive food intake disorder (ARFID) can be confused with anorexia nervosa, but distinguishing features include a lack of fear of weight gain in ARFID, no shape and weight concerns in ARFID, and no specific focus on weight loss in ARFID (option C is incorrect). **Chapter 18 (pp. 499, 507, 509)**

18.6   A 30-year-old obese man (BMI 36.4 kg/m^2) reports extremely low self-esteem from perceiving his body image to be "so overweight." He has tried exercising a bit, but finds it too painful on his joints. He has been suffering from low mood, anhedonia, avolition, and anergia over the past year or so. He blames his obesity on "these out-of-control episodes where I eat a ton and then feel horrible about it afterwards," which occur regularly. Because of other medical concerns, he is most interested in first stopping or decreasing the frequency of these episodes, rather than focusing on weight loss. Given this patient's current goal, which of the following is first-line treatment?

A. Cognitive-behavioral therapy or interpersonal therapy.
B. Lisdexamfetamine.
C. A selective serotonin reuptake inhibitor (SSRI).
D. Weight loss therapy.

The correct response is option A: Cognitive-behavioral therapy or interpersonal therapy.

At present, cognitive-behavioral therapy (CBT) and interpersonal therapy (IPT) are the recommended first-line treatments for binge-eating disorder (BED) for reducing binge eating (option A is correct), but they do not lead to weight loss. IPT has the advantage that essentially the same treatment used for BED can be used to treat depression and anxiety (this patient seems to suffer from depression; in BED as in the other eating disorders, the prevalence of lifetime comorbid major depressive disorder (MDD) is about 60%, and that of current MDD is about 25% [Grilo et al. 2009]).

Well-designed controlled studies have shown that both CBT and IPT are effective in reducing binge eating, with 50%–60% of patients achieving remission at end of treatment (Wilson et al. 2010). A third nonpharmacological treatment, behavioral weight loss therapy, has also been used to treat BED on the basis of the finding that binge eating decreases with weight loss; however, controlled comparisons of CBT with weight loss therapy have found that CBT is superior in reducing the frequency of binge eating (option D is incorrect).

Antidepressants, particularly SSRIs, used at dosages similar to those used for the treatment of depression, are effective in the treatment of BED, with response rates of about 40% (Stefano et al. 2008). Controlled studies suggest that CBT is more effective than antidepressants in treating BED (Ricca et al. 2001) (option C is incorrect).

More recently, several studies have examined the efficacy of lisdexamfetamine (LDX), a medication used in the treatment of attention-deficit/hyperactivity disorder, resulting in U.S. Food and Drug Administration approval of LDX for the treatment of BED in 2015 (McElroy 2017). In a further 6-month maintenance trial (Hudson et al. 2017), only 3.7% of patients on LDX relapsed to binge eating, compared with 32.1% of patients switched to placebo. Hence, LDX appears to be a promising medication for the treatment of BED (option B is incorrect). **Chapter 18 (pp. 506, 508)**

18.7 Which of the following is a characteristic of rumination syndrome?

    A. Effortful regurgitation of food.
    B. Association with developmental disability.
    C. Eating of nonnutritive substances.
    D. Self-worth dependent on weight.

The correct response is option B: Association with developmental disability.

DSM-5 criteria for rumination disorder include recurrent effortless (nonretching) regurgitation of food (option A is incorrect). Although its prevalence is unknown, rumination disorder appears to occur more often in individuals with intellectual disability (option B is correct). DSM-5 criteria for pica (not rumination) include eating of nonnutritive, nonfood substances (option C is incorrect). Dependence of self-worth on weight or body shape is not an essential feature of rumination syndrome (option D is incorrect). **Chapter 18 (pp. 510–511)**

18.8 Which of the following evidence-based treatments for binge-eating disorder (BED) reduces both binge eating and weight?

    A. Cognitive-behavioral therapy.
    B. Selective serotonin reuptake inhibitors (SSRIs).
    C. Interpersonal psychotherapy.
    D. Lisdexamfetamine.

The correct response is option D: Lisdexamfetamine.

Antidepressants, particularly SSRIs, used at dosages similar to those used for the treatment of depression, are effective in the treatment of BED, with response rates of about 40% (Stefano et al. 2008). Evidence supports a modest effect of antidepressants on binge eating but not on weight (McElroy 2017) (option B is incorrect).

    Well-designed controlled studies have shown that both cognitive-behavioral therapy (CBT) and interpersonal therapy (IPT) are effective in reducing binge eating, but do not lead to weight loss (options A and C are incorrect).

    More recently, several studies (McElroy 2017) have examined the efficacy of lisdexamfetamine (LDX), a medication used in the treatment of attention-deficit/hyperactivity disorder, resulting in U.S. Food and Drug Administration approval of LDX for the treatment of BED in 2015. In placebo-controlled trials of LDX (at dosages between 50 and 70 mg/day), approximately 50% of patients receiving LDX achieved abstinence from binge eating, compared with 21% of patients receiving placebo (McElroy et al. 2015). Moreover, unlike patients treated with psychotherapies such as CBT or IPT, patients on LDX showed an average weight loss of 5.0 kg, compared with little weight loss in the placebo group (McElroy et al. 2015) (option D is correct). **Chapter 18 (p. 508)**

18.9   While recommending treatment for a 14-year-old girl with anorexia nervosa, you indicate that one intervention appears to be most effective for patients in her age group. What is this intervention?

A. Residential treatment.
B. Cognitive-behavioral therapy.
C. Adolescent-focused therapy.
D. Family-based treatment.

The correct response is option D: Family-based treatment.

Findings from randomized controlled trials suggest that family approaches, particularly family-based treatment (FBT), are effective and superior to comparison individual therapies (option D is correct).

FBT is an outpatient, manualized intervention that consists of between 10 and 20 family meetings over a 6- to 12-month treatment course (Lock and Le Grange 2013). FBT helps parents learn how to disrupt their child's starvation and overexercise and to take charge of weight restoration. Although individual therapy was not as effective as FBT in these trials (options B and C are incorrect), individual approaches are nonetheless beneficial and could be offered to patients in cases in which FBT is not an acceptable or tenable option.

A recent uncontrolled study suggested that residential and day treatment may be useful in anorexia nervosa, but no randomized studies have compared residential or day treatment with outpatient treatment (Twohig et al. 2016) (option A is incorrect). **Chapter 18 (pp. 499–501)**

References

American Psychiatric Association: Diagnostic and Statistical Manual of Mental Disorders, 5th Edition. Arlington, VA, American Psychiatric Association, 2013

Grilo CM, White MA, Masheb RM: DSM-IV psychiatric disorder comorbidity and its correlates in binge eating disorder. Int J Eat Disord 42(3):228–234, 2009 18951458

Hudson JI, McElroy SL, Ferreira-Cornwell MC, et al: Efficacy of lisdexamfetamine in adults with moderate to severe binge-eating disorder: a randomized clinical trial. JAMA Psychiatry 74(9):903–910, 2017 28700805

Lock J, Le Grange D: Treatment Manual for Anorexia Nervosa: A Family Based Approach. New York, Guilford, 2013

McElroy SL: Pharmacologic treatments for binge-eating disorder. J Clin Psychiatry 78 (suppl 1):14–19, 2017 28125174

McElroy SL, Guerdjikova AI, Mori N, et al: Overview of the treatment of binge eating disorder. CNS Spectr 20(6):546–556, 2015 26594849

Ricca V, Mannucci E, Mezzani B, et al: Fluoxetine and fluvoxamine combined with individual cognitive-behaviour therapy in binge eating disorder: a one-year follow-up study. Psychother Psychosom 70(6):298–306, 2001 11598429

Stefano SC, Bacaltchuk J, Blay SL, Appolinário JC: Antidepressants in short-term treatment of binge eating disorder: systematic review and meta-analysis. Eat Behav 9(2):129–136, 2008 18329590

Twohig MP, Bluett EJ, Cullum JL, et al: Effectiveness and clinical response rates of a residential eating disorders facility. Eat Disord 24(3):224–239, 2016 26214231

Wilson GT, Wilfley DE, Agras WS, et al: Psychological treatments of binge eating disorder. Arch Gen Psychiatry 67(1):94–101, 2010 20048227

CHAPTER 19

Elimination Disorders

19.1 A 5-year-old boy with normal development stopped wetting his bed 6 months ago; however, 2 weeks ago, he began to wet the bed again (at a frequency of twice per week) after his family moved into a new house. He does not wet himself during the daytime. He is otherwise healthy and is not being treated with any medications. What is the most likely diagnosis?

A. Primary nocturnal enuresis.
B. Secondary enuresis.
C. Diurnal enuresis.
D. Retentive encopresis.

The correct response is option B: Secondary enuresis.

There are two clinical subtypes of enuresis based on the natural history of the disorder; those individuals who have never achieved continence have the subtype called *primary enuresis* (option A is incorrect because this boy previously achieved continence), whereas those who were able to achieve continence but subsequently resumed wetting have the subtype called *secondary enuresis*. A time period of 6 months to 1 year is usually accepted as the length of time continence must have been maintained before secondary enuresis is diagnosed (option B is correct). The word *diurnal* is used to describe events that occur during the day (option C is incorrect). *Encopresis* refers to the passage of feces, not the voiding of urine (as in bed wetting) (option D is incorrect). **Chapter 19 (pp. 517–518, 525)**

19.2 In comparison with children who have never had a period of sustained continence lasting at least 6 months, the patient described in question 19.1 is more likely to present with which of the following additional problems?

A. Urinary tract infection.
B. Diabetes insipidus.
C. Seizure disorder.
D. Comorbid psychiatric disorders.

The correct response is option D: Comorbid psychiatric disorders.

Potential medical causes of enuresis include urinary tract infection, diabetes insipidus, urethritis, seizure disorders, sickle cell trait, sleep apnea, neurogenic bladder, sleep disorders, genitourinary malformation or obstruction, and side effects or idiosyncratic reactions to a medication. (Apart from the enuresis, the patient is healthy and is on no medications; therefore, options A, B, and C are incorrect.)

Children with secondary enuresis are more apt than those with primary enuresis to present with comorbid psychiatric disorders (option D is correct). As might be expected, there is a high rate of comorbidity in children with a diagnosis of autism spectrum disorder (von Gontard et al. 2015). The psychiatric disorder with the most evidence of comorbidity is attention-deficit/hyperactivity disorder (ADHD) (von Gontard and Equit 2015). Shreeram et al. (2009) also found that ADHD was "strongly associated with enuresis." These studies support the hypothesis that enuresis is comorbid with ADHD and is not secondarily related to ADHD. Other than the association with ADHD, the primary finding has been that behavioral disorders in children with enuresis are nonspecific (von Gontard et al. 2011). **Chapter 19 (pp. 519–520)**

19.3   Which of the following is a treatment for primary nocturnal enuresis that minimizes both side effects and relapse risk after treatment cessation, and therefore should generally be tried first?

A. Bell-and-pad method.
B. Oral imipramine.
C. Nasal desmopressin.
D. Punitive response.

The correct response is option A: Bell-and-pad method.

Investigations that have compared the bell-and-pad method with both imipramine and desmopressin have demonstrated that the efficacy of the bell-and-pad approach is comparable to that of the pharmacological interventions, with virtually no side effects (option A is correct; options B and C are incorrect). Another advantage of the bell-and-pad method of conditioning is that the therapeutic effect is usually sustained after cessation of treatment, whereas relapse almost always occurs after cessation of treatment with imipramine or desmopressin (Kwak et al. 2010). On the basis of available research data, it appears that the bell-and-pad method of conditioning would be the most rational method to consider first, because it is just as effective as the pharmacological approaches, it has a much safer side-effect profile, and its effects are sustained once continence has developed and been sustained for a period of time.

It is extremely important that the parents realize that primary nocturnal enuresis is not volitional in nature and that a punitive response is counterproductive (option D is incorrect). **Chapter 19 (p. 524)**

19.4 A 4-year-old girl who had stopped wetting her bed for a month restarted bed wetting at a frequency of twice a week for the past month. Her developmental history has otherwise been normal, and she is on no medications. She does not seem bothered by her bed wetting, but her parents are concerned about this possible "behavioral regression" and seek clinical evaluation. A maternal history of primary nocturnal enuresis until age 6 years is noted. Her parents are coping with her bed wetting, but are still concerned. Which of the following options would be the most reasonable next step?

A. Start the patient on oral imipramine.
B. Refer the patient for cystoscopy.
C. Start the patient on nasal desmopressin.
D. Watch and wait.

The correct response is option D: Watch and wait.

Perhaps the most significant observation with regard to primary nocturnal enuresis (PNE) derives from the natural history of the disorder, which indicates that it is a self-limited condition that will eventually remit spontaneously (option D is correct). In general, the epidemiological studies are supportive of this observation, because they document that the incidence of PNE decreases in each advancing age group. Yearly remission rates of 14%–16% have been reported (Fritz et al. 2004). It can be helpful to ascertain the natural history of the enuretic events in family members with a childhood history of PNE. This information may lead to a better understanding of when spontaneous remission might be expected to occur in the child. An important part of the assessment will also include both the child's and the family's perceptions of the enuresis and the effect on both the child's self-esteem and the family's interpersonal dynamics.

The primary medical workup consists of a physical examination to rule out any obvious rare anatomical abnormalities, as well as a urinalysis to rule out a bladder infection, which can cause wetting, particularly in females. However, a bladder infection would result in a fairly abrupt and relatively recent onset of wetting. A urine dipstick test for glucose is also indicated if there has been a recent dramatic onset of polydipsia, which could be related to new-onset diabetes mellitus. More intrusive and potentially painful diagnostic interventions are not considered necessary, unless there is reason to suspect an anatomic abnormality (option B is incorrect).

The tricyclic antidepressant imipramine remained the primary pharmacological treatment for PNE for decades until the introduction of desmopressin. Although its use has diminished greatly, imipramine is still used for children whose symptoms do not respond to other forms of treatment (option A is incorrect).

The form of desmopressin initially used was a nasal preparation, which was reported as being safer than imipramine. However, beginning in the 1990s, a number of case reports of clinically significant hyponatremia, seizures, and related fatalities began to emerge. Eventually, excess fluid intake was identified as a contributing factor in the reported events, leading to the recommendation that children not ingest more than 8 ounces of fluid on nights when desmopressin was taken. It also appeared that younger children were at greater risk of experiencing clinically significant effects, and that these severe side effects were also more apt to occur during the initial phases of treatment. In 2007, the U.S. Food and Drug Administration issued a safety alert, and the use of the nasal spray became contraindicated for PNE in children (option C is incorrect). **Chapter 19 (pp. 521–523)**

19.5   A 6-year-old boy had soiled his undergarments three times in the past 3 months while at school, and once placed fecal matter in his mother's purse. The mother has found feces in a shoe box under her son's bed. The boy does not complain of abdominal pain or constipation, and he continues to have regular bowel movements. He eats a normal diet and has a normal weight and height for his chronological age. Which of the following would be the best next step in a comprehensive evaluation?

A. Bowel catharsis coupled with ongoing use of laxatives.
B. Fixed daily schedule of toileting.
C. Full psychological evaluation.
D. Watch and wait.

The correct response is option C: Full psychological evaluation.

Nonretentive encopresis involves the voluntary or involuntary passing of feces in inappropriate places (e.g., clothing, floor). Voluntary nonretentive encopresis is at times associated with the hoarding of feces. Children who voluntarily defecate in inappropriate places and/or hoard feces are in need of a psychological evaluation and will likely benefit from psychotherapeutic interventions (option C is correct). This pattern of encopresis represents underlying psychopathology that should be identified and addressed (option D is incorrect).

   The physiological mechanism of retentive encopresis begins with chronic constipation, which creates a bolus of feces in the colon, and the encopretic event actually represents overflow of loose fecal matter around the impacted bolus of feces. The long-standing conventional intervention for retentive encopresis involves bowel catharsis, coupled with the ongoing use of laxatives, for a period of time sufficient to develop a regular pattern of bowel movements, together with a fixed daily schedule of toileting in an effort to develop regular bowel habits. This patient does not complain of constipation, and he continues to have regular bowel movements; therefore, he does not have retentive encopresis (options A and B are incorrect). **Chapter 19 (pp. 526, 528)**

References

Fritz G, Rockney R, Bernet W, et al: Practice parameter for the assessment and treatment of children and adolescents with enuresis. J Am Acad Child Adolesc Psychiatry 43(12):1540–1550, 2004 15564822

Kwak KW, Lee YS, Park KH, et al: Efficacy of desmopressin and enuresis alarm as first and second line treatment for primary monosymptomatic nocturnal enuresis: prospective randomized crossover study. J Urol 184(6):2521–2526, 2010 20961574

Shreeram S, He JP, Kalaydjian A, et al: Prevalence of enuresis and its association with attention-deficit/hyperactivity disorder among U.S. children: results from a nationally representative study. J Am Acad Child Adolesc Psychiatry 48(1):35–41, 2009 19096296

von Gontard A, Equit M: Comorbidity of ADHD and incontinence in children. Eur Child Adolesc Psychiatry 24(2):127–140, 2015 24980793

von Gontard A, Heron J, Joinson C: Family history of nocturnal enuresis and urinary incontinence: results from a large epidemiological study. J Urol 185(6):2303–2306, 2011 21511300

von Gontard A, Pirrung M, Neimczyk J, Equit M: Incontinence in children with autism spectrum disorder. J Pediatr Urol 11(5):264.e1–264.e7, 2015 26052001

CHAPTER 20

Sleep–Wake Disorders

20.1 The normal onset of wakefulness is associated with which of the following patterns of hormonal changes and body temperature?

A. A fall in plasma melatonin and in body temperature.
B. A rise in plasma melatonin and in body temperature.
C. A rise in plasma cortisol and in body temperature.
D. A fall in plasma cortisol and in body temperature.

The correct response is option C: A rise in plasma cortisol and in body temperature.

Plasma cortisol secretion begins to increase before morning awakening (option D is incorrect) and peaks in the early morning. Growth hormone secretion peaks early in the night. Melatonin is secreted after dark and is suppressed by light (option B is incorrect). Body temperature peaks in the late afternoon to early evening and starts to decrease before sleep onset (option C is correct; option A is incorrect). **Chapter 20 (p. 536 [Figure 20–1])**

20.2 Older age is associated with which of the following changes (measured by electroencephalogram) in sleep latency, rapid eye movement (REM) sleep, and N3 (delta) non–REM (NREM) "deep sleep"?

A. Increased sleep latency and N3 NREM sleep and decreased REM sleep.
B. Decreased sleep latency, REM sleep, and N3 NREM sleep.
C. Decreased sleep latency and increased REM sleep and N3 NREM sleep.
D. Increased sleep latency and decreased REM sleep and N3 NREM sleep.

The correct response is option D: Increased sleep latency and decreased REM sleep and N3 NREM sleep.

Typically, N3 (delta) sleep begins to decrease with advancing age, possibly due in part to loss of ventrolateral preoptic nucleus neurons, decline in aerobic fitness, and perhaps other yet-uncertain mechanisms. Unfortunately, in the elderly, poor sleep is often the norm, with an increased sleep latency (time from lights off to sleep onset) (options B and C are incorrect), decreased amounts of NREM and

REM sleep (option D is correct; option A is incorrect), advanced sleep phase, and more sleep fragmentation due to medical, psychiatric, and sleep disorders, producing significant daytime sleepiness. **Chapter 20 (p. 545)**

20.3 Which of the following is the strongest risk factor for obstructive sleep apnea (OSA)?

A. Hypothyroidism.
B. Prader-Willi syndrome.
C. Obesity.
D. Neuromuscular disease.

The correct response is option C: Obesity.

Obesity is the strongest risk factor for OSA (option C is correct). The prevalence of OSA is much higher in patients with cardiac or metabolic disorders. Psychotropic medication–induced weight gain may also contribute to the development of OSA. Other conditions that increase the risk for OSA include hypothyroidism (option A is incorrect), Cushing's syndrome, acromegaly, cerebral palsy, Down syndrome, Prader-Willi syndrome (option B is incorrect), neuromuscular disease (option D is incorrect), Parkinson's disease, asthma, and sickle-cell disease. **Chapter 20 (p. 557)**

20.4 Which of the following medications does not cause or worsen restless legs syndrome (RLS)?

A. Bupropion.
B. Fluoxetine.
C. Amitriptyline.
D. Lithium.

The correct response is option A: Bupropion.

Medications that can precipitate or worsen RLS include most psychotropics—selective serotonin reuptake inhibitors (SSRIs) (option B is incorrect), tricyclic antidepressants (TCAs) (option C is incorrect), antipsychotics, and lithium (option D is incorrect)—and also antihistamines. Bupropion does not cause or worsen RLS or periodic limb movements of sleep, likely because it increases dopamine (option A is correct). **Chapter 20 (p. 564)**

20.5 Which of the following medications does not precipitate rapid eye movement (REM) sleep behavior disorder but treats it by reducing dream enactment?

A. Amitriptyline.
B. Phenelzine.
C. Clonazepam.
D. Fluoxetine.

The correct response is option C: Clonazepam.

In people of all ages, REM sleep behavior disorder can be precipitated by antidepressants (tricyclic antidepressants, selective serotonin reuptake inhibitors, and monoamine oxidase inhibitors) as well as by alcohol consumption or excessive caffeine use (options A, B, and D are incorrect). Nightly low-dose clonazepam (0.25 mg) reduces dream enactment but does not restore atonia (option C is correct). **Chapter 20 (p. 567)**

CHAPTER 21

Sexual Dysfunctions

21.1   Which of the following statements best describes the direct role of cyclic guanosine monophosphate (cGMP) in physiological arousal in men?

A. cGMP relaxes smooth musculature of corpora cavernosa.
B. cGMP activates guanylate cyclase to increase stimulation of nitric oxide.
C. cGMP triggers emission of semen.
D. cGMP stimulates production of dopamine by the nucleus accumbens.

The correct response is option A: cGMP relaxes smooth musculature of corpora cavernosa.

Men become aroused by visual stimuli (e.g., naked body, pictures), fantasies, or physical stimulation of the genitals. These stimuli lead to involuntary discharge in the parasympathetic nerves that control the diameter and valves of the penile blood vessels. Understanding of this process has increased in recent years with the elucidation of the mechanism of action of medications used to treat erectile disorder. The stimulation actually releases nitric oxide in the corpora cavernosa. Nitric oxide activates guanylate cyclase, leading to increased production of cGMP (option B is incorrect). The cGMP relaxes the smooth musculature of the corpora cavernosa (option A is correct) and thus facilitates the blood inflow into them. Increased blood inflow into the corpora cavernosa leads to their distention, which finally produces erection. Then, continued stimulation leads to emission of semen and ejaculation (option C is incorrect), which are controlled through sympathetic fibers and the pudendal nerve. Dopaminergic systems in the central nervous system (particularly the nucleus accumbens, which is responsible for pleasure and other structures) facilitate arousal and ejaculation, whereas serotonergic systems inhibit these functions (option D is incorrect). (These neurotransmitter systems play similar roles in women.) In addition, androgens expedite and modulate desire and, to some extent, erection and ejaculation. This description clearly demonstrates the delicate interplay of psychology and biology: stimuli lead to a biological processes cascade, which leads to erection and ejaculation, which are usually accompanied by psychological satisfaction. **Chapter 21 (pp. 576–577)**

21.2   Which of the following has been found to be associated with erectile dysfunction?

A. Depression.
B. Personality traits of dominance.
C. High levels of physical activity.
D. Low levels of anxiety.

The correct response is option A: Depression.

Numerous population studies have found *depression* to be strongly associated with erectile dysfunction. Similarly, men with depression have a high incidence of erectile dysfunction (option A is correct) that frequently resolves with the successful treatment of the depressive disorder.

Certain personality traits have been found to be associated with erectile problems. In British students, personality traits of neuroticism (*anxiety proneness*) (option D is incorrect) were significantly associated with the presence of erectile problems. In the Massachusetts Male Aging Study (Feldman et al. 1994), personality traits of *submissiveness* (option B is incorrect) were associated with the subsequent development of erectile dysfunction.

Population surveys have found relationships between the presence of erectile dysfunction in men 40 years and older and aging, vascular disease, smoking, and *inactivity* (option C is incorrect). **Chapter 21 (pp. 582–583)**

21.3   A 23-year-old man with a history of asthma, active nicotine use disorder, and anxiety disorder presents to a family medicine clinic for a routine checkup. He shares with his doctor that he's just recently started having sex and is worried that he may have erectile dysfunction. He is embarrassed that "most of the time" he has difficulty obtaining and maintaining an erection. What time duration and frequency of symptoms must be present to fulfill DSM-5 diagnostic criteria for erectile disorder?

A. Duration of at least 4 weeks, occurring more than 25% of the time.
B. Duration of at least 2 months, occurring more than 50% of the time.
C. Duration of at least 6 months, occurring more than 75% of the time.
D. No specific time duration is required, but the symptoms must have occurred every time penetrative sex has been attempted.

The correct response is option C: Duration of at least 6 months, occurring more than 75% of the time.

The DSM-IV (American Psychiatric Association 1994) diagnostic criteria for sexual dysfunctions were criticized as lacking precision and as not clearly differentiating normal variations in sexual function from sexual disorders that might merit medical intervention. Epidemiological data clearly indicated that problems occurring most of the time and persisting for 6 months or longer had a much lower prevalence than disorders occurring only some of the time and lasting less than 6 months (options A and B are incorrect) (e.g., Mercer et al. 2003). Thus, in DSM-

5 (American Psychiatric Association 2013), most of the diagnostic criteria include the requirement that symptoms be present for at least 6 months and occur on at least 75% of occasions to meet the threshold for diagnosis (option C is correct). The addition of the duration criterion makes the diagnosis of sexual dysfunctions more consistent with the rest of the DSM classification system (option D is incorrect). The diagnostic criteria for substance/medication-induced sexual dysfunction represent an exception; for this diagnosis, the decision was made to leave out a duration criterion so as to encourage recognition of iatrogenic sexual dysfunction. **Chapter 21 (p. 578)**

21.4 You are conducting an in-depth interview with a 35-year-old man with a medical history of Bechet's vasculitis and carotid stenosis who is experiencing new-onset erectile dysfunction. He denies low sexual desire. Which of the following would be the best initial step in terms of workup?

A. Nerve conduction studies.
B. Doppler ultrasound.
C. Serum free testosterone.
D. Lipid profile.

The correct response is option B: Doppler ultrasound.

The extent to which a clinician pursues possible medical etiologies to erectile problems is dependent on the patient's age, his overall health status and risk factors, and the presentation of the problem. In general, the clinical presentation provides clues regarding the etiology. An inconsistent problem, an acute onset following psychological stress, and a situational pattern (e.g., failure in partnered activities yet normal erections on awakening or with masturbation) are all strongly suggestive of a psychological etiology to the problem. If the clinician suspects a peripheral neuropathy, nerve conduction studies such as somatosensory evoked potentials can be performed (option A is incorrect). If a possible vascular etiology is suspected, Doppler ultrasonography (option B is correct) and intracavernosal injection of a vasoactive drug can be employed, as well as more invasive procedures such as dynamic infusion cavernosometry. Studies of serum lipid profiles (option D is incorrect) are also indicated because studies have found that the onset of erectile problems in men age 40 years and older was highly predictive of future coronary artery disease (Osondu et al. 2018). If a patient has a history compatible with low sexual desire, either bioavailable testosterone or free testosterone levels should be obtained to rule out hypogonadism (option C is incorrect). Some clinicians also routinely order serum glucose and thyroid-stimulating hormone levels. **Chapter 21 (pp. 581–582)**

21.5 Which of the following antipsychotics is associated with the lowest incidence of delayed ejaculation?

A. Ziprasidone.
B. Risperidone.

C. Haloperidol.
D. Fluphenazine.

The correct response is option A: Ziprasidone.

Antipsychotic agents, especially the traditional antipsychotics (options C and D are incorrect) and risperidone (option B is incorrect), are associated with delayed ejaculation. This side effect can usually be managed by dosage reduction or drug substitution. Agents such as quetiapine, ziprasidone (option A is correct), and aripiprazole have a lower incidence of delayed ejaculation. **Chapter 21 (p. 581)**

21.6   You are weighing the risks and benefits of prescribing tadalafil for your patient, a 63-year-old man with newly diagnosed erectile disorder and a history of coronary artery disease, diabetes, and benign prostatic hyperplasia. In regard to potential drug-drug interactions, which of the following medications, when taken in combination with a phosphodiesterase type 5 (PDE-5) inhibitor, can result in catastrophic hypotension?

A. Bupropion.
B. Nitroglycerin.
C. Amantadine.
D. Mirtazapine.

The correct response is option B: Nitroglycerin.

The treatment of erectile disorder has been revolutionized by the introduction of effective oral vasoactive drugs, the PDE-5 inhibitors such as avanafil, sildenafil, tadalafil, and vardenafil (others available outside of the United States include lodenafil and udenafil). All of these drugs inhibit the degradation of cyclic cGMP, thereby prolonging the action of cGMP in causing smooth muscle relaxation of the cavernosal muscle of the penile arteries. It is important to note that no head-to-head comparisons of these four medications have been reported to date. Their only differences are in the duration of their action: tadalafil acts longer (regular low-dose tadalafil has been approved by the U.S. Food and Drug Administration for erectile dysfunction and symptoms of benign prostatic hypertrophy). The PDE-5 inhibitors have all been shown to be effective in the treatment of psychogenic erectile problems, as well as those due to a general medical condition or substance use. They have also been shown to be effective in reversing erectile dysfunction caused by antidepressants and other psychiatric drugs. However, several lines of evidence suggest that the use of PDE-5 inhibitors alone is insufficient. A large number of PDE-5 inhibitor prescriptions are not refilled, for unknown reasons. Also, the use of PDE-5 inhibitors is not risk free.

Catastrophic hypotension can result if PDE-5 inhibitors are combined with nitrates (e.g., nitroglycerin, amyl nitrate) (option B is correct), and there is also a risk if these drugs are combined with other hypotensive agents (options A, C, and D are incorrect). **Chapter 21 (p. 583)**

21.7   A 54-year-old man with type 2 diabetes mellitus and obstructive sleep apnea (OSA) has used a phosphodiesterase type 5 (PDE-5) to treat erectile dysfunction but finds the side effects too burdensome. Which of the following would be the next best intervention that is reversible?

A. Over-the-counter preparations for erectile disorder (e.g., L-arginine).
B. Penile prosthetic devices.
C. Vacuum pump with constriction ring.
D. Oral papaverine.

The correct response is option C: Vacuum pump with constriction ring.

Additional options exist if the PDE-5 agents are unsuccessful. The vacuum pump combined with constriction devices or rings is useful as a reversible intervention (option C is correct).

Other second-line interventions include the use of intracavernosal injections or intra-urethral pellets of vasoactive agents such as alprostadil, papaverine (option D is incorrect), or VIP (vasoactive intestinal polypeptide)/phentolamine.

Surgical implantation of penile prosthetic devices (option B is incorrect) remains an option if other treatments are unsuccessful.

Patients should also be reminded that various over-the-counter preparations for erectile disorder and other male sexual dysfunctions are untested and ineffective (option A is incorrect). **Chapter 21 (p. 584)**

21.8   In regard to the etiology of female orgasmic disorder, approximately what percentage of the variability in frequency of orgasm during sexual contact is influenced by genetics?

A. 10%.
B. 20%.
C. 30%.
D. 40%.

The correct response is option C: 30%.

Twin studies have indicated that genetic influences account for approximately 30% (option C is correct; options A, B, and D are incorrect) of the variability in frequency of orgasm during sexual contact (Dawood et al. 2005). **Chapter 21 (p. 584)**

21.9   Which of the following therapies has been approved by the U.S. Food and Drug Administration (FDA) for use in the treatment of DSM-IV hypoactive sexual desire disorder in premenopausal women?

A. L-arginine.
B. Testosterone patches.
C. Flibanserin.
D. Bupropion.

The correct response is option C: Flibanserin.

The DSM-5 female sexual interest/arousal disorder (FSIAD) diagnosis basically combines features of two DSM-IV diagnoses—female hypoactive sexual desire disorder and female sexual arousal disorder. Depending on the underlying etiology (e.g., a hormonal deficit determined by measuring levels of hormones such as thyroid-stimulating hormone and estrogen) and the symptomatology (e.g., lack of lubrication accompanying absence of desire) and after lack of success with sex therapy and cognitive-behavioral therapy, various pharmacological options could be implemented. Although no pharmacological agents have received FDA approval specifically for use in treating FSIAD (understandably, because this is a new diagnostic entity) or for other sexual dysfunctions, pharmacotherapies used for this indication have included testosterone patches (option B is incorrect) (especially in women with bilateral oophorectomy), other hormones (local and systemic estrogens), bupropion (option D is incorrect), L-arginine (option A is incorrect), and phosphodiesterase type 5 inhibitors (Segraves and Balon 2003).

However, in 2015, the FDA approved flibanserin (a serotonin 1A receptor agonist and serotonin 2A receptor antagonist) for use in the treatment of DSM-IV hypoactive sexual desire disorder in premenopausal women (option C is correct) (the low desire must be acquired and generalized). Although this medication is indicated for DSM-IV hypoactive sexual desire disorder, it could probably be used for premenopausal women with acquired generalized FSIAD. Because of an increased risk of hypotension and syncope due to an interaction with alcohol, flibanserin is available only through an FDA-mandated risk evaluation and mitigation strategy (REMS) program—the Addyi REMS Program. **Chapter 21 (pp. 585, 586)**

21.10   A 28-year-old woman presents to her primary care physician reporting chronic pain during sexual activity. Upon further questioning, she describes sharp, burning pain with penetration, including when she uses masturbatory aids and even when she tries to insert a tampon. She has read about various treatments and is motivated to "try anything at this point." Which of the following would be the best initial step in treatment?

A. Vulvar hygiene (i.e., milder soap, cotton underwear).
B. Systematic desensitization using vaginal dilators.
C. Gabapentin.
D. Topical lidocaine.

The correct response is option A: Vulvar hygiene (i.e., milder soap, cotton underwear).

Various medical and psychological treatment modalities have been used in the management of sexual pain (for a review, see Boyer et al. 2011). An initial treatment step may involve vulvar hygiene (e.g., use of mild soap and cotton underwear) (option A is correct).

Medical modalities include systematic desensitization (option B is incorrect) (e.g., in the case of vaginal spasm, by first inserting dilators of gradually increasing size and then practicing guided penetration with the partner lying on his back and the patient controlling the insertion and the following movements), pelvic floor rehabilitation (applied, usually, by specialized physical therapists), pelvic floor exercises, manual therapy techniques (massage of various areas that may increase circulation and improve motility), topical medication (botulotoxin, anesthetics such as lidocaine [option D is incorrect] [the efficacy remains unclear]), systemic medications (e.g., tricyclic antidepressants, anticonvulsants including gabapentin [option C is incorrect] [however, these medications could themselves be associated with various sexual dysfunctions]), sitz baths, biofeedback, electrotherapeutic modalities (intravaginal electrical stimulation), and surgery (removal of the hypersensitive tissue causing painful intercourse actually has the highest success rate among the current treatments for provoked vestibulodynia). Psychological modalities include using various cognitive-behavioral models (including group cognitive-behavioral therapy) and sex therapy. Alternative modalities such as hypnosis and acupuncture have also been studied. **Chapter 21 (p. 588)**

References

American Psychiatric Association: Diagnostic and Statistical Manual of Mental Disorders, 4th Edition. Washington, DC, American Psychiatric Association, 1994

American Psychiatric Association: Diagnostic and Statistical Manual of Mental Disorders, 5th Edition. Arlington, VA, American Psychiatric Association, 2013

Boyer SC, Goldfinger C, Thibault-Gagnon S, et al: Management of female sexual pain disorders. Adv Psychosom Med 31:83–104, 2011 22005206

Dawood K, Kirk K, Bailey J, et al: Genetic and environmental influences on the frequency of orgasm in women. Twin Res Hum Genet 8(1):27–33, 2005 15836807

Feldman HA, Goldstein I, Hatzichristou DG, et al: Impotence and its medical and psychological correlates: results of the Massachusetts Male Aging Study. J Urol 151(1):54–61, 1994 8254833

Mercer CH, Fenton KA, Johnson AM, et al: Sexual function problems and help seeking behaviour in Britain: national probability sample survey. BMJ 327(7412):426–427, 2003 12933730

Osondu CU, Vo B, Oni ET, et al: The relationship of erectile dysfunction and subclinical cardiovascular disease: a systematic review and meta-analysis. Vasc Med 23(1):9–20, 2018 29243995

Segraves RT, Balon R: Sexual Pharmacology: Fast Facts. New York, WW Norton, 2003

CHAPTER 22

Gender Dysphoria

22.1 A 40-year-old transgender woman presents to your outpatient practice for an initial evaluation. You have never received training in gender-affirming therapy and have not had significant experience treating gender-diverse individuals. You are unsure about your ability to treat her. What is the most appropriate next step?

A. Invite the patient's friends and family to a session to provide collateral information.
B. Assess for a mood disorder as the cause of the patient's gender dysphoria.
C. Provide supportive interventions to help the patient process ambivalence and cope with the stressors of being transgender.
D. Help guide the patient toward identifying long-term as male to minimize the risk of future distress and psychiatric symptoms.

The correct response is option C: Provide supportive interventions to help the patient process ambivalence and cope with the stressors of being transgender.

Clinicians trained in the art and practice of psychiatry are able to help even if they lack specific knowledge about gender-affirming care. Psychiatrists trained in psychotherapy can help patients to process ambivalence and existential crises and can provide supportive interventions as patients move through uncharted territory (option C is correct).

Gender-affirming therapy becomes more complicated with the influences of the outside world. Family, friends, and work colleagues can question the person's treatment plans, creating ambivalence and triggering fears that they may be making the "wrong" choices. A gender-affirming therapist will weed through all of these external relationships and make space for the person sitting in front of them (option A is incorrect).

Conversion therapy is considered unethical and can lead to worsening of symptoms and suicide. Patients should be told that the goal of gender-affirming therapy is not to change their gender identity, but rather to help them express who they feel their true self to be (option D is incorrect).

It is rare for psychiatric illness to cause symptoms of gender dysphoria (option B is incorrect). **Chapter 22 (pp. 603–604)**

22.2   Which of the following patient presentations would meet criteria for a DSM-5
        gender dysphoria diagnosis?

        A. A patient who is biologically male but portrays themselves as female for sex-
           ual pleasure.
        B. A patient who is biologically male but for the past month has felt that they
           identify more as female.
        C. A patient who is biologically male but has experienced distress for several
           years because they strongly identify as female.
        D. A patient who is biologically male but does not identify as exclusively male or
           female in gender.

**The correct response is option C: A patient who is biologically male but has ex-
perienced distress for several years because they strongly identify as female.**

The DSM-5 (American Psychiatric Association 2013) gender dysphoria diagnosis
focuses on the individual's personal, interior identity and how they view themselves. To meet criteria for the diagnosis, a person must have "a marked incongruence between their experienced/expressed gender and their assigned gender, of at
least 6 months' duration" (DSM-5, p. 452) (option C is correct; option B is incorrect).

   In DSM-IV (American Psychiatric Association 1994), gender dysphoria was a
specifier applied to the diagnosis of transvestic fetishism, a paraphilia in which
people dress up as the opposite sex largely for sexual pleasure, and not because
they feel themselves to *be* the opposite gender (option A is incorrect).

   Being diverse in one's gender presentation is not in itself a mental illness, but
having dysphoric feelings about one's primary and secondary sex characteristics
as well as about being labeled as "the wrong gender" can lead to psychiatric
symptoms (Berlin 2016) (option D is incorrect). **Chapter 22 (pp. 599–600)**

22.3   A 30-year-old woman of transgender experience presents to the psychiatric emer-
        gency room after a suicide attempt. On evaluation, she is found to have an exten-
        sive trauma history as well as a history of suicidality, interpersonal conflicts, and
        mood lability. She reports ongoing daily alcohol use and frequent cannabis use.
        On exam, the patient is irritable and continues to endorse suicidal ideation. What
        is the most appropriate diagnosis?

        A. Borderline personality disorder.
        B. Gender dysphoria secondary to a primary mood disorder.
        C. Gender identity disorder.
        D. Defer diagnosis and monitor longitudinally.

The correct response is option D: Defer diagnosis and monitor longitudinally.

The presence of comorbid psychiatric disorders alongside gender dysphoria is
common. It is generally believed that the high levels of comorbidity among gender-diverse people are largely attributable to the hostile and unaccepting environ-

ments in which many transgender people grow up. In comparison with the general population, transgender individuals report higher stress, trauma, depression, anxiety, substance use, suicidal ideation, and suicide attempts. Knowing about transgender mental health is necessary so as not to overdiagnose common experiences as a disorder. Because of the frequency of traumatic reactions and suicidal ideation, many transgender people are diagnosed with borderline personality disorder, particularly in an emergency department, where they are at their most vulnerable. Mood lability, impulsivity, and suicidal ideation are common symptoms of a personality disorder, but such symptoms could also affect anyone exposed to the daily threats faced by those in the lesbian, gay, bisexual, transgender, and queer (LGBTQ) population (Budge et al. 2013). Typically, a person who is in a stage of coming out or transitioning is more susceptible to these symptoms; however, the symptoms often resolve once the person is in a more stable place (Bariola et al. 2015). Anyone who is LGBTQ would need a more extensive observation over time before a diagnosis such as a personality disorder could be made (option D is correct; option A is incorrect). Clinicians might be quick to identify a mood disorder as the "cause" of someone's gender diversity. It is rare for psychiatric illness to cause symptoms of gender dysphoria (option B is incorrect). In DSM-5, gender identity disorder was changed to gender dysphoria in an effort to depathologize gender diversity (option C is incorrect). **Chapter 22 (pp. 600, 603)**

22.4   Which of the following statements regarding gender-affirming surgery is *correct*?

A. Patients who receive this surgery are at high risk of regretting their decision.
B. Insurance will not pay for any of the cost of the surgery.
C. Gender-affirming surgery is associated with positive mental health outcomes.
D. A high percentage of individuals who receive gender-affirming surgical procedures opt to "de-transition" and reverse the surgery.

The correct response is option C: Gender-affirming surgery is associated with positive mental health outcomes.

There is evidence that gender-affirming surgical procedures have a positive impact on a person's mental health in the long term (option C is correct). Any dissatisfaction with surgical procedures may be due not to regret but rather to unhappiness with the quality of the procedure (option A is incorrect). Public and private insurance companies are starting to cover the procedures (option B is incorrect). Whereas some people may "de-transition," this phenomenon is relatively rare among those who are happy with surgical outcomes (option D is incorrect). **Chapter 22 (p. 605)**

22.5   Which of the following statements about hormone therapy is *true*?

A. The effects of hormones will be seen immediately.
B. Most individuals who take hormones are ultimately dissatisfied with the results.

C. There are no contraindications to hormone therapy.

D. Individuals who start hormone therapy often find that strangers are beginning to recognize and address them as their self-identified gender.

The correct response is option D: Individuals who start hormone therapy often find that strangers are beginning to recognize and address them as their self-identified gender.

Hormones change the body in such a way that strangers may start to refer to a person by the gender they identify as (option D is correct). This experience can be very validating.

Traditionally, hormones have fallen outside of the purview of psychiatrists, but gender dysphoria and gender-affirming care are slowly changing the psychiatrist's scope of practice regarding hormone prescribing. With an understanding of dosing and monitoring standards, psychiatrists are in a unique place to provide these types of treatment to transgender individuals who lack access to them (Thomas and Safer 2015).

Providing hormones should be viewed from an informed consent model. The clinician should ensure that the patient understands the risks and benefits of the treatment, both short-term and long-term (Deutsch 2012). Armed with this information, patients can make a decision that is best for them and their bodies. The changes that take place with hormones occur over months to years (option A is incorrect). These slow changes can frustrate patients. General lab work is done prior to starting treatment and quarterly thereafter.

There are a few contraindications to hormone treatment (e.g., clotting disorders, certain cancers, liver dysfunction), but they are generally rare (Ettner et al. 2007), and ultimately the patient and the prescriber must weigh the risks and benefits of treatment (option C is incorrect). Lab work and general primary care follow-up will usually identify any potential adverse reactions; however, the majority of people who take hormones are quite happy with the results (White Hughto and Reisner 2016) (option B is incorrect). **Chapter 22 (pp. 604–605)**

22.6 A 23-year-old patient presents to your office reporting symptoms of gender dysphoria and expressing a desire to transition. The patient discloses that his mother feels negatively about his desire to do so, and states she "does not understand" why he feels this way. How would you counsel this patient and his mother?

A. Gender-diverse individuals should try to portray themselves within cultural norms of masculinity and femininity.

B. Gender is assigned and constant from birth.

C. Masculinity and femininity are largely rooted in biological factors.

D. Gender exists on a continuum rather than as an either/or dichotomy.

The correct response is option D: Gender exists on a continuum rather than as an either/or dichotomy.

Conceptually, gender-affirming therapy is simple to understand. It involves taking the stance that gender diversity is not pathological and that the gender spectrum has many presentations. The most difficult conceptual benchmark that clinicians struggle with when working with gender-diverse patients is the understanding that gender exists on a continuum rather than as an either/or dichotomy (option D is correct).

Male or female sex is identified on the basis of the external genitalia at birth, but what comes after that largely depends on when and where one is born. Gender resides in the mind, not in the genitals. Most of our understanding about what makes people masculine or feminine is a social construct (option C is incorrect).

Grasping that gender is neither assigned nor constant from birth will ease the process of working with gender-diverse people (option B is incorrect).

Gender-diverse individuals are people who fall outside the typical cultural norms of what we call masculine and feminine and of how we perceive these traits to relate to the male or female sex (option A is incorrect). **Chapter 22 (p. 599)**

22.7 Which of the following statements regarding gender diversity and gender-affirming care is *correct*?

A. The number of people seeking gender-affirming treatment is decreasing.
B. Individuals living outside traditional gender stereotypes is a relatively new social occurrence which only began in the past decade.
C. Gender-diverse people are more comfortable coming out and publicly expressing who they are.
D. There is no central leading authority that defines standards for gender-affirming care.

The correct response is option C: Gender-diverse people are more comfortable coming out and publicly expressing who they are.

There have always been people who lived outside of traditional gender stereotypes (option B is incorrect). The World Professional Association of Transgender Health is seen as the leading authority in regard to defining the standards of gender-affirming care (option D is incorrect). The number of people seeking gender-affirming treatment has skyrocketed since 2010, mainly because society has become slightly more accepting (option A is incorrect). Gender-diverse people are more comfortable coming out and publicly expressing who they are (option C is correct). **Chapter 22 (p. 601)**

22.8 A 34-year-old gender-diverse patient who recently started hormone treatment, presents to your office reporting anxiety, depression, and intermittent suicidality. He discloses that his family remains unsupportive of his transition and that he feels hopeless about things ever improving. He also endorses feeling uncomfortable at work, where many of his colleagues have asked probing questions. Which of the following statements represents the most accurate understanding of this patient's symptoms?

A. The patient should stop the hormones immediately, as anxiety and depression among transgender individuals is most commonly due to side effects of hormone treatment.
B. Hostile environments, which many gender-diverse individuals are exposed to, can lead to the development of psychiatric symptoms.
C. Although transgender individuals are exposed to heightened discrimination, rates of suicide do not differ compared with the general population.
D. The patient's symptoms are likely to worsen over the course of his lifetime.

The correct response is option B: Hostile environments, which many gender-diverse individuals are exposed to, can lead to the development of psychiatric symptoms.

High levels of psychiatric comorbidity among gender-diverse people are largely attributable to the hostile and unaccepting environments in which many transgender people grow up (option A is incorrect). The added daily stressors, best explained by the minority stress model, can lead to development and/or worsening of symptoms that might not emerge in people who are not exposed to such stressors (option B is correct). Compared with the general population, transgender people report higher levels of stress, trauma, depression, anxiety, substance use, suicidal ideation, and suicide attempts (option C is incorrect). Typically, a person who is in a stage of coming out or transitioning is more susceptible to symptoms; however, the symptoms often resolve once the person is in a more stable place (option D is incorrect). **Chapter 22 (p. 603)**

References

American Psychiatric Association: Diagnostic and Statistical Manual of Mental Disorders, 4th Edition. Washington, DC, American Psychiatric Association, 1994
American Psychiatric Association: Diagnostic and Statistical Manual of Mental Disorders, 5th Edition. Arlington, VA, American Psychiatric Association, 2013
Bariola E, Lyons A, Leonard W, et al: Demographic and psychosocial factors associated with psychological distress and resilience among transgender individuals. Am J Public Health 105(10):2108–2116, 2015 26270284
Berlin FS: A conceptual overview and commentary on gender dysphoria. J Am Acad Psychiatry Law 44(2):246–252, 2016 27236181
Budge SL, Adelson JL, Howard KA: Anxiety and depression in transgender individuals: the roles of transition status, loss, social support, and coping. J Consult Clin Psychol 81(3):545–557, 2013 23398495
Deutsch M: Use of the informed consent model in the provision of cross-sex hormone therapy: a survey of the practices of selected clinics. International Journal of Transgenderism 13(3):140–146, 2012
Ettner R, Monstrey S, Coleman E: Principles of Transgender Medicine and Surgery. New York, Haworth, 2007
Thomas DD, Safer JD: A simple intervention raised resident-physician willingness to assist transgender patients seeking hormone therapy. Endocr Pract 21(10):1134–1142, 2015 26151424
White Hughto JM, Reisner SL: A systematic review of the effects of hormone therapy on psychological functioning and quality of life in transgender individuals. Transgend Health 1(1):21–31, 2016 27595141

CHAPTER 23

Disruptive, Impulse-Control, and Conduct Disorders

23.1   A 6-year-old boy is brought to the doctor by his parents because of his persistently disruptive behavior over the past year. The patient's teacher reports that he frequently ends up in conflict with peers and refuses to follow along with class activities. At home, he refuses to do his assigned chores and instigates arguments with his siblings over his toys every night. His parents are worried that he will not be able to graduate to the next grade because of his constant disputes with others. This child's symptom profile suggests a potential future risk of developing which of the following disorders?

A. Major depressive disorder.
B. Attention-deficit/hyperactivity disorder (ADHD).
C. Conduct disorder.
D. Antisocial personality disorder.

The correct response is option B: Attention-deficit/hyperactivity disorder (ADHD).

DSM-5 (American Psychiatric Association 2013) separates oppositional defiant disorder (ODD) symptoms into clusters based on whether they have an emotional component (e.g., angry, irritable, resentful behaviors), a behavioral element (e.g., argumentative, defiant behaviors), or a spiteful/vindictive aspect to them. This classification structure emerged on the basis of empirical findings suggesting that these three clusters are associated with unique predictive outcomes. Specifically, whereas the emotional symptoms of ODD (angry and irritable) are associated with the development of future mood and anxiety disorders (option A is incorrect), the headstrong symptoms (i.e., argumentative and defiant) are more likely to be predictive of a later diagnosis of ADHD (option B is correct), and the spiteful or vindictive behaviors (e.g., aggression) are associated with an increased risk of a conduct disorder diagnosis (option C is incorrect) and development of other delinquent behaviors (Rowe et al. 2010; Stringaris and Goodman 2009).

The stability of ODD symptoms over time correlates with the severity of the symptoms; furthermore, higher numbers of ODD symptoms are associated with greater risk for later development of conduct disorder. Early-onset ODD is likewise predictive of future conduct disorder and constitutes a risk factor for a later diagnosis of ADHD. A child with ODD is also more likely to progress to conduct disorder if he or she is of low socioeconomic status and has parents with substance use disorders. Notably, although ODD is usually a predecessor of conduct disorder, the majority of children with ODD do not go on to develop conduct disorder or antisocial behaviors in adulthood (Loeber et al. 2000) (option D is incorrect). **Chapter 23 (pp. 615, 618)**

23.2   An 8-year-old boy is brought to the doctor by his parents because of his persistently disruptive behavior over the past year. The boy's teacher reports that he has been generally irritable during class and becomes upset easily when teachers call on him. He lashes out when he feels that his peers are playing without him. The parents recall that their son was always a happy, easy-going child until the past year; however, he has become increasingly irritable, and lately, any small matter can cause him to explode into a tantrum. This child's symptom profile suggests a potential future risk of developing which of the following disorders?

A. Major depressive disorder.
B. Attention-deficit/hyperactivity disorder (ADHD).
C. Conduct disorder.
D. Antisocial personality disorder.

The correct response is option A: Major depressive disorder.

DSM-5 separates oppositional defiant disorder (ODD) symptoms into clusters based on whether they have an emotional component (e.g., angry, irritable, resentful behaviors), a behavioral element (e.g., argumentative, defiant behaviors), or a spiteful/vindictive aspect to them. This classification structure emerged on the basis of empirical findings suggesting that these three clusters are associated with unique predictive outcomes. Specifically, whereas the emotional symptoms of ODD (angry and irritable) are associated with the development of future mood and anxiety disorders (option A is correct), the headstrong symptoms (i.e., argumentative and defiant) are more likely to be predictive of a later diagnosis of ADHD (option B is incorrect), and the spiteful or vindictive behaviors (e.g., aggression) are associated with an increased risk of a conduct disorder diagnosis (option C is incorrect) and development of other delinquent behaviors (Rowe et al. 2010; Stringaris and Goodman 2009).

Notably, although ODD is usually a predecessor of conduct disorder, the majority of children with ODD do not go on to develop conduct disorder or antisocial behaviors in adulthood (Loeber et al. 2000) (option D is incorrect). **Chapter 23 (pp. 615–618)**

23.3   A 6-year-old boy is brought to the doctor by his parents because of his persistently disruptive behavior over the past year. The boy's teacher reports that he has been provoking his peers and getting in physical altercations several times a week. At home, his parents have noticed that he frequently lashes out vindictively. Last week, he intentionally threw his mother's favorite glass vase on the floor after being chastised for not doing his chores. This child's symptom profile suggests a potential future risk of developing which of the following disorders?

A. Major depressive disorder.
B. Attention-deficit/hyperactivity disorder (ADHD).
C. Conduct disorder.
D. Antisocial personality disorder.

The correct response is option C: Conduct disorder.

DSM-5 separates oppositional defiant disorder (ODD) symptoms into clusters based on whether they have an emotional component (e.g., angry, irritable, resentful behaviors), a behavioral element (e.g., argumentative, defiant behaviors), or a spiteful/vindictive aspect to them. This classification structure emerged on the basis of empirical findings suggesting that these three clusters are associated with unique predictive outcomes. Specifically, whereas the emotional symptoms of ODD (angry and irritable) are associated with the development of future mood and anxiety disorders (option A is incorrect), the headstrong symptoms (i.e., argumentative and defiant) are more likely to be predictive of a later diagnosis of ADHD (option B is incorrect), and the spiteful or vindictive behaviors (e.g., aggression) are associated with an increased risk of a conduct disorder diagnosis (option C is correct) and development of other delinquent behaviors (Rowe et al. 2010; Stringaris and Goodman 2009).

Notably, although ODD is usually a predecessor of conduct disorder, the majority of children with ODD do not go on to develop conduct disorder or antisocial behaviors in adulthood (Loeber et al. 2000) (option D is incorrect). **Chapter 23 (pp. 615–618)**

23.4   A 10-year-old boy is brought to clinic by his mother because of frequent aggressive outbursts. His mother says that over the last several months, her son has been fighting with peers, is openly rude to his teachers, and actively ignores his parents' rules. She reports that he goes out of his way to bully his younger sister. A week ago, he stole his classmate's backpack. The classmate began crying, but her son did not return the backpack, apologize, or appear remorseful. The mother says she is worried that if this behavior continues, her son will soon be suspended from school. Which of the following traits displayed by this patient is more suggestive of a diagnosis of conduct disorder than of oppositional defiant disorder (ODD)?

A. Frequent verbal fights with peers.
B. Ignoring rules at home and at school.

C. Bullying of a younger sibling.
D. Lack of remorse over stolen backpack.

The correct response is option D: Lack of remorse over stolen backpack.

Whether ODD can manifest concurrently with conduct disorder has been a question of debate, given that ODD and conduct disorder encompass similar features. For example, both disorders consist of behaviors that are vastly negative, including disobedient, angry (option C is incorrect), defiant (option B is incorrect), rebellious, and resentful (option A is incorrect) behavior. ODD differs from conduct disorder, however, in that children with conduct disorder fail to recognize societal rules and personal rights, resulting in aggression that may cause physical injury to people or animals and/or deliberate destruction of property. Table 23–1 outlines differences and similarities between ODD and conduct disorder in terms of their behavioral characteristics, age at onset, and unique specifiers (option D is correct). As can be seen, the age at onset for ODD is younger than that for conduct disorder, and in fact, ODD is often a precursor to a diagnosis of conduct disorder at a later age. DSM-5 allows for the concurrent diagnosis of ODD and conduct disorder and emphasizes the prognostic value of ODD symptoms in predicting future clinical outcomes (e.g., depression, anxiety, substance use, attention-deficit/hyperactivity disorder) in individuals diagnosed with conduct disorder comorbid with ODD (American Psychiatric Association 2013). **Chapter 23 (Table 23–2 [p. 617])**

23.5   Which of the following statements about the course of oppositional defiant disorder (ODD) is *false*?

A. Onset is usually between 6 and 8 years.
B. Symptoms typically first emerge at home before presenting in other settings.
C. Lower socioeconomic status and having parents with substance use disorders are correlated with increased risk of developing conduct disorder.
D. The majority of children with ODD will go on to develop conduct disorder.

The correct response is option D: The majority of children with ODD will go on to develop conduct disorder.

The age at onset of ODD is usually between 6 and 8 years (option A is incorrect), after typical normative oppositional behaviors diminish. The onset of symptoms is gradual and develops over the course of months or even years. Symptoms commonly first materialize in the home setting and may then emerge in other settings and circumstances (option B is incorrect). When symptoms extend to multiple settings, they can lead to severe impairment in social, educational, and other important areas of functioning. The stability of ODD symptoms over time correlates with the severity of the symptoms; furthermore, higher numbers of ODD symptoms are associated with greater risk for later development of conduct disorder. Early-onset ODD is likewise predictive of future conduct disorder and constitutes a risk factor for a later diagnosis of attention-deficit/hyperactivity disorder. A

TABLE 23–1. Comparison of DSM-5 diagnostic features for oppositional defiant disorder and conduct disorder

	Oppositional defiant disorder	Conduct disorder
Age at onset (years)	6–8	9–17
Behavioral features	Verbal arguments and temper tantrums expressed as the following: Angry/irritable mood (loses temper, easily annoyed) Argumentative/defiant behavior (argues, deliberately annoys others, defies rules/requests) Spite/vindictiveness	Lack of recognition of societal rules and personal rights, engaging in the following: Aggression toward people or animals Destruction of property Deceitfulness or theft Serious violations of rules
Specifiers	**Current severity** Mild: symptoms occur in one setting Moderate: some symptoms present in at least two settings Severe: some symptoms present in at least three settings	**Current severity** Mild: symptoms occur in one setting Moderate: some symptoms present in at least two settings Severe: some symptoms present in at least three settings **Onset type** Childhood onset: before age 10 years Adolescent onset: at or after age 10 years **With limited prosocial emotions**— persistently displays 2 or more of the following: Lack of remorse or guilt Callousness—lack of empathy Lack of concern about performance Shallow/deficient affect

Note. For the complete diagnostic criteria for oppositional defiant disorder and conduct disorder, please refer to pp. 462–463 and pp. 469–471, respectively, in DSM-5 (American Psychiatric Association 2013).

child with ODD is also more likely to progress to conduct disorder if he or she is of low socioeconomic status and has parents with substance use disorders (option C is incorrect). Notably, although ODD is usually a predecessor of conduct disorder, the majority of children with ODD do not go on to develop conduct disorder or antisocial behaviors in adulthood (Loeber et al. 2000) (option D is correct). **Chapter 23 (p. 618)**

23.6   Which of the following strategies for the treatment of school-age children with oppositional defiant disorder (ODD) has the greatest amount of empirical support?

A. Group-based treatments.
B. Combining selective serotonin reuptake inhibitors (SSRIs) with individual cognitive-behavioral therapy (CBT).
C. Combining parent management training with individual CBT.
D. Combining a mood stabilizer with parent management training.

The correct response is option C: Combining parent management training with individual CBT.

When school age is reached, parent management training and individual cognitive-based strategies are the programs with the greatest amount of empirical support. Combining parent management training and individual problem-solving approaches has been shown to be more effective than using either treatment alone (Kazdin et al. 1992) (option C is correct). School-based programs, such as those aimed at resisting negative peer influences and reducing bullying and antisocial behavior, may also be effective for this age group. For adolescents, cognitive-based techniques and vocational and skills training, as well as parent management tools, are recommended. Group-based treatments for adolescents can have negative outcomes (option A is incorrect), particularly if the group participants engage in discussions of oppositional behaviors (Barlow and Stewart-Brown 2000). In regard to pharmacological treatment options, no medication has been approved to specifically treat the symptoms of ODD (options B and D are incorrect). Medications are nonetheless used in children with ODD to treat coexisting conditions (e.g., attention-deficit/hyperactivity disorder, depression, anxiety) and may also be effective in improving oppositional behaviors. **Chapter 23 (p. 619)**

23.7   Multiple studies in patients with intermittent explosive disorder (IED) have found functional alterations in which of the following neurotransmitters?

A. Serotonin.
B. Dopamine.
C. Glutamate.
D. GABA.

The correct response is option A: Serotonin.

Research supports the presence of altered serotonin function in individuals with IED. For example, subjects with IED have been shown to have decreased numbers of platelet serotonin transporters as well as differences in the availability of the serotonin transporter and serotonin type 2A receptors compared with healthy control subjects (Coccaro et al. 2010a, 2010b; Frankle et al. 2005; Rosell et al. 2010) (option A is correct).

Psychostimulants such as methylphenidate and amphetamine prescribed for the treatment of attention-deficit/hyperactivity disorder exert their effects in part through inhibition of dopamine reuptake. However, more research is needed on the effects of dopamine and psychostimulants on impulsivity comorbid with aggression (option B is incorrect).

Glutamate and GABA (γ-aminobutyric acid) have been hypothesized to play a role in schizophrenia, but not in IED (options C and D are incorrect). **Chapter 23 (pp. 620–621); see also Chapter 10 ("Schizophrenia Spectrum and Other Psychotic Disorders"; p. 275) and Chapter 29 ("Psychopharmacology"; p. 840)**

23.8   Which of the following medications has been found to be effective in reducing aggression in patients with intermittent explosive disorder (IED) and comorbid Cluster B personality disorder features?

A. Fluoxetine.
B. Divalproex.
C. Phenytoin.
D. Risperidone.

The correct response is option B: Divalproex.

Symptoms of IED may respond to selective serotonin reuptake inhibitors (SSRIs), anticonvulsants, antipsychotics, phenytoin, β-blockers, and α_2-agonists (Dell' Osso et al. 2006). SSRIs show some short-term effects (Dell'Osso et al. 2006) but often fail to produce long-term remission of aggressive symptoms (option A is incorrect). Certain temperamental factors, such as neuroticism and harm avoidance, may be predictive of SSRI treatment response (Phan et al. 2011).

Divalproex has shown promise as an option for the treatment of aggression because it was superior to placebo in treating impulsive aggression in persons with borderline personality disorder (Hollander et al. 2005). However, divalproex did not have significant antiaggressive effects in IED patients without Cluster B personality disorders or posttraumatic stress disorder. For this reason, divalproex may be preferentially effective in highly aggressive individuals with personality disorders (Hollander et al. 2003, 2005) (option B is correct).

Studies have shown that phenytoin, carbamazepine, and valproate all can reduce impulsive aggression (Stanford et al. 2005) (option C is incorrect).

Risperidone can lead to improvement in clinical severity and produces relatively few side effects during treatment (Buitelaar et al. 2001) (option D is incorrect). **Chapter 23 (pp. 621–622; Table 23–3 [p. 622])**

23.9 A 15-year-old boy presents to the emergency department with his mother for treatment of smoke inhalation. According to his mother, he has recently become obsessed with fire after spending a week with his uncle, a firefighter. He has told his family he hopes to become a firefighter like his uncle. He spends his free time excitedly lighting various objects on fire, including pens, kitchen utensils, and most recently his father's watch. He accidentally set off a large fire on the stove top in the kitchen this morning. The patient does not appear particularly disturbed despite his mother's exasperation. He is otherwise a pleasant teenager. He has a few friends, and he does reasonably well in school. This patient's symptom profile is suggestive of which of the following disorders?

A. Pyromania.
B. Kleptomania.
C. Bipolar disorder.
D. Psychotic disorder.

The correct response is option A: Pyromania.

The primary feature of pyromania is deliberate and purposeful fire setting that recurs on multiple occasions. In addition to this hallmark behavior, DSM-5 criteria require that the individual must experience tension or affective arousal before setting the fire; must have a fascination with or attraction to fire; and must feel pleasure, gratification, or relief when setting or witnessing fires or when participating in their aftermath. Furthermore, the fire setting must not be done for monetary gain, as an expression of sociopolitical ideology or anger, to conceal criminal activity, or to improve one's living circumstances (option A is correct).

In addition, the fire setting cannot be a response to a delusion or hallucination (option D is incorrect), a result of impaired judgment, or attributable to a manic episode (option C is incorrect) or another disorder.

The defining feature of kleptomania is the inability to resist recurrent impulses to steal specific objects that are not required for personal use or for their monetary value (American Psychiatric Association 2013) (option B is incorrect). **Chapter 23 (pp. 628, 632)**

23.10 Which of the following impulse-control disorders is more common in women than in men?

A. Pyromania.
B. Kleptomania.
C. Gambling disorder.
D. Intermittent explosive disorder.

The correct response is option B. Kleptomania.

Kleptomania appears to be more prevalent in women than in men, with an estimated female-to-male ratio of 3 to 1 (American Psychiatric Association 2013). This reported female predominance in kleptomania may be biased, because courts are more likely to require female shoplifters to present for a psychiatric evaluation and women may be more likely to independently seek psychiatric evaluation. The severity and clinical presentation of kleptomania do not seem to differ between males and females (Grant and Kim 2002; McElroy et al. 1991) (option B is correct).

Juvenile fire setting is more common in males than in females, with male fire setters outnumbering female fire setters by approximately three to one (Lambie et al. 2013) (option A is incorrect).

The 12-month prevalence of gambling disorder is about 0.2% (American Psychiatric Association 2013). Males are about three times more likely to have a gambling disorder than females (option C is incorrect).

Sociodemographic correlates of lifetime intermittent explosive disorder (IED) include being male, young, unemployed, and divorced or separated and having low educational attainment (Scott et al. 2016). The age at onset for males is typically earlier than that for females, but overall, females are as likely as males to develop IED (Coccaro et al. 2005) (option D is incorrect). **Chapter 23 (pp. 620, 629, 632); see also Chapter 24 ("Substance-Related and Addictive Disorders"; p. 662)**

23.11 Studies in patients with kleptomania have identified primary neurotransmitter alterations in which of the following brain areas?

A. Nucleus ambiguous.
B. Amygdala.
C. Nucleus accumbens.
D. Hippocampus.

The correct response is option C: Nucleus accumbens.

Dopaminergic systems that affect reinforcement and reward may influence kleptomania pathogenesis. Changes in dopaminergic pathways have been implicated as the underlying cause of increased reward-seeking behavior, such as shoplifting, which may trigger dopamine release and produce pleasurable feelings. The function and structure of dopamine neurons within the mesocorticolimbic system, concurrent with intrinsic GABAergic and afferent glutamatergic activity, seem to adjust in response to these rewarding experiences, thereby influencing the nucleus accumbens. Later behavior may therefore be influenced by earlier rewarding experiences through neuroplastic alterations within the nucleus accumbens (option C is correct). These alterations may explain why many individuals with kleptomania describe shoplifting as "a habit" without feeling overt urges or cravings beforehand (Hollander et al. 2008).

Humans and other mammals have two functionally distinct vagal circuits. One vagal circuit is phylogenetically older and unmyelinated. It originates in a brain-stem area called the dorsal motor nucleus of the vagus. The other vagal circuit is uniquely mammalian and myelinated. It originates in the brain-stem area called the *nucleus ambiguous* (option A is incorrect).

The amygdala is central in the neural circuit involved in regulating fear conditioning (option B is incorrect). Emerging data suggest interesting relationships between facial emotional recognition in subjects with intermittent explosive disorder (IED) and amygdala–orbitofrontal cortex dysfunction. Specifically, individuals with IED show exaggerated amygdala reactivity and diminished orbitofrontal cortex activation in response to angry faces (Coccaro et al. 2007). A study that used high-resolution 3.0 Tesla structural magnetic resonance imaging found that IED was associated with structural abnormalities as well as a significant loss of neurons in both the amygdala and the hippocampus (Coccaro et al. 2015).

The hippocampus is important in recognizing context and limiting conditioned stimulus overgeneralization. Although research to date suggests that most of the functional and structural brain abnormalities in posttraumatic stress disorder (PTSD) are acquired following the traumatic event, the hippocampus appears to be at least a partial exception. Research in identical twins discordant for combat exposure suggests that lower hippocampal volume confers risk for PTSD following traumatic exposure (Gilbertson et al. 2002) (option D is incorrect). **Chapter 23 (pp. 621, 633–634); see also Chapter 15 ("Trauma- and Stressor-Related Disorders"; pp. 396, 397 [Figure 15–1]) and Chapter 37 ("Complementary and Integrative Therapies"; p. 1068)**

References

American Psychiatric Association: Diagnostic and Statistical Manual of Mental Disorders, 5th Edition. Arlington, VA, American Psychiatric Association, 2013

Barlow J, Stewart-Brown S: Behavior problems and group-based parent education programs. J Dev Behav Pediatr 21(5):356–370, 2000 11064964

Buitelaar JK, van der Gaag RJ, Cohen-Kettenis P, Melman CT: A randomized controlled trial of risperidone in the treatment of aggression in hospitalized adolescents with subaverage cognitive abilities. J Clin Psychiatry 62(4):239–248, 2001 11379837

Coccaro EF, Posternak MA, Zimmerman M: Prevalence and features of intermittent explosive disorder in a clinical setting. J Clin Psychiatry 66(10):1221–1227, 2005 16259534

Coccaro EF, McCloskey MS, Fitzgerald DA, Phan KL: Amygdala and orbitofrontal reactivity to social threat in individuals with impulsive aggression. Biol Psychiatry 62(2):168–178, 2007 17210136

Coccaro EF, Lee R, Kavoussi RJ: Aggression, suicidality, and intermittent explosive disorder: serotonergic correlates in personality disorder and healthy control subjects. Neuropsychopharmacology 35(2):435–444, 2010a 19776731

Coccaro EF, Lee R, Kavoussi RJ: Inverse relationship between numbers of 5-HT transporter binding sites and life history of aggression and intermittent explosive disorder. J Psychiatr Res 44(3):137–142, 2010b 19767013

Coccaro EF, Lee R, McCloskey M, et al: Morphometric analysis of amygdala and hippocampus shape in impulsively aggressive and healthy control subjects. J Psychiatr Res 69:80–86, 2015 26343598

Dell'Osso B, Altamura AC, Allen A, et al: Epidemiologic and clinical updates on impulse control disorders: a critical review. Eur Arch Psychiatry Clin Neurosci 256(8):464–475, 2006 16960655

Frankle WG, Lombardo I, New AS, et al: Brain serotonin transporter distribution in subjects with impulsive aggressivity: a positron emission study with [11C]McN 5652. Am J Psychiatry 162(5):915–923, 2005 15863793

Gilbertson MW, Shenton ME, Ciszewski A, et al: Smaller hippocampal volume predicts pathologic vulnerability to psychological trauma. Nat Neurosci 5(11):1242–1247, 2002 12379862

Grant JE, Kim SW: Clinical characteristics and associated psychopathology of 22 patients with kleptomania. Compr Psychiatry 43(5):378–384, 2002 12216013

Hollander E, Tracy KA, Swann AC, et al: Divalproex in the treatment of impulsive aggression: efficacy in cluster B personality disorders. Neuropsychopharmacology 28(6):1186–1197, 2003 12700713

Hollander E, Swann AC, Coccaro EF, et al: Impact of trait impulsivity and state aggression on divalproex versus placebo response in borderline personality disorder. Am J Psychiatry 162(3):621–624, 2005 15741486

Hollander E, Berlin HA, Stein DJ: Impulse-control disorders not elsewhere classified, in The American Psychiatric Publishing Textbook of Psychiatry, 5th Edition. Edited by Hales RE, Yudofsky SC, Gabbard GO. Arlington, VA, American Psychiatric Publishing, 2008, pp 777–820

Kazdin AE, Siegel T, Bass D: Cognitive problem-solving skills training and parent management training in the treatment of antisocial behavior in children. J Consult Clin Psychol 60(5):733–747, 1992 1401389

Lambie I, Ioane J, Randell I, et al: Offending behaviours of child and adolescent firesetters over a 10-year follow-up. J Child Psychol Psychiatry 54(12):1295–1307, 2013 23927002

Loeber R, Green SM, Lahey BB, et al: Findings on disruptive behavior disorders from the first decade of the developmental trends study. Clin Child Fam Psychol Rev 3(1):37–60, 2000 11228766

McElroy SL, Pope HG Jr, Hudson JI, et al: Kleptomania: a report of 20 cases. Am J Psychiatry 148(5):652–657, 1991 2018170

Phan KL, Lee R, Coccaro EF: Personality predictors of antiaggressive response to fluoxetine: inverse association with neuroticism and harm avoidance. Int Clin Psychopharmacol 26(5):278–283, 2011 21795983

Rosell DR, Thompson JL, Slifstein M, et al: Increased serotonin 2A receptor availability in the orbitofrontal cortex of physically aggressive personality disordered patients. Biol Psychiatry 67(12):1154–1162, 2010 20434136

Rowe R, Costello EJ, Angold A, et al: Developmental pathways in oppositional defiant disorder and conduct disorder. J Abnorm Psychol 119(4):726–773, 2010 21090876

Scott KM, Lim CC, Hwang I, et al: The cross-national epidemiology of DSM-IV intermittent explosive disorder. Psychol Med 46(15):3161–3172, 2016 27572872

Stanford MS, Helfritz LE, Conklin SM, et al: A comparison of anticonvulsants in the treatment of impulsive aggression. Exp Clin Psychopharmacol 13(1):72–77, 2005 15727506

Stringaris A, Goodman R: Longitudinal outcome of youth oppositionality: irritable, head-strong, and hurtful behaviors have distinctive predictions. J Am Acad Child Adolesc Psychiatry 48(4):404–412, 2009 19318881

CHAPTER 24

Substance-Related and Addictive Disorders

24.1 Which of the following substances produces its effects by increasing dopamine either through direct action or through disinhibition via GABAergic receptors?

A. Cocaine.
B. Opioids.
C. Stimulants.
D. Alcohol.

The correct response is option D: Alcohol.

Kosten et al. (2014) has outlined the target neurotransmitters and mechanisms of action for commonly used substances. Alcohol's primary mechanism of action is increase of dopamine either by direct action or possibly by disinhibition via GABAergic receptors (option D is correct).

Cocaine's primary mechanism of action is binding to presynaptic monoamine transporters and blocking their reuptake, thereby increasing synaptic levels (option A is incorrect).

Opioids' primary mechanism of action is increasing dopamine release by disinhibition of inhibitory GABAergic neurons through μ-opioid receptors (option B is incorrect).

Stimulants' primary mechanism of action is induction of norepinephrine and dopamine presynaptic release, reversing transporters (option C is incorrect). **Chapter 24 (Table 24–1 [p. 646])**

24.2 A patient comes to your office and says, "I'm considering cutting down on my drinking soon. Do you have any suggestions?" According to the Transtheoretical Model of Change, what is this patient's stage of change?

A. Precontemplation.
B. Contemplation.
C. Preparation.
D. Action.

The correct response is option C: Preparation.

In the Transtheoretical Model of Change (Prochaska and DiClemente 1982), patients have different levels of motivation for changing their substance use and may not always be ready to engage with the clinician. The five stages of change are 1) precontemplation—"I don't need to change" (option A is incorrect); 2) contemplation—"Maybe in the future I will quit using" (option B is incorrect); 3) preparation—"I'm considering planning to change soon" (option C is correct); 4) action—"I have stopped using and plan to continue sober" (option D is incorrect); and 5) maintenance—"Now that I have been sober for months, I want to continue to be abstinent." Although patients may progress sequentially through the stages of change from precontemplation to maintenance, patients often do not follow this pattern. **Chapter 24 (pp. 649–650)**

24.3   An intoxicated patient presents to the emergency department with pupillary dilation, elevated blood pressure, psychomotor agitation, chest pain, and confusion. The patient appears quite thin. Which of the following substances is most likely the cause of these symptoms?

A. Cannabis.
B. Stimulant.
C. Opioid.
D. Phencyclidine.

The correct response is option B: Stimulant.

Most substances produce clinically significant intoxication states, characterized by problematic behavioral and psychological changes that develop shortly after use of a substance. Type of substance, route of self-administration, amount used, and characteristics of the individual using the substance, such as body weight, determine whether use of a substance will result in clinically significant intoxication. Cannabis intoxication signs/symptoms include conjunctival injection, increased appetite, dry mouth, and tachycardia (option A is incorrect).

Stimulant intoxication signs/symptoms include tachycardia or bradycardia, pupillary dilation, elevated or lowered blood pressure, perspiration or chills, nausea or vomiting, evidence of weight loss, psychomotor agitation or retardation, muscular weakness, respiratory depression, chest pain, arrhythmias, confusion, seizures, dyskinesias, dystonias, and coma (option B is correct).

Opioid intoxication signs/symptoms include pupillary constriction, drowsiness, coma, slurred speech, and impairment in attention or memory (option C is incorrect).

Phencyclidine intoxication signs/symptoms include vertical or horizontal nystagmus, hyperacusis, hypertension or tachycardia, numbness or diminished responsiveness to pain, ataxia, dysarthria, muscle rigidity, seizures, and coma (option D is incorrect). **Chapter 24 (pp. 654–655; Table 24–5 [p. 655])**

24.4   A patient presents to your office reporting new-onset visual and auditory hallu-
       cinations over the past 24 hours. On examination you observe a bilateral hand
       tremor and psychomotor agitation. Vitals are significant for tachycardia and hy-
       pertension. This patient is most likely experiencing withdrawal from which of the
       following substances?

       A. Cannabis.
       B. Opioid.
       C. Alcohol.
       D. Stimulant.

       The correct response is option C: Alcohol.

       Most drugs can produce clinically significant withdrawal leading to impairment
       in social, occupational, or other important areas of functioning. These withdrawal
       states generally occur after the cessation of heavy and prolonged use of a sub-
       stance. Withdrawal symptoms associated with cannabis include irritability, anger,
       aggression, nervousness, anxiety, sleep difficulty, decreased appetite, weight loss,
       restlessness, depressed mood, abdominal pain, tremors, sweating, fever, chills,
       and headache (option A is incorrect).
           Withdrawal symptoms associated with opioids include dysphoric mood, nau-
       sea or vomiting, muscle aches, lacrimation or rhinorrhea, pupillary dilation, pilo-
       erection, and sweating (option B is incorrect).
           Withdrawal symptoms associated with alcohol include autonomic hyperactiv-
       ity; hand tremor; insomnia; nausea or vomiting; transient visual, tactile, or audi-
       tory hallucinations or illusions; psychomotor agitation; anxiety; and generalized
       tonic-clonic seizures (option C is correct).
           Acute alcohol withdrawal may lead to seizures and hallucinations (especially
       in the first 48 hours) and more severe states, such as delirium tremens (character-
       ized by disorientation, agitation, psychosis, autonomic hyperactivity, and a 5%
       mortality rate). Withdrawal symptoms associated with stimulants include fa-
       tigue; vivid, unpleasant dreams; insomnia or hypersomnia; increased appetite;
       and psychomotor retardation or agitation (option D is incorrect). **Chapter 24
       (pp. 654, 656; Table 24–6 [p. 656])**

24.5   Which of the following is a partial opioid agonist that can be administered to in-
       dividuals with opioid use disorder for opioid maintenance treatment?

       A. Buprenorphine.
       B. Benzodiazepines.
       C. Clonidine.
       D. Methadone.

       The correct response is option A: Buprenorphine.

Opioid withdrawal is treated with an induction into opioid maintenance treatment. Outcomes appear best when an individual with an opioid use disorder is provided with opioid maintenance treatment with buprenorphine (a partial opioid agonist) (option A is correct) or methadone (a long-acting full opioid agonist) (option D is incorrect).

There are nonopioid options for managing opioid withdrawal, including the α_2-adrenergic agonist clonidine (option C is incorrect).

Withdrawal syndromes from sedative, hypnotic, and anxiolytic medications, such as alprazolam or phenobarbital, are similar to alcohol withdrawal syndromes and are treated similarly with long-acting benzodiazepines or barbiturates, which also activate the GABA system (option B is incorrect). **Chapter 24 (pp. 655–656)**

24.6   According to epidemiological data, which of the following is the most frequently used illicit substance in the United States and around the world?

A. MDMA (3,4-methylenedioxymethamphetamine).
B. Cocaine.
C. Cannabis.
D. LSD (lysergic acid diethylamide).

The correct response is option C: Cannabis.

Epidemiological data consistently show that cannabinoids are the most frequently used illicit substance in the United States and around the world (option C is correct). The 12-month prevalence rates of cannabis use disorder have risen in recent years and are approximately 3.5% in adolescents and 1.5% in adults, with rates two or three times higher in men than in women (American Psychiatric Association 2013).

Many substances produce alterations in perception, mood, and cognition similar to those produced by phencyclidine. These "other hallucinogens" include phenylalkylamines, such as MDMA; the indoleamines, such as psilocybin; and the ergolines, such as LSD. Among the substance use disorders listed in DSM-5, other hallucinogen use disorder is the rarest, with an estimated 12-month prevalence rate of less than 0.5% (American Psychiatric Association 2013) (options A and D are incorrect).

Stimulant use disorder is a pattern of amphetamine-type substance, cocaine, or other stimulant use that leads to clinically significant impairment or distress. The 12-month prevalence rates for amphetamine-type stimulant use disorder and cocaine use disorder are about 0.2% for each disorder in adolescents and adults. Use is most common in younger adults and in males (especially for intravenous misuse). Males and females have similar rates of noninjection stimulant use disorders (American Psychiatric Association 2013) (option B is incorrect). **Chapter 24 (pp. 657–660)**

24.7   Which of the following psychosocial treatments for substance-related and addictive disorders conceptualizes relapse as a process while improving the ability to identify its warning signs?

A. Relapse prevention.
B. Cognitive-behavioral therapy.
C. Dialectical behavior therapy.
D. Contingency management.

The correct response is option A: Relapse prevention.

Relapse prevention conceptualizes relapse as a process while improving the ability to identify its warning signs (option A is correct). Cognitive-behavioral therapy (CBT) utilizes cognitive and behavioral techniques to help patients identify and cope with the thoughts, feelings, behaviors, and high-risk situations that can lead to relapse (option B is incorrect). Dialectical behavioral therapy combines CBT techniques for relapse with distress tolerance, acceptance, and mindfulness (option C is incorrect). Contingency management uses contingent-based reinforcements to change behavior (option D is incorrect). **Chapter 24 (Table 24–9 [p. 664])**

24.8   Which of the following is a U.S. Food and Drug Administration (FDA)–approved medication for treating opioid use disorder?

A. Acamprosate (Campral).
B. Varenicline (Chantix).
C. Bupropion (Wellbutrin, Zyban).
D. Naltrexone (ReVia, Vivitrol).

The correct response is option D: Naltrexone (ReVia, Vivitrol).

Acamprosate (Campral) is FDA approved for treating alcohol use disorder (option A is incorrect). Varenicline (Chantix) and bupropion (Wellbutrin, Zyban) are FDA approved for use in the treatment of tobacco use disorder (options B and C are incorrect). Naltrexone (ReVia, Vivitrol) is FDA approved for treating opioid use disorder (option D is correct). **Chapter 24 (Table 24–10 [p. 665])**

24.9   Which of the following is an aldehyde dehydrogenase inhibitor that is used to treat alcohol use disorder?

A. Naltrexone (ReVia).
B. Disulfiram (Antabuse).
C. Acamprosate (Campral).
D. Varenicline (Chantix).

The correct response is option B: Disulfiram (Antabuse).

There are several medications for alcohol use disorder. Disulfiram is an aldehyde dehydrogenase inhibitor, which blocks the metabolism of alcohol (option B is correct). If a person drinks alcohol while taking disulfiram, she or he experiences the disulfiram reaction, an agonizing and (ultimately) aversive syndrome characterized by increased heart rate, flushing, headache, nausea, and vomiting.

Oral naltrexone (ReVia) and long-acting injectable naltrexone (Vivitrol), which are opioid antagonists (option A is incorrect), help to reduce craving and increase the ability to maintain abstinence from or moderation in alcohol use. Acamprosate, an N-methyl-D-aspartate (NMDA) receptor modulator (option C is incorrect) also used in the treatment of alcohol use disorder, has the advantage of being metabolized by the kidney, although the evidence supporting its use is not as strong as that for naltrexone (Gueorguieva et al. 2010).

The first-line pharmacological interventions for tobacco use disorder are nicotine replacement therapy (available in many forms [e.g., gum, patch]), varenicline (a partial nicotinic receptor agonist), and bupropion (an antidepressant that inhibits the reuptake of dopamine and norepinephrine) (option D is incorrect). **Chapter 24 (p. 665)**

24.10 Which of the following medications or medication classes is considered the mainstay treatment for alcohol withdrawal?

A. Thiamine.
B. Barbiturates.
C. Clonidine.
D. Benzodiazepines.

The correct response is option D: Benzodiazepines.

In addition to addressing co-occurring medical conditions and providing vitamin supplementation, such as thiamine to prevent Wernicke's encephalopathy and Korsakoff's psychosis, the mainstay of treatment for alcohol withdrawal is administration of oral or intravenous benzodiazepines (option D is correct; option A is incorrect). Withdrawal syndromes from sedative, hypnotic, and anxiolytic medications are similar to alcohol withdrawal syndromes and are treated similarly with long-acting benzodiazepines or barbiturates (option B is incorrect). The α_2-adrenergic agonist clonidine is used for managing opioid withdrawal (option C is incorrect). **Chapter 24 (pp. 654–655, 656)**

References

American Psychiatric Association: Diagnostic and Statistical Manual of Mental Disorders, 5th Edition. Arlington, VA, American Psychiatric Association, 2013

Gueorguieva R, Wu R, Donovan D, et al: Naltrexone and combined behavioral intervention effects on trajectories of drinking in the COMBINE study. Drug Alcohol Depend 107(2–3):221–229, 2010 19969427

Kosten TR, Newton TF, De La Garza R, Haile CN: Substance-related and addictive disorders, in The American Psychiatric Publishing Textbook of Psychiatry, Sixth Edition. Edited by Hales RE, Yudofsky SC, Roberts LW. Arlington, VA, American Psychiatric Association, 2014, pp 735–814

Prochaska JO, DiClemente CC: Transtheoretical therapy: toward a more integrative model of change. Psychotherapy: Theory, Research, and Practice 19(3):276–288, 1982

CHAPTER 25

Neurocognitive Disorders

25.1   A 47-year-old man has a remote past psychiatric history of depression treated with psychotherapy. He uses marijuana occasionally. His wife brings him for a psychiatric consultation because has been showing odd behavior, with worsening over the past 5 months. He has lost interest in spending time with his children, has been making sexually inappropriate comments, and has been eating large amounts of junk food. On examination, the patient denies any recent mood or behavioral change and exhibits a flat affect and indifference to his symptoms. His memory is intact, and he has a grasp reflex on physical exam. Urine toxicology is negative. What is the most likely diagnosis?

A. Cannabis use disorder.
B. Mild neurocognitive disorder.
C. Frontotemporal lobar dementia.
D. Alzheimer's disease.

The correct response is option C: Frontotemporal lobar dementia.

Symptoms associated with cannabis intoxication include conjunctival injection, increased appetite, dry mouth, and tachycardia. Urine toxicology can detect cannabis for 3 days to 1 month, depending on amount and time course of use. There is extensive debate on the functional consequences of cannabis use disorder for people who have the disorder. While there appears to be evidence that use may lead to an amotivational syndrome and may have a "gateway" effect, for example, the data are mixed. It does appear, however, that heavy use may impair cognitive abilities and school and work functioning, and co-occurring use of other substances is quite common (Volkow et al. 2014) (option A is incorrect).

The major subcategories within the neurocognitive disorder (NCD) category in DSM-5 are delirium and mild and major NCDs. The major and mild NCDs differ in severity. Until DSM-5, psychiatrically diagnosable conditions needed to cause "clinically significant distress or impairment in social, occupational, or other important areas of functioning" (American Psychiatric Association 2000, p. 8). This level of disability is now classified as major NCD. In contrast, mild NCD involves symptoms that are minimally disabling or disruptive. The diagnosis of mild NCD indicates that the person is able to maintain independence despite the presence of impaired cognition (option B is incorrect).

The prototypical behavioral variant of frontotemporal lobar dementia presents as personality change with progressive impairment of judgment, loss of social graces, lack of self-awareness, disinhibition, stimulus boundedness, and a craving for sweets. Patients' impaired judgment, irritability, impulsiveness, and total lack of self-awareness often lead to a misdiagnosis of bipolar disorder (option C is correct).

The clinical illness of Alzheimer's disease usually manifests in the late 60s or early 70s with impairment of short-term memory that may or may not be noticed by the patient. In many cases, the disease first comes to medical attention with the advent of executive impairment. In addition to impaired recent memory, common additional findings on mental status examination are reduced attention and verbal fluency, word (noun)–finding difficulties, ideational dyspraxia (e.g., when asked to "show me how you turn a key in a lock"), constructional dyspraxia (e.g., when copying a drawing of intersecting pentagons), impaired clock drawing, and impaired abstract reasoning. Neuropsychiatric symptoms in early disease tend to be apathy and depression (option D is incorrect). **Chapter 25 (pp. 674, 690–691, 694, 696); see also Chapter 24 ("Substance-Related and Addictive Disorders"; pp. 654 [Table 24–4], 655 [Table 24–5], 658)**

25.2 Which of the following cognitive changes can be associated with normal aging?

A. Decreased vocabulary.
B. Decreased general knowledge.
C. Decreased processing speed.
D. Increased vocabulary.

The correct response is option C: Decreased processing speed.

Because many of the NCDs occur in older adults, the clinician's familiarity with known patterns of typical age-related cognitive dysfunction is important. Whereas there is a vast amount of individual variability in age-related declines, there are certain typical patterns (Institute of Medicine 2015). Vocabulary and general knowledge tend to remain stable with aging, although word-finding difficulty is common (options A, B, and D are incorrect).

Speed of information processing and psychomotor performance decline with age (option C is correct). Older adults typically take longer to respond to and process information; therefore, clinicians must adjust their evaluations to accommodate patients and to ensure that they understand what is expected of them. **Chapter 25 (p. 676)**

25.3 Which of the following is the most appropriate initial medication regimen for a patient newly diagnosed with Alzheimer's disease in keeping with the standard of care for patients with moderate to severe Alzheimer's disease?

A. An atypical antipsychotic.
B. A cholinesterase inhibitor.
C. An *N*-methyl-D-aspartate (NMDA) receptor antagonist.
D. Combination of a cholinesterase inhibitor and an NMDA receptor antagonist.

The correct response is option D: Combination of a cholinesterase inhibitor and an NMDA receptor antagonist.

Antipsychotic medications should not be routinely used to treat neuropsychiatric symptoms related to dementia because these agents are associated with an increased risk of mortality (Reus et al. 2016) (option A is incorrect).

Acetylcholinesterase inhibitors have been used with some success in patients with all stages of Alzheimer's disease and Lewy body disease, as well as in cognitive impairment associated with vascular disease (option B is incorrect).

Memantine theoretically blocks the action of NMDA-type glutamate receptors, improving synaptic transmission and/or preventing calcium release, which may provide neuroprotection. Memantine has been approved by the U.S. Food and Drug Administration for use in the treatment of moderate to severe Alzheimer's disease. Although it is frequently used in patients with early Alzheimer's disease, there are no convincing efficacy data for this use of memantine (option C is incorrect).

Cholinesterase inhibitors and memantine have different mechanisms of action; thus, combination therapy could confer additional benefits (Tariot et al. 2004). The combination of a cholinesterase inhibitor and an NMDA receptor antagonist has become the standard of care in clinical practice for patients with moderate to severe Alzheimer's disease (option D is correct). **Chapter 25 (pp. 701–702, 703)**

25.4   A 75-year-old woman is brought to the emergency department (ED) by her husband because she is displaying confusion. He reports that for months, his wife has been talking about seeing "little animals" in their bedroom at night, has had difficulty walking, and has experienced sleep problems. She becomes agitated in the ED and is given an oral medication to calm her down. An hour later, she develops severe rigidity and tremor in her arms, as well as worsening mental status. Which of the following medications is most likely to have caused these symptoms?

A. Haloperidol.
B. Quetiapine.
C. Lorazepam.
D. Diphenhydramine.

The correct response is option A: Haloperidol.

Lewy body disease often clinically resembles Alzheimer's disease; however, there are certain key features—including visual and tactile hallucinations with sudden onset and frequent remission and recurrence; marked fluctuations in cognition, with episodes of confusion lasting hours or days followed by relative clarity; and motor features of Parkinson's disease—that occur early in the disease. Antipsychotic medications should be avoided in patients with Lewy body disease when possible, because they place patients at risk for neuroleptic sensitivity or neuroleptic malignant syndrome, a condition characterized by worsening cognition, sedation, and increased or possibly irreversible acute-onset parkinsonism.

In general, high-potency first-generation antipsychotics (e.g., haloperidol) carry the greatest risk for extrapyramidal side effects (EPS) (option A is correct), whereas low-potency phenothiazines (e.g., chlorpromazine) and second-generation antipsychotics (except risperidone) carry a significantly lower risk (option B is incorrect).

The benzodiazepine lorazepam (option C is incorrect) and the anticholinergic agent diphenhydramine (option D is incorrect) are not likely to cause parkinsonism or EPS; in fact, both are used as treatments for EPS. **Chapter 25 (p. 697); see also Chapter 29 ("Psychopharmacology"; pp. 804, 809 [Table 29–4])**

25.5   Ms. C is an 80-year-old woman with a diagnosis of moderate neurocognitive disorder due to Alzheimer's disease. Her son, who is her caregiver, notices that although she is usually a very pleasant person, she has become more irritable out of frustration over her increasing limitations, such as inability to drive or cook for herself. She is occasionally agitated, and last week she yelled at him and stomped her foot. She complains of feeling "down" and "bored" at times, and has some trouble sleeping, but she denies persistent depressed mood. Which of the following would be the most appropriate first-line medication treatment for Ms. C's low mood and irritability?

A. Quetiapine.
B. Sertraline.
C. Clonazepam.
D. Valproic acid.

The correct response is option B: Sertraline.

Antipsychotic medications should not routinely be used to treat neuropsychiatric symptoms related to dementia because these agents are associated with an increased risk of mortality (option A is incorrect). Serotonin reuptake inhibitors can reduce agitation and irritability in depressed or nondepressed persons with Alzheimer's disease (Porsteinsson et al. 2014). Serotonin reuptake inhibitors should be preferred over other antipsychotic medications and sedative medication for treating behavior problems (option B is correct). Conventional hypnotics (i.e., benzodiazepines) are generally avoided in patients with dementia because of their tendency to cause oversedation and confusion (option C is incorrect). There is evidence supporting the use of valproic acid to reduce aggression in young to middle-aged adults with brain injury, but not in older adults with dementia (option D is incorrect). **Chapter 25 (pp. 703–705)**

25.6   A 72-year-old man is hospitalized for cellulitis in his leg. Psychiatry is consulted because the man's daughter is worried that her father seems "a little off." On examination, the patient is well-appearing, alert, and attentive, with a euthymic reactive affect. He denies any complaints aside from leg pain. Although he is oriented to person, place, and month and year, he is unable to remember the exact date. He is able to recall only two out of three words on a short-term memory test. The patient's daughter notes that although her father lives independently, he has "slowed down a little" over the past few months and takes "a long time" to balance his checkbook, which surprises her because he worked as an accountant until a year ago. What is the most likely diagnosis?

A. Delirium.
B. Normal aging.
C. Mild neurocognitive disorder.
D. Major neurocognitive disorder.

The correct response is option C: Mild neurocognitive disorder.

Delirium typically has an abrupt onset and a course of fluctuating severity rather than a subacute onset and persistent course (option A is incorrect). Normal aging can entail gradual slowing of processing speed and word-finding difficulties but does not usually involve a rapid decline in memory relative to premorbid status (option B is incorrect). Mild cognitive problems requiring increased effort with instrumental activities of daily living but not causing significant functional impairment are most consistent with a DSM-5 (American Psychiatric Association 2013) diagnosis of mild neurocognitive disorder (option C is correct). Major neurocognitive disorder involves significant cognitive decline from previous performance levels and deficits severe enough to interfere with the capacity for independence in everyday activities (option D is incorrect). **Chapter 25 (pp. 674, 676, 689, 691)**

25.7   A 65-year-old war veteran with a history of alcohol use was witnessed by his neighbor to fall down the stairs, sustaining a head strike but no loss of consciousness. In the emergency department, the patient's computed tomography head scan results are unremarkable, but X ray reveals a fracture in the left hip. Following hip surgery, the patient receives a single dose of alprazolam for sleep. He appears confused the following day and is not oriented to place (he believes he is in a hotel) or time (he states the year as 1898). In the following days, the patient is noted to show unusual eye movements. He tells nurses stories about himself that are inconsistent with information in the chart. He does not appear to remember the names of nurses or doctors or their directions regarding his activities. Neurological exam findings are otherwise nonfocal. Based on this patient's symptom profile, which of the following is the most likely underlying diagnosis?

A. Wernicke-Korsakoff syndrome.
B. Benzodiazepine-induced delirium.
C. Dissociative amnesia.
D. Postoperative cognitive dysfunction.

The correct response is option A: Wernicke-Korsakoff syndrome.

Korsakoff's syndrome results from thiamine deficiency, typically associated with malnutrition accompanying long-term alcohol abuse, and is often preceded by the delirium, ophthalmoplegia, and ataxia of Wernicke's encephalopathy. In DSM-5, the amnestic confabulatory disorder known as Korsakoff's syndrome would receive a diagnosis of alcohol-induced major neurocognitive disorder, amnestic-confabulatory type, persistent (option A is correct).

In contrast to the persistence of Korsakoff's syndrome, the amnestic episodes that occur with short-acting benzodiazepines (option B is incorrect) are transient.

In dissociative amnesia (see Chapter 16, "Dissociative Disorders"), which can be associated with trauma and head injury, individuals lose the ability to recall what happened during a specific period of time, which can range from minutes to years (option C is incorrect). People with dissociative amnesia demonstrate not vagueness or spotty memory, but rather a loss of *any* autobiographical–episodic memory for a finite period. Dissociative amnesia does not, however, involve a difficulty in memory storage, as in Wernicke-Korsakoff syndrome.

Postoperative cognitive dysfunction is characterized as a chronic level of dysfunction that manifests after a medical/surgical procedure that is followed by a delirium (option D is incorrect). **Chapter 25 (pp. 681, 699–700); see also Chapter 16 ("Dissociative Disorders"; p. 461)**

25.8 Which of the following strategies for the prevention of dementia has been shown to have cognitive benefits?

A. Physical exercise.
B. Vitamin E.
C. Nonsteroidal anti-inflammatory drugs (NSAIDs).
D. Cognitive exercises.

The correct response is option A: Physical exercise.

Vitamin E has been studied extensively in the treatment of mild cognitive impairment (MCI) and Alzheimer's dementia. However, evidence for its benefit in MCI or Alzheimer's disease is lacking (option B is incorrect).

NSAIDs have been associated with decreased dementia risk, but randomized clinical trials have not supported their preventive ability (Wang et al. 2015) (option C is incorrect).

Evidence that cognitive exercises have a preventive effect in dementia is mixed at best, with the strongest criticism being that skills fail to generalize beyond the task learned (Simons et al. 2016) (option D is incorrect).

In contrast, there appear to be a variety of cognitive and brain-based benefits from physical exercise that endure if exercise is maintained (Erickson et al. 2014; Oberlin et al. 2016) (option A is correct). **Chapter 25 (pp. 702, 705)**

25.9   A 60-year-old woman is diagnosed with a nonfluent aphasia after a stroke. Which of the following tasks would present the *least* amount of difficulty for this patient?

A. Writing a sentence.
B. Repeating a phrase.
C. Following simple commands.
D. Reading aloud.

The correct response is option C: Following simple commands.

Patients with nonfluent aphasia generally understand what is said to them and can obey simple commands (option C is correct), but they have difficulty with repetition (option B is incorrect), reading aloud (option D is incorrect), and writing (option A is incorrect). **Chapter 25 (p. 679)**

25.10   Which of the following positron emission tomography (PET) scan findings is most typical of Lewy body disease?

A. Reduced temporoparietal and posterior cingulate metabolism.
B. Reduced frontotemporal metabolism.
C. Reduced temporoparietal and occipital metabolism.
D. Reduced metabolism in the area of a prior stroke.

The correct response is option C: Reduced temporoparietal and occipital metabolism.

Lewy body disease often clinically resembles Alzheimer's disease, but certain key features—including visual and tactile hallucinations with sudden onset and frequent remission and recurrence; marked fluctuations in cognition, with episodes of confusion lasting hours or days followed by relative clarity; and motor features of Parkinson's disease—can help differentiate the two conditions. Patients with Lewy body disease show reduced temporoparietal and occipital metabolism on PET scan (option C is correct).

Reduced temporoparietal and posterior cingulate metabolism is more commonly associated with Alzheimer's disease (option A is incorrect).

Reduced frontotemporal metabolism is more commonly associated with frontotemporal lobar degeneration (option B is incorrect).

Reduced metabolism in the area of a stroke or strokes is more commonly associated with cerebrovascular disease (option D is incorrect). **Chapter 25 (pp. 693 [Table 25–9], 697)**

References

American Psychiatric Association: Diagnostic and Statistical Manual of Mental Disorders, 4th Edition, Text Revision. Washington, DC, American Psychiatric Association, 2000
American Psychiatric Association: Diagnostic and Statistical Manual of Mental Disorders, 5th Edition. Arlington, VA, American Psychiatric Association, 2013

Erickson KI, Leckie RL, Weinstein AM: Physical activity, fitness, and gray matter volume. Neurobiol Aging 35 (suppl 2):S20–S28, 2014 24952993

Institute of Medicine: Cognitive Aging: Progress in Understanding and Opportunities for Action. Washington, DC, National Academies Press, 2015

Oberlin LE, Verstynen TD, Burzynska AZ, et al: White matter microstructure mediates the relationship between cardiorespiratory fitness and spatial working memory in older adults. Neuroimage 131:91–101, 2016 26439513

Porsteinsson AP, Drye LT, Pollock BG, et al: Effect of citalopram on agitation in Alzheimer disease: the CitAD randomized clinical trial. JAMA 311(7):682–691, 2014 24549548

Reus VI, Fochtmann LJ, Eyler AE, et al: The American Psychiatric Association practice guideline on the use of antipsychotics to treat agitation or psychosis in patients with dementia. Am J Psychiatry 173(5):543–546, 2016 27133416

Simons DJ, Boot WR, Charness N, et al: Do "brain-training" programs work? Psychol Sci Public Interest 17(3):103–186, 2016 27697851

Tariot PN, Farlow MR, Grossberg GT, et al; Memantine Study Group: Memantine treatment in patients with moderate to severe Alzheimer disease already receiving donepezil: a randomized controlled trial. JAMA 291(3):317–324, 2004 14734594

Volkow ND, Baler RD, Compton WM, et al: Adverse health effects of marijuana use. N Engl J Med 370(23):2219–2227, 2014 24897085

Wang J, Tan L, Wang HF, et al: Anti-inflammatory drugs and risk of Alzheimer's disease: an updated systematic review and meta-analysis. J Alzheimers Dis 44(2):385–396, 2015 25227314

CHAPTER 26

Personality Pathology and Personality Disorders

26.1 Studies indicate that at least what percentage of patients evaluated in clinical settings have a personality disorder?

   A. 15%.
   B. 30%.
   C. 50%.
   D. 70%.

The correct response is option C: 50%.

Studies indicate that at least 50% of patients evaluated in clinical settings have a personality disorder (Zimmerman et al. 2005) (option C is correct; options A, B, and D are incorrect), often co-occurring with other mental disorders, and many more patients have significant personality problems that do not meet criteria for a personality disorder diagnosis, making personality pathology one of the most common psychopathologies encountered by mental health care professionals. Personality disorders are also common in the general population, with an estimated prevalence of about 11% (Torgersen 2014). **Chapter 26 (p. 711)**

26.2 Section III of DSM-5 includes the Alternative DSM-5 Model for Personality Disorders (AMPD). Which of the following is included as a specific personality disorder in this model?

   A. Schizotypal personality disorder.
   B. Schizoid personality disorder.
   C. Dependent personality disorder.
   D. Histrionic personality disorder.

The correct response is option A: Schizotypal personality disorder.

In the DSM-5 (American Psychiatric Association 2013) AMPD, only six distinct personality disorders were retained: antisocial, avoidant, borderline, narcissistic, obsessive-compulsive, and schizotypal (option A is correct).

Growing evidence suggests that the other four categories—dependent, histrionic, paranoid, and schizoid personality disorders—might be better represented as impairments in personality functioning and pathological personality traits (i.e., as personality disorder—trait specified [PD-TS], a diagnosis applicable for individuals who have moderate or greater impairment in personality functioning but do not meet criteria for a specific personality disorder) (options B, C, and D are incorrect). **Chapter 26 (pp. 728, 740)**

26.3   Which of the following statements about treatment of obsessive-compulsive personality disorder (OCPD) is *true*?

A. Patients with OCPD do not usually respond to any type of treatment.
B. Patients with OCPD often respond well to serotonin reuptake inhibitor medications.
C. Patients with OCPD often respond well to dialectical behavior therapy.
D. Patients with OCPD often respond well to psychoanalytic psychotherapy or psychoanalysis.

The correct response is option D: Patients with OCPD often respond well to psychoanalytic psychotherapy or psychoanalysis.

Persons with OCPD may seem difficult to treat because of their excessive intellectualization and difficulty expressing emotion. However, these patients often respond well to psychoanalytic psychotherapy or psychoanalysis (option D is correct; option A is incorrect). Cognitive techniques may also be used to diminish the patient's excessive need for control and perfection. Although patients may resist group treatment because of their need for control, dynamically oriented groups that focus on feelings may provide insight and increase patients' comfort with exploring and expressing new affects.

The serotonin reuptake inhibitors represent the first-line pharmacotherapy intervention for obsessive-compulsive disorder (Bandelow et al. 2008) (option B is incorrect).

Dialectical behavior therapy, a behavioral treatment consisting of once-weekly individual psychotherapy and twice-weekly group skills training, can effectively diminish the self-destructive behaviors and hospitalizations of patients with borderline personality disorder (Linehan et al. 2006) (option C is incorrect). **Chapter 26 (pp. 735, 738); see also Chapter 14 ("Obsessive-Compulsive and Related Disorders"; p. 375)**

26.4   A 32-year-old man presents to your office for a consultation after being fired from his third job in 2 years. Evaluation reveals impulsivity, separation insecurity, emotional lability, hostility, and heightened anxiety. Which of the following diagnoses is suggested by this symptom profile?

A. Antisocial personality disorder.
B. Borderline personality disorder.
C. Narcissistic personality disorder.
D. Histrionic personality disorder.

The correct response is option B: Borderline personality disorder.

Borderline personality disorder is defined by characteristic impairments in personality functioning that are at a severe level and by four or more of the following seven pathological personality traits: emotional lability, anxiousness, separation insecurity, depressivity, impulsivity, risk taking, and hostility (option B is correct).

The diagnostic algorithm requires at least one of the latter three traits, because borderline personality disorder has traits from both the negative affectivity and the disinhibition or antagonism domains and is not typically represented by only emotional dysregulation. Antisocial personality disorder is characterized by specific impairments in personality functioning at a moderate or greater level and by six or more of the following seven pathological personality traits: manipulativeness, callousness, deceitfulness, hostility, risk taking, impulsivity, and irresponsibility (option A is incorrect).

Narcissistic personality disorder is characterized by grandiosity and attention seeking, inflated or deflated self-appraisal, and feelings of entitlement (option C is incorrect).

Histrionic personality disorder, characterized by excessive emotionality and attention seeking (option D is incorrect), is one of four DSM-5 Section II personality disorders not included as specific diagnoses in the Alternative DSM-5 Model for Personality Disorders (the other three are). **Chapter 26 (pp. 718 [Table 26–3], 729, 732, 735–736)**

26.5   Which of the following statements about diagnosing personality disorders in children and adolescents is *true*?

A. Personality disorders are usually diagnosed by late childhood or early adolescence, as personality traits remain stable over time.
B. Personality disorders should be diagnosed sparingly in children, whose personalities are still developing, but can be diagnosed in adolescents, whose personalities are fully formed.
C. Personality disorders should be diagnosed sparingly in children and adolescents, as their personalities are still developing.
D. Personality disorders should be diagnosed only in late adulthood, to ensure stability of symptoms over time prior to diagnosis.

The correct response is option C: Personality disorders should be diagnosed sparingly in children and adolescents, as their personalities are still developing.

Because the personalities of children and adolescents are still developing, personality disorders should be diagnosed sparingly in this age group (option C is correct). Early diagnoses may prove to be wrong, given that stage-specific difficulties of childhood or adolescence, such as submissiveness and dependency or hostility and risk taking, often resolve as the person matures (options A and B are incorrect).

It is often preferable to defer diagnosis until early adulthood, at which time a personality disorder diagnosis may be appropriate if the features appear to be more pervasive and stable (option D is incorrect). **Chapter 26 (pp. 723–724)**

26.6   What is the prevalence of personality disorders in the general population?

   A. 7.5%.
   B. 11%.
   C. 22%.
   D. 31%.

The correct response is option B: 11%.

Personality disorders are common in the general population, with an estimated prevalence of about 11% (Torgersen 2014) (option B is correct; options A, C, and D are incorrect). **Chapter 26 (p. 711)**

26.7   Which of the following personality disorders is most prevalent in the general population?

   A. Borderline personality disorder.
   B. Schizotypal personality disorder.
   C. Antisocial personality disorder.
   D. Obsessive-compulsive personality disorder.

The correct response is option D: Obsessive-compulsive personality disorder.

Obsessive-compulsive personality disorder is one of the most common personality disorders in the general population, with a prevalence of about 2.5% (option D is correct). The prevalences of the other three personality disorders listed as options are as follows: antisocial personality disorder, 1.8%; borderline personality disorder, 1.6%; schizotypal personality disorder, 1.3% (Torgersen 2014) (options A, B, and C are incorrect). **Chapter 26 (pp. 730, 733, 737, 739)**

References

American Psychiatric Association: Diagnostic and Statistical Manual of Mental Disorders, 5th Edition. Arlington, VA, American Psychiatric Association, 2013

Bandelow B, Zohar J, Hollander E, et al: World Federation of Societies of Biological Psychiatry (WFSBP) guidelines for the pharmacological treatment of anxiety, obsessive-compulsive and post-traumatic stress disorders—first revision. World J Biol Psychiatry 9(4):248–312, 2008 18949648

Linehan MM, Comtois KA, Murray AM, et al: Two-year randomized controlled trial and follow-up of dialectical behavior therapy vs. therapy by experts for suicidal behaviors and borderline personality disorder. Arch Gen Psychiatry 63(7):757–766, 2006 16818865

Torgersen S: Prevalence, sociodemographics, and functional impairment, in Textbook of Personality Disorders, 2nd Edition. Edited by Oldham JM, Skodol AE, Bender DS. Washington, DC, American Psychiatric Publishing, 2014, pp 109–130

Zimmerman M, Rothchild L, Chelminski I: The prevalence of DSM-IV personality disorders in psychiatric outpatients. Am J Psychiatry 162(10):1911–1918, 2005 16199838

CHAPTER 27

Paraphilic Disorders

27.1 A colleague asks your advice concerning a 20-year-old student who told her that a man had rubbed his genitals on her arm during a crowded bus ride. Your colleague notes that she has heard of similar incidents from other students and does not recall whether this behavior has a specific name. You reply that this behavior is most consistent with which of the following?

A. Fetishistic disorder.
B. Frotteuristic disorder.
C. Sexual masochism disorder.
D. Exhibitionistic disorder.

The correct response is option B: Frotteuristic disorder.

Frotteuristic disorder involves touching or rubbing against a nonconsenting person, or having fantasies about or urges to do so (Långström 2010) (option B is correct).

The main feature of *fetishistic disorder* is sexual arousal that often involves the use of nonliving objects, such as women's underpants, bras, stockings, shoes, boots, or other apparel, but may also include a highly specific focus on nongenital body parts (option A is incorrect).

The DSM-5 diagnostic criteria for *sexual masochism disorder* require intense sexually arousing fantasies, urges, or behaviors involving the act of being humiliated, beaten, bound, or otherwise made to suffer (option C is incorrect).

Exhibitionistic disorder is identified as either the exposure of one's genitals to an unsuspecting person or the manifestation of urges to do so in the form of fantasy (option D is incorrect). **Chapter 27 (pp. 751–752)**

27.2 The mother of an 18-year-old man requests a consultation. She recently discovered that her son is in a consensual sexual relationship with a 16-year-old boy. She is employed as a court reporter and says she recently heard of a similar relationship where the older partner was convicted of a crime and labeled a "sexual offender" by the state. She shares her concern that her son might be a "pedophile" and requests an evaluation for him. Which of the following would be the most appropriate response?

A. Recommend that the son receive treatment for pedophilic disorder.
B. Suggest a phallometric assessment to gather more information.
C. Suggest visual reaction time testing with the Abel Assessment for Sexual Interest.
D. Advise the mother that an 18-year-old man's consensual sexual relationship with a 16-year-old partner does not meet criteria for any psychiatric disorder.

The correct response is option D: Advise the mother that an 18-year-old man's consensual sexual relationship with a 16-year-old partner does not meet criteria for any psychiatric disorder.

Pedophilic disorder is defined as intense, recurrent, sexually arousing fantasies, urges, or behaviors involving a prepubescent child or children (generally age 13 years or younger) over a period of at least 6 months. To receive a diagnosis of pedophilic disorder, an individual must be at least 16 years of age and at least 5 years older than the child (option A is incorrect). An 18-year-old man in a consensual sexual relationship with a 16-year old boy is not indicative of a paraphilic disorder (option D is correct). However, it is important to realize that the legal and medical definitions of what constitutes paraphilic behavior or pedophilia/pedophilic disorder can sometimes differ. The DSM-5 criterion specifying that the individual diagnosed with pedophilic disorder be at least 5 years older than the child does not necessarily hold in the legal system, and thus a 16- or 17-year-old who has sex with a 15-year-old may still be labeled as a sexual offender.

Phallometric assessments (i.e., measurements of penile erection) have been used to objectively assess the sexual arousal of individuals who have engaged in paraphilic behavior. Although phallometric assessments can show the degree of sexual preference among various stimulus categories, they cannot determine whether someone has engaged in paraphilic behavior or has committed a sexual offense (option B is incorrect).

The Abel Assessment for Sexual Interest (Abel et al. 2001) is used to measure the subject's viewing time of specially designed photographs of clothed models. Tests of visual reaction time are based on the assumption that the length of viewing time of stimuli may correlate to degree of sexual interest (option C is incorrect). **Chapter 27 (pp. 752–753, 756–758)**

27.3 Which of the following statements regarding biological treatments of paraphilic disorders is *true*?

A. Surgical castration (orchiectomy) should be used for violent sexual offenders, because it is a permanent and irreversible treatment.
B. No medications on the market in the United States have been approved by the U.S. Food and Drug Administration (FDA) for treating paraphilic disorders or for reducing paraphilic fantasy and behavior.
C. Hormonal treatment should be used for all sexual offenders, given that these agents are effective and risk-free.
D. Hormonal treatment should be used only for sexual offenders who meet criteria for antisocial personality disorder.

The correct response is option B: No medications on the market in the United States have been approved by the U.S. Food and Drug Administration (FDA) for treating paraphilic disorders or for reducing paraphilic fantasy and behavior.

No medications on the market in the United States have been approved by the FDA for treating paraphilic disorders or for reducing paraphilic fantasy and behavior (option B is correct). Although orchiectomy can reduce sexual desire, the effects can be reversed by testosterone replacement (option A is incorrect). Hormonal treatment can be reversed through testosterone replacement and may have some risk (option C is incorrect). The presence of antisocial personality disorder is not known to increase the risk of sexual offending, and hormonal treatment is not a recognized treatment for antisocial personality disorder (option D is incorrect). **Chapter 27 (pp. 760–761)**

27.4   A 23-year-old man comes to your office requesting treatment. He tells you that while vacationing in Europe, he visited a public beach where some women were topless, and he became sexually aroused. He noted that the beach was crowded and that other visitors did not seem surprised that the women were topless. He is worried that something may be wrong with him, and he has "diagnosed" himself with voyeuristic disorder after doing some research on the internet. After completing a full history, you decide which of the following?

A. He meets criteria for voyeuristic disorder.
B. He has an unspecified paraphilic disorder.
C. He meets criteria for exhibitionistic disorder.
D. Sexual arousal after incidental exposure to naked people in a public area is normal.

The correct response is option D: Sexual arousal after incidental exposure to naked people in a public area is normal.

The desire to view naked individuals is not necessarily unusual, but the professional should be looking for qualitative and quantitative differences from normal behavior, fantasy, or urges (option D is correct).

Voyeuristic disorder is commonly viewed as the act of becoming sexually aroused by fantasy or the actual viewing of unsuspecting and nonconsenting people who are naked, disrobing, or engaging in sexual activity when they do not realize they are being watched or have not given permission (Långström 2010) (option A is incorrect).

The diagnosis *unspecified paraphilic disorder* is used in situations where a paraphilic disorder appears to be present but does not meet full criteria for any of the listed disorders and either the clinician chooses not to specify why the disorder does not meet full criteria or there is not enough information to make a more specific diagnosis (option B is incorrect).

Exhibitionistic disorder is identified as either the exposure of one's genitals to an unsuspecting person or the manifestation of urges to do so in the form of fantasy (option C is incorrect). **Chapter 27 (pp. 750–751, 754)**

27.5   A mother brings in her 12-year-old son for an assessment. She explains that she recently found some printouts of photographs in her son's room that showed women in various states of undress. During the interview with the son, he adamantly denies any history of sexual activity. In documenting the case afterward, which of the following would be the best working diagnosis?

A. Pedophilic disorder.
B. Fetishistic disorder.
C. Pedophilic disorder, exclusive type.
D. Normal sexual interest.

The correct response is option D: Normal sexual interest.

The desire to view naked individuals is not necessarily unusual; the professional should be looking for qualitative and quantitative differences from normal behavior, fantasy, or urges. The above child does not meet criteria for any condition listed above nor any other specific sexual/paraphilic disorder (option D is correct).

Pedophilic disorder is defined as intense, recurrent, sexually arousing fantasies, urges, or behaviors involving a prepubescent child or children (generally age 13 years or younger) over a period of at least 6 months. A diagnosis is suggested if an individual has acted on these urges or if the urges or fantasies caused marked distress. To receive a diagnosis of pedophilic disorder, the individual must have been at least age 16 years and at least 5 years older than the child (option A is incorrect).

The DSM-5 criteria for pedophilic disorder include specifiers for an *exclusive type* (only attracted to children) versus a *nonexclusive type* (attracted to both adults and children) (option C is incorrect).

The main feature of *fetishistic disorder* is sexual arousal that often involves the use of nonliving objects, such as women's underpants, bras, stockings, shoes, boots, or other apparel, but may also include a highly specific focus on nongenital body parts (option B is incorrect). **Chapter 27 (pp. 751–754)**

27.6   A 55-year-old woman brings her 92-year-old father in for an evaluation. She is seeking advice because her father recently exposed himself to other patients and staff at the assisted living facility where he resides. During the patient evaluation, it is clear that the man shows a pattern of progressive memory loss over the last several years. More recently, he has been having difficulty performing some self-care tasks without assistance. There is no previous history of sexual inappropriateness. The woman is distraught, fearing that her father will be evicted from the facility if he exposes himself again. Which of the following statements represents the most accurate understanding of this patient's symptoms?

A. This patient has exhibitionistic disorder.
B. This patient's behavior may be the result of cognitive impairment and not represent a paraphilic disorder.

C. This patient should be prescribed hormonal treatment to lower his testosterone level.

D. This patient should be prescribed high-dosage selective serotonin reuptake inhibitor (SSRI) treatment.

The correct response is option B: This patient's behavior may be the result of cognitive impairment and not represent a paraphilic disorder.

Inappropriate sexual behavior is not always the result of a paraphilia. A patient with dementia can behave in a sexually inappropriate manner (e.g., masturbate in a room full of people) because of cognitive impairment. In this specific example, it is likely that the patient's new pattern of exposing himself is related to cognitive impairment, as suggested by his history of progressive memory loss (option B is correct).

Exhibitionistic disorder is identified as either the exposure of one's genitals to an unsuspecting person or the manifestation of urges to do so in the form of fantasy (option A is incorrect).

The main target of hormonal treatment has been the lowering of testosterone levels. Some studies (e.g., Studer et al. 2005) demonstrated a relationship between high testosterone and sexual violence. Although these results suggest that there may be cases in which medical lowering of testosterone levels may be helpful in decreasing the risk of recidivism in men with paraphilic disorders, one has to keep in mind that even if sexual desire is decreased pharmacologically, this does not necessarily change the patients' sexual interest or their behavior (option C is incorrect).

Treatment using SSRIs (typically at higher dosages than those used for other disorders) may be applicable to different types of sexually inappropriate behaviors; however, for various reasons (e.g., difficulty in recruitment, stigma, ethical issues), there have been no double-blind, placebo-controlled studies to test the efficacy of SSRIs in treating paraphilic disorders (option D is incorrect). **Chapter 27 (pp. 750–751, 756, 760, 762)**

27.7 A 23-year-old man is directed to your office by his parole officer. He shares that he has been arrested several times for theft of women's undergarments. During further review of his history, he shares that he has a difficult time achieving orgasm when masturbating unless he is looking at the undergarments. After completing a review of his sexual and psychiatric history, you establish a diagnosis of which of the following?

A. Transvestic disorder.
B. Fetishistic disorder.
C. Other specified paraphilic disorder.
D. Sexual sadism disorder.

The correct response is option B: Fetishistic disorder.

The main feature of *fetishistic disorder* is sexual arousal that often involves the use of nonliving objects, such as women's underpants, bras, stockings, shoes, boots, or other apparel, but may also include a highly specific focus on nongenital body parts (option B is correct).

DSM-5 *transvestic disorder* involves cross-dressing, in most cases producing sexual arousal (option A is incorrect).

The diagnosis *other specified paraphilic disorder* is used in cases where the clinician can specify the reason that full criteria are not met. Presentations for which the "other specified" designation would be appropriate include—but are not limited to—recurrent and intense sexual arousal involving telephone scatologia (obscene phone calls), necrophilia (corpses), zoophilia (animals), coprophilia (feces), klismaphilia (enemas), or urophilia (urine) (option C is incorrect).

Sexual sadism involves real acts (not simulated) in which sexual arousal is achieved from the psychological or physical suffering of another nonconsenting individual (option D is incorrect). **Chapter 27 (pp. 752, 753, 754)**

27.8   You are asked by a local prosecutor to evaluate a 25-year-old man who was arrested and charged with a criminal offense after making several obscene telephone calls to a woman. The prosecutor explains that the patient was observed masturbating while peering through the window of the woman, who was changing at the time. While taking a sexual history, the man shares that since puberty he has been making similar phone calls, where he would repeatedly curse or graphically describe sexual practices. He explains he initially found the calls quite sexually arousing but has found that making these calls, while observing the recipient either undressing or engaged in sexual activity, is even more arousing. You establish a diagnosis of which of the following?

A. Sexual sadism disorder.
B. Exhibitionistic disorder.
C. Antisocial personality disorder.
D. Telephone scatologia with voyeuristic disorder.

The correct response is option D: Telephone scatologia with voyeuristic disorder.

The diagnosis *other specified paraphilic disorder* is used in cases where the clinician can specify the reason that full criteria are not met. Presentations for which the "other specified" designation would be appropriate include—but are not limited to—recurrent and intense sexual arousal involving telephone scatologia (obscene phone calls) (option D is correct).

Sexual sadism involves real acts (not simulated) in which sexual arousal is achieved from the psychological or physical suffering of another nonconsenting individual (option A is incorrect).

Exhibitionistic disorder is identified as either the exposure of one's genitals to an unsuspecting person or the manifestation of urges to do so in the form of fantasy. When the behavior does occur, it may involve masturbation during the exposure, and in some cases the individual tries to surprise or shock the observer (option B is incorrect).

Although some individuals with antisocial personality disorder also commit deviant sexual acts, such behaviors usually are part of the individuals' overall disregard for societal norms and sanctions and are not necessarily indicative of a deviant sexual interest (option C is incorrect). **Chapter 27 (pp. 751, 752, 754, 756)**

27.9 While attending a conference, you have the opportunity to hear a lecture by a prominent forensic psychiatrist. During the lecture, he speaks about Jeffrey Dahmer, who at age 16 reported fantasies of attacking an unsuspecting runner, then having sex with the subdued victim. You learn that Mr. Dahmer eventually was arrested for serial murder and revealed that he would often masturbate while standing over the corpses of his victims. After the lecture concludes, you decide that Mr. Dahmer most likely had which of the following disorders?

A. Sexual masochism disorder.
B. Sexual sadism disorder.
C. Voyeuristic disorder.
D. Exhibitionistic disorder.

The correct response is option B: Sexual sadism disorder.

Sexual sadism involves real acts (not simulated) in which sexual arousal is achieved from the psychological or physical suffering of a nonconsenting individual (option B is correct).

The DSM-5 diagnostic criteria for *sexual masochism disorder* require intense sexually arousing fantasies, urges, or behaviors involving the act of being humiliated, beaten, bound, or otherwise made to suffer (option A is incorrect).

Voyeuristic disorder is commonly viewed as the act of becoming sexually aroused by fantasy or the actual viewing of unsuspecting and nonconsenting people who are naked, disrobing, or engaging in sexual activity when they do not realize they are being watched or have not given permission (Långström 2010) (option C is incorrect).

Exhibitionistic disorder is identified as either the exposure of one's genitals to an unsuspecting person or the manifestation of urges to do so in the form of fantasy (option D is incorrect). **Chapter 27 (pp. 750–751, 752)**

References

Abel GG, Jordan A, Hand CG, et al: Classification models of child molesters utilizing the Abel Assessment for sexual interest. Child Abuse Negl 25(5):703–718, 2001 11428430
American Psychiatric Association: Diagnostic and Statistical Manual of Mental Disorders, 5th Edition. Arlington, VA, American Psychiatric Association, 2013
Långström N: The DSM diagnostic criteria for exhibitionism, voyeurism, and frotteurism. Arch Sex Behav 39(2):317–324, 2010 19924524
Studer LH, Aylwin AS, Reddon JR: Testosterone, sexual offense recidivism, and treatment effect among adult male sex offenders. Sex Abuse 17(2):171–181, 2005 15974423

CHAPTER 28

Precision Psychiatry

28.1   What large-scale U.S. research project was the first to bridge the gap between scientific and technological advances and their clinical applications in the field of cardiology?

A. The Precision Medicine Initiative.
B. The BRAIN Initiative.
C. The Framingham study.
D. The Research Domain Criteria (RDoC) project.

The correct response is option C: The Framingham study.

The Framingham study, which was inspired by Franklin Delano Roosevelt's death from cardiovascular disease (Mahmood et al. 2014), spawned the assessment of standard vital signs and a subsequent range of imaging techniques capable of linking precise insights about the organ of interest (the heart) to treatment indications and even prevention (option C is correct).

In 2015, the Obama administration launched the Precision Medicine Initiative, a major research effort aimed at improving health and changing the way we treat disease (Office of the Press Secretary 2015). In the press release announcing this initiative, *precision medicine* was defined as "an innovative approach that takes into account individual differences in people's genes, environments, and lifestyles," thereby allowing doctors to tailor treatment to individual patients (option A is incorrect).

This federal Precision Medicine Initiative is paralleled by two federal research efforts focused specifically on psychiatry and neurosciences. First, the "BRAIN Initiative" is aimed at developing neurotechnologies for demystifying brain disorders, including psychiatric disorders (Markoff 2013) (option B is incorrect).

Second, the National Institute of Mental Health (NIMH) is pioneering the RDoC project (Insel et al. 2010), which has initiated a research approach to generating a neurobiologically valid framework for classifying psychiatric disorders and for generating novel interventions related to neurobiological underpinnings (option D is incorrect). Together, the Precision Medicine, BRAIN, and RDoC initiatives will support and promote significant advances in precision psychiatry.
Chapter 28 (pp. 772–773)

28.2   Which of the following terms refers to the relationships among brain regions in the brain at rest?

A. Default mode.
B. Functional connectivity.
C. Biotype.
D. Stratified medicine.

The correct response is option B: Functional connectivity.

Modern imaging technologies allow researchers to see the brain at work, examine differences in how an individual's brain is functioning, and use those differences to predict what treatments may work best for that individual. Researchers using modern imaging technologies have identified an intrinsic neural architecture of large-scale circuits, and meta-analyses examining the relationships among brain regions in the brain at rest—termed *functional connectivity* (Cole et al. 2014) (option B is correct)—have demonstrated the universality of this intrinsic architecture. There is converging evidence that these same intrinsic circuits are disrupted in psychiatric disorders (Williams 2016). For example, the *default mode* circuit, which has core nodes in the anterior and posterior cingulate cortex, has been implicated in self-reflective thought (option A is incorrect).

Biotypes are subtype profiles that coherently map neurobiological disruptions onto symptoms and behaviors, take into account life experience and context, and are relevant to guiding treatment choices (Williams 2016) (option C is incorrect).

Stratified medicine focuses on identifying subgroups of patients who will benefit from treatments as a step toward a fully personalized approach that tailors treatments to individual people (option D is incorrect). **Chapter 28 (pp. 771–772, 775)**

28.3   High functional connectivity in which of the following intrinsic circuits is hypothesized to reflect maladaptive self-referential thoughts such as rumination and worry?

A. The attention circuit.
B. The default mode circuit.
C. The salience circuit.
D. The reward circuit.

The correct response is option B: The default mode circuit.

The *default mode circuit* has core nodes in the anterior and posterior cingulate cortex and has been implicated in self-reflective thought. High functional connectivity in this circuit is thought to reflect maladaptive self-referential thought such as rumination and worry (Hamilton et al. 2015) (option B is correct).

The *salience circuit* has core nodes in the anterior cingulate cortex, amygdala, and anterior insula and is thought to detect salient internal sensations and external changes. Low functional connectivity in this circuit has been associated with social anxiety disorder and may reflect anxious avoidance (reviewed in Williams 2016) (option C is incorrect).

The *attention circuit* has core nodes in the medial superior frontal cortex, anterior inferior parietal lobe, anterior insula, and precuneus. Low functional connectivity in this circuit is thought to reflect the inattention symptoms common across psychiatric disorders (Williams 2016) (option A is incorrect).

Large-scale circuits related to specific processing of threat, reward, and cognitive load have also been identified. The extent to which these circuits are engaged by threatening, rewarding, or cognitively challenging tasks varies across individuals and may be associated with specific biomarkers of psychopathology. For example, decreased activation in the ventral striatum, a core node of the *reward circuit*, has been associated with anhedonia (Der-Avakian and Markou 2012) (option D is incorrect). **Chapter 28 (pp. 775–776)**

28.4   Which of the following symptoms is associated with decreased activation in the ventral striatum?

A. Anhedonia.
B. Inattention.
C. Anxiety.
D. Rumination.

The correct response is option A: Anhedonia.

Meta-analyses examining the relationships among brain regions in the brain at rest, termed *functional connectivity* (Cole et al. 2014), have demonstrated the universality of an intrinsic neural architecture of large-scale circuits, and there is converging evidence that these intrinsic circuits are disrupted in psychiatric disorders (Williams 2016). The *default mode*, *salience*, and *attention* circuits are of particular interest.

The *default mode circuit* has core nodes in the anterior and posterior cingulate cortex and has been implicated in self-reflective thought (option D is incorrect). High functional connectivity in this circuit is thought to reflect maladaptive self-referential thought such as rumination and worry (Hamilton et al. 2015). The *salience circuit* has core nodes in the anterior cingulate cortex, amygdala, and anterior insula and is thought to detect salient internal sensations and external changes. Low functional connectivity in this circuit has been associated with social anxiety disorder and may reflect anxious avoidance (reviewed in Williams 2016). The *attention circuit* has core nodes in the medial superior frontal cortex, anterior inferior parietal lobe, anterior insula, and precuneus. Low functional connectivity in this circuit is thought to reflect the inattention symptoms common across psychiatric disorders (Williams 2016) (option B is incorrect).

Decreased activation in the ventral striatum, a core node of the reward circuit, has been associated with anhedonia (Der-Avakian and Markou 2012) (option A is correct), whereas increased activation in the amygdala in response to threatening stimuli has been associated with heightened anxiety (Shin and Liberzon 2010) (option C is incorrect). **Chapter 28 (pp. 775–776)**

28.5 For which of the following disorders is there active pursuit of translation of genetic insights into genetic tests for screening and diagnosis?

A. Major depressive disorder.
B. Autism spectrum disorder.
C. Attention-deficit/hyperactivity disorder.
D. Bipolar disorder.

The correct response is option B: Autism spectrum disorder.

Psychiatric disorders that have been studied intensively in genome-wide analyses (Sullivan et al. 2012) and in studies of candidate genetic variants (Gatt et al. 2015) include major depressive disorder, bipolar disorder, schizophrenia, attention-deficit/hyperactivity disorder, and autism spectrum disorder (Psychiatric Genomics Consortium 2016). It is worth noting one area of direct clinical application: for autism spectrum disorder, there is active pursuit of the translation of genetic insights into genetic tests for screening and diagnosis (Schaefer et al. 2008), especially in regard to genomic structural variation (option B is correct; options A, C, and D are incorrect). **Chapter 28 (p. 776)**

28.6 Which of the following variables was found to predict better response of depression to venlafaxine in the international Study to Predict Optimized Treatment for Depression (iSPOT-D) trial?

A. Early life stress.
B. High levels of anxious arousal.
C. More responsive threat circuitry.
D. Higher body mass index.

The correct response is option D: Higher body mass index.

The iSPOT-D trial (Williams et al. 2011) uncovered several promising predictors of treatment response. The trial found that clinical variables such as early-life stress (Williams et al. 2016) and high levels of anxious arousal (Saveanu et al. 2015) predicted poorer treatment response to any medication (options A and B are incorrect), while higher body mass index predicted better response specifically to venlafaxine (Green et al. 2017) (option D is correct). Functional neuroimaging analyses have suggested that intact cognitive control circuitry (Gyurak et al. 2016) and less-responsive threat circuitry (Williams et al. 2015) are predictive of good antidepressant outcomes (option C is incorrect). **Chapter 28 (p. 777)**

28.7 Which of the following biomarkers confers an increased risk of agranulocytosis in patients taking clozapine?

A. The *ABCB1* gene.
B. The *SLC6AF* gene.
C. The *HLA-DQB1* gene.
D. The *HTR2A* gene.

The correct response is option C: The *HLA-DQB1* gene.

A review of potential biomarkers of psychosis identified a pharmacogenetic biomarker in the *HLA-DQB1* gene that predicts significantly greater risk for clozapine-induced agranulocytosis (Prata et al. 2014) (option C is correct).

A single-nucleotide polymorphism in the *ABCB1* gene (which plays a role in controlling antidepressant concentrations in the brain) predicts good response to escitalopram and sertraline for individuals with the common variant and good response to venlafaxine for those with the more rare variant (Schatzberg et al. 2015) (option A is incorrect).

Mayo Clinic researchers are working with industry partners to evaluate the utility of individualized genetic prediction of antidepressant choice in practice and have focused on candidate genes identified in the literature, including *SLC6AF* and *HTR2A* (Hodgson et al. 2012) (options B and D are incorrect). **Chapter 28 (pp. 777–778)**

28.8 For which of the following tools in precision psychiatry is it more challenging to define normal functioning than it is to define abnormal functioning?

A. Genomic data.
B. Neuroimaging.
C. Cognitive testing.
D. Self-report scales.

The correct response is option B: Neuroimaging.

In order to incorporate pathophysiology into psychiatric diagnoses, we must be able to define for each person whether they have normal or abnormal functioning. This task is straightforward for self-report scales and cognitive testing, for which population norms are often available (options C and D are incorrect).

Genomic data, being inherently categorical, can also be clearly separated into normal and abnormal risk/variants (option A is incorrect).

Neuroimaging, however, poses more of a challenge (option B is correct). It will therefore be important to define the normative distribution of neural circuit function in healthy individuals (as in Ball et al. 2017) and to identify thresholds for overt disorder and failures of function. **Chapter 28 (p. 779)**

28.9 Which of the following "re-purposed" medications is currently being evaluated for the treatment of bipolar disorder as a result of findings from genome-wide association studies?

A. Isradipine.
B. D-cycloserine.
C. Glucocorticoids.
D. Cannabinoids.

The correct response is option A: Isradipine.

As etiologically based subtypes of psychiatric disorders are discovered, new medications can be developed to target specific deficits. For example, based on results from genome-wide association studies, Drs. Michael Ostacher and Roy Perlis and their colleagues are evaluating the "re-purposing" of isradipine (a U.S. Food and Drug Administration–approved antihypertensive drug that interacts with the protein product of CAC-NA1C) for the treatment of bipolar disorder. Preliminary proof-of-concept findings are promising (Ostacher et al. 2014) (option A is correct).

New medications designed to boost psychotherapy efficacy are also being developed; several compounds (e.g., D-cycloserine, glucocorticoids, cannabinoids) are candidates that may improve learning in exposure therapy for anxiety disorders based on their ability to induce cellular learning in animal models (options B, C, and D are incorrect). **Chapter 28 (pp. 781–782)**

28.10 Which of the following is a potential beneficial social consequence of precision psychiatry?

A. Quick dissemination of findings by researchers.
B. Low costs and easy adoption by clinicians.
C. Less stigmatizing discussions about psychiatry and mental health.
D. Decreased disparities in health outcomes.

The correct response is option C: Less stigmatizing discussions about psychiatry and mental health.

Because precision psychiatry is based on a deep biological understanding of psychiatric disorders, it offers a model for patients to understand their experiences from an external perspective, rather than as an internal character flaw. A tangible model of understanding that is shared by the patient and the clinician can lead to a new perspective on the illness that diminishes the patient's shame and self-blame. Brain-based models of mental illness are rapidly being infused into the public consciousness, fostering more open and less stigmatizing discussions about psychiatry and mental health (option C is correct).

Many promising findings in precision psychiatry rely on techniques that are currently not widely available, in part because of relatively high costs and other logistical hurdles (option B is incorrect).

Too often, innovative new technologies and biomedical advances initially widen disparities in health outcomes, such that individuals with resources are able to take advantage of these advances while those without resources are left out (option D is incorrect).

Precision psychiatry as we are envisioning it requires continuous integration and updating of disease models and treatment planning based on emerging neuroscience and other research findings. A major challenge to this continual updating is that researchers are often hesitant to disseminate findings without an extremely high level of certainty, and providers are often hesitant to adopt new approaches (option A is incorrect). **Chapter 28 (pp. 782–785)**

References

Ball TM, Goldstein-Piekarski AN, Gatt JM, et al: Quantifying person-level brain network functioning to facilitate clinical translation. Transl Psychiatry 7(10):e1248, 2017 29039851

Cole MW, Bassett DS, Power JD, et al: Intrinsic and task-evoked network architectures of the human brain. Neuron 83(1):238–251, 2014 24991964

Der-Avakian A, Markou A: The neurobiology of anhedonia and other reward-related deficits. Trends Neurosci 35(1):68–77, 2012 22177980

Gatt JM, Burton KLO, Williams LM, et al: Specific and common genes implicated across major mental disorders: a review of meta-analysis studies. J Psychiatr Res 60(October):1–13, 2015 25287955

Green E, Goldstein-Piekarski AN, Schatzberg AF, et al: Personalizing antidepressant choice by sex, body mass index, and symptom profile: an iSPOT-D report. Personalized Medicine in Psychiatry 1–2(March–April):65–73, 2017

Gyurak A, Patenaude B, Korgaonkar MS, et al: Frontoparietal activation during response inhibition predicts remission to antidepressants in patients with major depression. Biol Psychiatry 79(4):274–281, 2016 25891220

Hamilton JP, Farmer M, Fogelman P, et al: Depressive rumination, the default-mode network, and the dark matter of clinical neuroscience. Biol Psychiatry 78(4):224–230, 2015 25861700

Hodgson K, Mufti SJ, Uher R, et al: Genome-wide approaches to antidepressant treatment: working towards understanding and predicting response. Genome Med 4(6):52, 2012 22738351

Insel T, Cuthbert B, Garvey M, et al: Research domain criteria (RDoC): toward a new classification framework for research on mental disorders. Am J Psychiatry 167(7):748–751, 2010 20595427

Mahmood SS, Levy D, Vasan RS, et al: The Framingham Heart Study and the epidemiology of cardiovascular disease: a historical perspective. Lancet 383(9921):999–1008, 2014 24084292

Markoff J: Obama seeking to boost study of human brain. The New York Times, February 17, 2013. Available at: http://www.nytimes.com/2013/02/18/science/project-seeks-to-build-map-of-human-brain.html. Accessed March 14, 2018.

Office of the Press Secretary: Fact Sheet: President Obama's Precision Medicine Initiative. Washington, DC, The White House, January 30, 2015. Available at: https://obamawhitehouse.archives.gov/the-press-office/2015/01/30/fact-sheet-president-obama-s-precision-medicine-initiative. Accessed March 14, 2018.

Ostacher MJ, Iosifescu DV, Hay A, et al: Pilot investigation of isradipine in the treatment of bipolar depression motivated by genome-wide association. Bipolar Disord 16(2):199–203, 2014 24372835

Prata D, Mechelli A, Kapur S: Clinically meaningful biomarkers for psychosis: a systematic and quantitative review. Neurosci Biobehav Rev 45:134–141, 2014 24877683

Psychiatric Genomics Consortium: Psychiatric Genomics Consortium: What is the PGC? (website). Chapel Hill, University of North Carolina School of Medicine, 2016. Available at: http://www.med.unc.edu/pgc/. Accessed March 14, 2018.

Saveanu R, Etkin A, Duchemin AM, et al: The international Study to Predict Optimized Treatment in Depression (iSPOT-D): outcomes from the acute phase of antidepressant treatment. J Psychiatr Res 61:1–12, 2015 25586212

Schaefer GB, Mendelsohn NJ; Professional Practice and Guidelines Committee: Clinical genetics evaluation in identifying the etiology of autism spectrum disorders. Genet Med 10(4):301–305, 2008 18414214

Schatzberg AF, DeBattista C, Lazzeroni LC, et al: ABCB1 genetic effects on antidepressant outcomes: a report from the iSPOT-D trial. Am J Psychiatry 172(8):751–759, 2015 25815420

Shin LM, Liberzon I: The neurocircuitry of fear, stress, and anxiety disorders. Neuropsychopharmacology 35(1):169–191, 2010 19625997

Sullivan PF, Daly MJ, O'Donovan M: Genetic architectures of psychiatric disorders: the emerging picture and its implications. Nat Rev Genet 13(8):537–551, 2012 22777127

Williams LM: Precision psychiatry: a neural circuit taxonomy for depression and anxiety. Lancet Psychiatry 3(5):472–480, 2016 27150382

Williams LM, Rush AJ, Koslow SH, et al: International Study to Predict Optimized Treatment for Depression (iSPOT-D), a randomized clinical trial: rationale and protocol. Trials 12(1):4, 2011 21208417

Williams LM, Korgaonkar MS, Song YC, et al: Amygdala reactivity to emotional faces in the prediction of general and medication-specific responses to antidepressant treatment in the randomized iSPOT-D trial. Neuropsychopharmacology 40(10):2398–2408, 2015 25824424

Williams LM, Debattista C, Duchemin A-M, et al: Childhood trauma predicts antidepressant response in adults with major depression: data from the randomized international study to predict optimized treatment for depression. Transl Psychiatry 6:e799, 2016 27138798

CHAPTER 29

Psychopharmacology

29.1   Which of the following statements accurately describes how drugs that are inducers of phase I metabolism by a specific cytochrome P450 (CYP) enzyme affect levels and rate of metabolism of that CYP enzyme?

A. Inducers increase CYP enzyme levels and rate of metabolism almost immediately.
B. Inducers decrease CYP enzyme levels and rate of metabolism almost immediately.
C. Inducers increase CYP enzyme levels and rate of metabolism over a period of
weeks.
D. Inducers decrease CYP enzyme levels and rate of metabolism over a period of
weeks.

**The correct response is option C: Inducers increase CYP enzyme levels and rate
of metabolism over a period of weeks.**

The majority of psychotropic drugs are *substrates* for phase I (oxidative) metabolism by one or more CYP enzymes. The most common pharmacokinetic drug–
drug interaction involves changes in the CYP-mediated metabolism of the substrate drug by an interacting drug. The interacting drug may be either an inducer
or an inhibitor of the specific CYP enzymes involved in the substrate drug's metabolism. In the presence of an inducer, CYP enzyme activity and the rate of metabolism of the substrate are increased (options B and D are incorrect).

Enzyme induction is not an immediate process but occurs over several weeks
(option A is incorrect; option C is correct). Induction will decrease the amount of
circulating parent drug and may reduce or abolish therapeutic efficacy. **Chapter 29
(p. 793)**

29.2 Which of the following statements about pharmacodynamic drug interactions is *true*?

A. Pharmacodynamic interactions occur when drugs with similar or opposing effects are combined.
B. Pharmacodynamic interactions occur when an interacting substance alters a drug's concentration due to a change in cytochrome P450 (CYP)–mediated metabolism of the substrate drug by the interacting drug.
C. Pharmacodynamic interactions occur when an interacting substance alters a drug's concentration due to a change in drug protein binding.
D. Pharmacodynamic interactions occur when an interacting substance increases or decreases the oral bioavailability of a poorly bioavailable drug.

The correct response is option A: Pharmacodynamic interactions occur when drugs with similar or opposing effects are combined.

A *drug interaction* is the alteration of the pharmacological effect of one drug by another concurrently administered drug or substance (the term *drug interaction* refers to all types of drug interactions—both pharmacodynamic and pharmacokinetic). *Pharmacodynamic* interactions occur when drugs with similar or opposing effects are combined (option A is correct). By contrast, *pharmacokinetic* interactions occur when an interacting substance alters a drug's concentration due to a change in its absorption, distribution, metabolism, or excretion. Changes in the CYP-mediated metabolism of a substrate drug by an interacting drug (a change affecting drug *metabolism*), changes in drug protein binding (a change affecting drug *distribution*), and changes in the oral bioavailability of poorly bioavailable drugs (a change affecting drug *absorption*) are examples of *pharmacokinetic*, not *pharmacodynamic*, drug interactions (options B, C, and D are incorrect). **Chapter 29 (pp. 792–795)**

29.3 Which of the following statements accurately describes the appropriate use of oral antipsychotics in patients with impaired enteral absorption?

A. Patients with impaired enteral absorption can absorb oral antipsychotics normally, so this is not a concern.
B. Patients with impaired enteral absorption can absorb only orally dissolvable formulations of antipsychotics normally, and these must be used in place of normal formulations.
C. Patients with impaired enteral absorption can absorb only sublingual asenapine among oral antipsychotics because of its unique property of being bucally absorbed.
D. Patients with impaired enteral absorption must have all antipsychotics provided parenterally.

The correct response is option C: Patients with impaired enteral absorption can absorb only sublingual asenapine among oral antipsychotics because of its unique property of being bucally absorbed.

Orally dissolving formulations are available for aripiprazole, clozapine, olanzapine, and risperidone, but they require swallowing and are absorbed enterally (option B is incorrect). Because it has no significant enteral absorption, asenapine is the only antipsychotic available as a sublingual preparation (option C is correct; options A and D are incorrect). **Chapter 29 (p. 804)**

29.4   Which of the following statements accurately describes the effect of lithium on the kidneys?

A. Lithium causes sodium retention and free water diuresis secondary to the syndrome of inappropriate antidiuretic hormone (SIADH) secretion.
B. Lithium causes sodium and free water retention leading to oliguria.
C. Lithium causes free water retention and salt wasting.
D. Lithium causes free water and sodium diuresis and can lead to nephrogenic diabetes insipidus.

The correct response is option D: Lithium causes free water and sodium diuresis and can lead to nephrogenic diabetes insipidus.

Lithium causes water and sodium diuresis and may precipitate nephrogenic diabetes insipidus (option D is correct; options B and C are incorrect).
Carbamazepine, not lithium, can cause SIADH, with resultant hyponatremia. The elderly, patients with alcohol use disorder, and patients receiving selective serotonin reuptake inhibitors may be at greater risk of developing carbamazepine-induced SIADH (option A is incorrect). **Chapter 29 (pp. 817, 823)**

29.5   Which of the following statements accurately describes how carbamazepine and valproate affect lamotrigine levels?

A. Carbamazepine increases lamotrigine levels, whereas valproate does not affect lamotrigine levels.
B. Valproate increases lamotrigine levels, whereas carbamazepine decreases them.
C. Valproate decreases lamotrigine levels, whereas carbamazepine increases them.
D. Valproate decreases lamotrigine levels, whereas carbamazepine does not affect lamotrigine levels.

The correct response is option B: Valproate increases lamotrigine levels, whereas carbamazepine decreases them.

Valproate can inhibit hepatic enzymes (UDP-glucuronosyltransferase [UGT] and cytochrome P450), leading to elevated levels of other medications, particularly lamotrigine, thereby increasing the risk of lamotrigine-induced rash (current lamotrigine product labeling provides specific lamotrigine dosing guidelines for patients who are taking valproate) (option B is correct; options A, C, and D are incorrect). Concurrent treatment with valproate will increase lamotrigine levels, and concurrent treatment with carbamazepine will decrease lamotrigine levels (option C is incorrect). **Chapter 29 (pp. 822, 824)**

29.6   Which of the following statements most accurately describes the contribution of bupropion dosage and formulation to seizure risk?

A. Seizure risk is dose-dependent, and the immediate-release formulation of bupropion confers higher risk than the sustained-release formulation.
B. Seizure risk is idiosyncratic and dose-independent, and the immediate-release formulation of bupropion confers higher risk than the sustained-release formulation.
C. Seizure risk is dose-dependent, and the sustained-release formulation of bupropion confers higher risk than the immediate-release formulation.
D. Seizure risk is idiosyncratic and dose-independent, and the sustained-release formulation of bupropion confers higher risk than the immediate-release formulation.

The correct response is option A: Seizure risk is dose-dependent, and the immediate-release formulation of bupropion confers higher risk than the sustained-release formulation.

Bupropion causes a dosage-related lowering of the seizure threshold and may precipitate seizures in susceptible patients receiving dosages greater than 450 mg/day (options B and D are incorrect).

Sustained-release dosage forms are associated with a lower seizure risk than are immediate-release bupropion products (option A is correct; option C is incorrect). **Chapter 29 (p. 830)**

29.7   Which of the following statements accurately describes how buspirone and benzodiazepines differ in their mechanism of action and effects?

A. Both buspirone and benzodiazepines affect GABA receptors, but buspirone does not have the potential for abuse, tolerance, and withdrawal.
B. Buspirone is a 5-HT_{1A} receptor partial agonist and does not have the potential for abuse, tolerance, and withdrawal carried by benzodiazepines, which work on GABA receptors.
C. Buspirone and benzodiazepines both work on GABA receptors, and both carry a potential for abuse, tolerance, and withdrawal.
D. Although buspirone and benzodiazepines both have a potential for abuse, tolerance, and withdrawal, buspirone works as a 5-HT_{1A} receptor partial agonist whereas benzodiazepines work on the GABA receptor.

The correct response is option B: Buspirone is a 5-HT_{1A} receptor partial agonist and does not have the potential for abuse, tolerance, and withdrawal carried by benzodiazepines, which work on GABA receptors.

Buspirone is a 5-HT_{1A} receptor partial agonist (options A and C are incorrect). Because it does not affect GABA receptors or chloride ion channels, buspirone does not possess many of the major concerns associated with benzodiazepines—namely, the potential for abuse, tolerance, and withdrawal (option B is correct; option D is incorrect). Buspirone is not cross-tolerant with benzodiazepines; thus, a rapid switch from a benzodiazepine to buspirone is likely to precipitate benzodiazepine withdrawal. **Chapter 29 (pp. 836–837)**

29.8 Which of the following antipsychotics has the lowest placental transfer?

A. Haloperidol.
B. Quetiapine.
C. Risperidone.
D. Olanzapine.

The correct response is option B: Quetiapine.

A small study found that placental passage of antipsychotics was highest for olanzapine and haloperidol, followed by risperidone (options A, C, and D are incorrect), with quetiapine having the least placental transfer (Kulkami et al. 2015) (option B is correct). **Chapter 29 (p. 852)**

29.9 Which of the following statements about the combined use of memantine and a cholinesterase inhibitor for treatment of Alzheimer's disease is *true*?

A. Memantine and cholinesterase inhibitors have dangerous effects on each other's pharmacokinetics and should never be used in tandem.
B. Although memantine and cholinesterase inhibitors are safe to use together, no clinical benefit is obtained from their combination.
C. Memantine and cholinesterase inhibitors used in tandem can significantly slow the disease trajectory of Alzheimer's dementia and improve functional performance.
D. Memantine and cholinesterase inhibitors do not interact pharmacokinetically; used in tandem, they may modestly improve cognition and behavior, but not functional performance.

The correct response is option D: Memantine and cholinesterase inhibitors do not interact pharmacokinetically; used in tandem, they may modestly improve cognition and behavior, but not functional performance.

Because of the differing mechanisms of action of cholinesterase inhibitors and memantine, it has been suggested that use of the two classes in combination might provide synergistic benefit for patients with moderate to severe Alzheimer's disease (data do not support memantine's use in mild Alzheimer's disease). A systematic review of pooled data from three 6-month trials in patients with moderate to severe Alzheimer's disease receiving memantine plus a cholinesterase inhibitor (mainly donepezil) concluded that combination therapy resulted in small improvements in cognition, clinical global scores, and behavior but had no effect on functional performance in activities of daily living (Farrimond et al. 2012) (option B is incorrect).

There is no evidence that memantine prevents or slows neurodegeneration or alters the course of the underlying disease process (option C is incorrect).

Memantine has no effect on the pharmacokinetics of cholinesterase inhibitors and thus may be used in combination with these agents without dosage adjustment (option A is incorrect; option D is correct). **Chapter 29 (pp. 849–851)**

29.10 An elderly patient has been taking metoprolol as part of her cardiac regimen. Her psychiatrist prescribes paroxetine to treat a major depressive episode. Two weeks after starting paroxetine, the patient returns to the office reporting dizziness and is found to be bradycardic and hypotensive. Which of the following types of pharmacokinetic drug interaction is most likely responsible for this effect?

A. Drug absorption.
B. Drug distribution.
C. Drug metabolism.
D. Drug elimination.

The correct response is option C: Drug metabolism.

The patient described in this case is likely experiencing beta-blocker toxicity, a pharmacokinetic drug interaction involving alteration in a drug's concentration due to a change in its metabolism caused by paroxetine-induced increases in metoprolol concentration. Like all beta-blockers, metoprolol is primarily metabolized by the cytochrome P450 (CYP) 2D6 isozyme. The addition of a potent CYP2D6 inhibitor, such as paroxetine, will inhibit metoprolol metabolism. Without a compensatory reduction in metoprolol dosage, drug levels will rise and toxicity (hypotension) may result. Paroxetine's effects in this scenario are not mediated by changes in metoprolol's absorption, distribution, or elimination (options A, B, and D are incorrect). **Chapter 29 (p. 794)**

29.11 What is the primary mechanism of action by which first-generation antipsychotics (FGAs) are thought to exert their therapeutic effects?

A. Antagonism of dopamine D_2 receptors.
B. Partial agonism of dopamine D_2 receptors.
C. Antagonism of serotonin $5-HT_{2A}$ receptors.
D. Partial agonism of $5-HT_{1A}$ receptors.

The correct response is option A: Antagonism of dopamine D_2 receptors.

The FGAs, most prominently the phenothiazines (e.g., chlorpromazine) and the butyrophenones (e.g., haloperidol), have heterogeneous receptor effects; however, their primary therapeutic effect is via nonspecific blockade of the dopamine D_2 receptor subtype (option A is correct).

The second-generation antipsychotics (SGAs) are a heterogeneous group of medications that are thought to exert more specific mesolimbic dopamine receptor blockade compared with the FGAs, combined with 5-HT$_{2A}$ receptor antagonism (option C is incorrect).

Three SGAs—aripiprazole, brexpiprazole, and cariprazine—work as partial agonists at both D$_2$ receptors (option B is incorrect) and 5-HT$_{1A}$ receptors (option D is incorrect) in addition to acting as antagonists at 5-HT$_{2A}$ receptors. **Chapter 29 (pp. 795–796)**

29.12 Which of the following potential side effects of clozapine prompted implementation of a federally mandated monitoring program for patients taking this drug?

A. Seizures.
B. Myocarditis.
C. Bowel obstruction.
D. Neutropenia.

The correct response is option D: Neutropenia.

Clozapine carries a risk of severe neutropenia (defined as an absolute neutrophil count less than 500/µL), with cumulative incidence estimated at 0.8% of patients receiving clozapine over a 15-month period (Raja 2011). Because neutropenia can potentially lead to fatal infections, the U.S. Food and Drug Administration mandated implementation of a Risk Evaluation and Mitigation Strategy (REMS) program to ensure optimal patient monitoring for and management of this serious complication (option D is correct).

Clozapine dispensing is linked to weekly absolute neutrophil counts during the first 6 months of treatment, biweekly (every 2 weeks) counts for the next 6 months, and monthly counts thereafter. Seizures, myocarditis, and bowel obstruction are other potentially fatal complications of clozapine therapy, but there is no mandatory monitoring system associated with these complications (options A, B, and C are incorrect). **Chapter 29 (pp. 814–815)**

29.13 Which of the following mood stabilizers is U.S. Food and Drug Administration (FDA) approved for both acute-phase and maintenance-phase treatment of bipolar disorder?

A. Lamotrigine.
B. Lithium.
C. Carbamazepine.
D. Valproate.

The correct response is option B: Lithium.

Lithium is the only medication listed that is FDA approved both for treatment of acute mania and for maintenance therapy in bipolar disorder (option B is correct). Lamotrigine is approved for use in the maintenance treatment in bipolar disorder and may have a role in acute bipolar depression, but it is not FDA approved for this indication (option A is incorrect). Carbamazepine is approved for acute treatment of manic and mixed episodes, and although some evidence supports its use for maintenance therapy, it is not approved for this indication (option C is incorrect). Valproate is approved only for the treatment of acute mania (option D is incorrect). **Chapter 29 (pp. 816–824)**

29.14 The presence of which of the following signs may help distinguish serotonin syndrome from neuroleptic malignant syndrome?

A. Rigidity.
B. Hyperreflexia.
C. Hyperthermia.
D. Autonomic disturbances.

The correct response is option B: Hyperreflexia.

Hyperreflexia and clonus are signs that often can be seen in serotonin syndrome but are not typically seen in neuroleptic malignant syndrome (option B is correct). Rigidity, hyperthermia, and autonomic disturbances are seen in both conditions (options A, C, and D are incorrect). **Chapter 29 (pp. 831–832)**

29.15 Which of the following off-label uses of antipsychotics carries a U.S. Food and Drug Administration (FDA) black-box warning for increased mortality risk?

A. Adjunctive treatment for refractory obsessive-compulsive disorder (OCD).
B. Dementia-related psychosis.
C. Severe anxiety/agitation.
D. Delirium-related psychosis.

The correct response is option B: Dementia-related psychosis.

Use of antipsychotics in elderly patients with dementia and psychotic symptoms is associated with an increased mortality risk secondary to cardiovascular events and infections, leading to an FDA black-box warning (option B is correct). Use of antipsychotics in the treatment of severe anxiety/agitation or delirium-related psychosis, or in the adjunctive treatment of refractory OCD, are off-label uses that are not associated with increased mortality risk (options A, C, and D are incorrect). **Chapter 29 (p. 796)**

29.16 You are choosing an initial antidepressant for a healthy young man who is not taking any other medications. The patient notes that in the past he has had trouble remembering to take his medications every day. Which of the following antidepressants would be *least* likely to produce a withdrawal syndrome if a dose was missed?

A. Fluvoxamine.
B. Fluoxetine.

C. Paroxetine.

D. Venlafaxine.

The correct response is option B: Fluoxetine.

Among the antidepressants, fluoxetine has one of the longest half-lives, making it least likely to cause a withdrawal syndrome if abruptly stopped, or if doses are missed (option B is correct). Fluvoxamine, paroxetine, and venlafaxine all have comparatively short half-lives, and can often be implicated in serotonin reuptake inhibitor withdrawal syndromes (options A, C, and D are incorrect). **Chapter 29 (pp. 827, 834)**

29.17 Which of the following benzodiazepines does not undergo phase I oxidative metabolism and therefore may be safer to use in patients with liver disease?

A. Lorazepam.

B. Diazepam.

C. Clonazepam.

D. Alprazolam.

The correct response is option A: Lorazepam.

All benzodiazepines are metabolized by the liver and therefore increase the risk of sedation, confusion, and hepatic encephalopathy in patients with hepatic failure. In such patients, lorazepam, oxazepam, and temazepam are the preferred agents because they undergo hepatic conjugation and renal excretion and have no active metabolites (option A is correct), whereas other benzodiazepines undergo phase I hepatic metabolism and may have long-acting active metabolites (options B, C, and D are incorrect). **Chapter 29 (p. 836)**

29.18 A 30-year-old woman with a history of bipolar disorder who is being maintained on lithium is planning to conceive. She asks you how to proceed with psychotropics during pregnancy. Which of the following statements best describes the relationship, in women with a previous mood disorder diagnosis, of risk of relapse with mood stabilizer use in pregnancy?

A. Continuation of mood stabilizers during pregnancy increases the risk of relapse.

B. Continuation of mood stabilizers during pregnancy does not change the risk of relapse.

C. Gradual tapering of mood stabilizers decreases the risk of relapse compared with abrupt cessation.

D. Gradual tapering of mood stabilizers increases the risk of relapse compared with abrupt cessation.

The correct response is option C: Gradual tapering of mood stabilizers decreases the risk of relapse compared with abrupt cessation.

Women with a history of a mood disorder who discontinue mood stabilizers during pregnancy are at greatly increased risk of relapse. Prospective studies found that 80% of women with bipolar disorder who discontinued mood stabilizers during pregnancy experienced recurrence of a mood episode (Viguera et al. 2007). In women with severe psychiatric disorders, the decision of whether to continue mood-stabilizing or antidepressant treatment during the first trimester and throughout pregnancy should be carefully balanced against the risks of discontinuation and should be discussed with the patient, her psychiatrist, and her obstetrician.

Continuation of mood stabilizers during pregnancy helps to prevent relapse (options A and B are incorrect). In women with mild mental illness and low relapse risk, the mood stabilizer or antidepressant may be tapered off or continued during efforts to conceive, and the patient can be monitored closely for relapse of mood symptoms. Compared with gradual tapering, abrupt cessation of mood stabilizers greatly increases the risk of relapse (50% within 2 weeks) (Viguera et al. 2007) (option C is correct; option D is incorrect). **Chapter 29 (pp. 851–852)**

29.19 Which of the following has *not* been reported as a risk associated with maternal use of selective serotonin reuptake inhibitors (SSRIs) during pregnancy?

A. Increased rate of stillbirth.
B. Increased rate of pre-eclampsia.
C. Increased rates of persistent pulmonary hypertension in the newborn.
D. Increased rate of prematurity.

The correct response is option A: Increased rate of stillbirth.

The risks of antidepressant exposure during pregnancy continue to be debated. SSRIs are not associated with an increased rate of stillbirths or major physical malformations (Wisner et al. 2009) (option A is correct).

Increased risks for premature birth, small-for-gestational-age birth, pre-eclampsia, and persistent pulmonary hypertension in the newborn have been reported in association with SSRI exposure during pregnancy; however, study results are conflicting, and the risk of one or more of these conditions occurring in association with SSRI exposure may be no worse than the risk of untreated depression in pregnancy (Altemus and Occhiogrosso 2017) (options B, C, and D are incorrect). **Chapter 29 (p. 853)**

References

Altemus M, Occhiogrosso M: Obstetrics and gynecology, in Clinical Manual of Psychopharmacology in the Medically Ill, 2nd edition. Edited by Levenson JL, Ferrando SJ. Washington, DC, American Psychiatric Publishing, 2017, pp 429–470

Farrimond LE, Roberts E, McShane R: Memantine and cholinesterase inhibitor combination therapy for Alzheimer's disease: a systematic review. BMJ Open 2(3):2, 2012 22689908

Kulkarni J, Storch A, Baraniuk A, et al: Antipsychotic use in pregnancy. Expert Opin Pharmacother 16(9):1335–1345, 2015 26001182

Raja M: Clozapine safety, 35 years later. Curr Drug Saf 6(3):164–184, 2011 22122392

Viguera AC, Whitfield T, Baldessarini RJ, et al: Risk of recurrence in women with bipolar disorder during pregnancy: prospective study of mood stabilizer discontinuation. Am J Psychiatry 164(12):1817–1824, quiz 1923, 2007 18056236

Wisner K, Sit D, Hanusa B, et al: Major depression and antidepressant treatment: impact on pregnancy and neonatal outcomes. Am J Psychiatry 166(5):557–566, 2009 19289451

CHAPTER 30

Brain Stimulation Therapies

30.1 Which of the following brain stimulation therapies predated the use of psychiatric medications?

A. Focused ultrasound.
B. Electroconvulsive therapy.
C. Epidural cortical stimulation.
D. Repetitive transcranial magnetic stimulation.

The correct response is option B: Electroconvulsive therapy.

Brain stimulation therapies, specifically electroconvulsive therapy (ECT), preceded the discovery of psychiatric medications. ECT was first used in 1938 for catatonic schizophrenia. ECT quickly became widely adopted throughout the world as the first bona fide treatment in modern psychiatry and saved the lives of numerous patients during a time when there were no effective treatments for psychiatric disorders (option B is correct). Also, for decades ECT remained the only brain stimulation treatment in psychiatry (options A, C, and D are incorrect).

Repetitive transcranial magnetic stimulation (rTMS) was first introduced in 1985. The first successful randomized controlled studies of rTMS in depression took place in the mid-1990s, and in 2008, following a key multisite study (O'Reardon et al. 2007), the first rTMS device received U.S. Food and Drug Administration (FDA) approval for acute treatment of depression (option D is incorrect).

High-frequency magnetic resonance–guided focused ultrasound targeting the thalamus is an FDA-approved treatment for essential tremor in Parkinson's disease (Magara et al. 2014), but focused ultrasound is still an investigational technique (option A is incorrect).

Although case series suggest that epidural cortical stimulation may have an antidepressant effect (Williams et al. 2016), this technique remains investigational at present (option C is incorrect). **Chapter 30 (pp. 861, 864, 870–871, 886)**

30.2   A patient with obsessive-compulsive disorder (OCD) spends all his waking hours cleaning despite having received adequate trials of clomipramine, sertraline, risperidone augmentation, and exposure and response prevention therapy. What brain stimulation therapy would be a U.S. Food and Drug Administration (FDA)–cleared next step in treatment?

A. Deep brain stimulation.
B. Epidural cortical stimulation.
C. Responsive neurostimulation.
D. Transcranial direct current stimulation.

The correct response is option A: Deep brain stimulation.

In 2008, deep brain stimulation (DBS) for treatment-resistant OCD was approved by the FDA under a humanitarian device exemption. Despite its invasive nature, DBS is relatively safe, adjustable, and reversible in comparison with other ablative neurosurgical methods used in OCD, such as capsulotomy (option A is correct).

Neurosurgically implanted responsive neurostimulation (RNS) was the first closed-loop treatment FDA approved for use in epilepsy. Given the episodic nature of pathological mental states in many psychiatric disorders, a closed-loop RNS system may provide a novel brain stimulation technology to individualize and enhance psychiatric treatments; however, RNS remains investigational at present (option C is incorrect).

Although early case series studying the effect of dorsolateral prefrontal epidural cortical stimulation in depressed patients suggested an antidepressant effect (Williams et al. 2016), the technique remains investigational at present (option B is incorrect).

Transcranial direct current stimulation (tDCS), a newer form of neurostimulation involving application of low-intensity direct current to modulate neuronal activity, has gained much interest as a potential treatment for depression and other psychiatric disorders. However, a double-blind noninferiority antidepressant trial demonstrated that whereas tDCS and escitalopram were each superior to placebo, tDCS did not show noninferiority to escitalopram and was associated with more adverse events (Brunoni et al. 2017). Although more studies are needed, to date tDCS has shown minimal clinical utility in depression and other psychiatric disorders, and therefore it is still investigational at this time (option D is incorrect). **Chapter 30 (pp. 861, 882, 885–887)**

30.3   Which of the following medications can improve outcomes in electroconvulsive therapy (ECT)?

A. Diazepam.
B. Clozapine.
C. Valproic acid.
D. Theophylline.

The correct response is option B: Clozapine.

Noradrenergic agents such as tricyclic antidepressants and serotonin-norepinephrine reuptake inhibitors (Sackeim et al. 2009), lithium, and antipsychotics (particularly clozapine) may be used to augment the therapeutic effects of ECT (option B is correct).

As a general rule, anticonvulsants are to be avoided with ECT, because their use will directly interfere with the ability to induce a seizure, thereby disrupting the therapeutic effects of ECT (Sienaert and Peuskens 2007) (option C is incorrect).

Benzodiazepines should likewise be avoided with ECT, but if they are necessary, short-acting benzodiazepines are recommended, which are less likely to interfere with the induction of a therapeutic seizure. Given this recommendation, diazepam, a long-acting benzodiazepine, would be very unlikely to improve outcomes for ECT (option A is incorrect).

Most nonanticonvulsant medications can be safety coadministered with ECT except for theophylline, which is rarely used. Use of theophylline during ECT can lead to prolonged seizures and result in status epilepticus (Rasmussen and Zorumski 1993) (option D is incorrect). **Chapter 30 (p. 866)**

30.4 Which of the following repetitive transcranial magnetic stimulation (rTMS) targets is most commonly used in the treatment of major depressive disorder (MDD)?

A. The ventral striatum.
B. The frontopolar cortex.
C. The orbitofrontal cortex.
D. The dorsolateral prefrontal cortex.

The correct response is option D: The dorsolateral prefrontal cortex.

In the treatment of MDD, by far the most commonly used rTMS stimulation target (as per the U.S. Food and Drug Administration (FDA)–approved protocol) is the dorsolateral prefrontal cortex (DLPFC), specifically the left side, using high-frequency stimulation, usually at 10 Hz (option D is correct).

Converging evidence from lesion, stimulation, neuroimaging, and connectivity studies suggests that several other rTMS-accessible regions may also be important in MDD, including the dorsomedial prefrontal cortex, the orbitofrontal cortex, and the frontopolar cortex (Downar and Daskalakis 2013). These alternative targets are now being studied in MDD; however, given the fairly embryonic evidence base to date, these new targets will require further study under randomized conditions (options B and C are incorrect).

Multiple targets for deep brain stimulation (DBS) have been explored for treatment of a range of psychiatric disorders. The FDA-approved target for use in obsessive-compulsive disorder (OCD) is the ventral capsule/ventral striatum. Ventral capsule/ventral striatum DBS is thought to target dysfunctional cortico-striato-thalamo-cortical circuits specific to OCD that connect the orbitofrontal cortex, medial prefrontal cortex, basal ganglia, and thalamus (Greenberg et al. 2010) (option A is incorrect). **Chapter 30 (pp. 874, 880, 882–884)**

30.5   A moderately depressed patient had no response to trials of sertraline (at a dosage of 200 mg/day for 3 months) and venlafaxine (at a dosage of 225 mg/day for 5 months). On the basis of research evidence for efficacy, which of the following interventions would be the best next step in treatment for this patient?

A. Deep brain stimulation (DBS).
B. Vagus nerve stimulation (VNS).
C. Switching to bupropion.
D. Repetitive transcranial magnetic stimulation (rTMS).

The correct response is option D: Repetitive transcranial magnetic stimulation (rTMS).

High-frequency (most often, 10 Hz) left dorsolateral prefrontal cortex rTMS is the most widely used and widely studied protocol in depression, with efficacy supported by several meta-analyses and more than 100 studies to date. The most recent trials using optimized stimulation parameters and adequate (20–30 sessions) course lengths reported response in 45%–55% and remission in 30%–40% of patients with medication-resistant depression (Blumberger et al. 2018; Levkovitz et al. 2015). Similar outcomes were reported in naturalistic case series in the community (Carpenter et al. 2012) (option D is correct).

For context in interpreting treatment outcomes for rTMS, it is worth reviewing outcomes for other types of interventions in treatment-resistant depression (usually defined as failure of two or more medication trials of adequate dosage and duration). After two failed medication trials, remission rates for subsequent medication trials are as low as 10%–15% in published studies of sequential treatment, such as the landmark STAR*D trial (Rush et al. 2006) (option C is incorrect).

Although DBS remains a promising tool for deep, targeted brain stimulation, it does not show a clear and consistent benefit in depression (option A is incorrect).

A 10-week sham-controlled VNS study in patients with treatment-resistant unipolar and bipolar depression failed to show an antidepressant effect after several weeks (Rush et al. 2005), but long-term, open-label trials have demonstrated long-term antidepressant effects (Nahas et al. 2005). However, these data do not suggest that VNS would produce higher remission rates than rTMS (option B is incorrect). **Chapter 30 (pp. 874–875, 881, 884)**

30.6   Subsequent repetitive transcranial magnetic stimulation (rTMS) treatments are most likely contraindicated after which of the following adverse events?

A. Seizure.
B. Syncope.
C. Headache.
D. Hearing loss.

The correct response is option A: Seizure.

The most serious adverse event with rTMS is induction of a generalized tonic-clonic seizure during stimulation. Patients suffering a seizure during rTMS normally should not undergo further rTMS treatment (option A is correct).

Transient headache or fatigue may occur after electroconvulsive therapy (ECT) stimulation sessions (reported by 25%–30% of patients); these symptoms diminish over time and typically respond well to over-the-counter analgesia. Although about 2%–4% of patients discontinue treatment due to pain, headache is not considered a possible contraindication (option C is incorrect).

Vasovagal syncope (reported by ~1% of patients) is another adverse event that can occur during ECT, particularly during the initial sessions of treatment (Rossi et al. 2009). Patients experiencing syncopal episodes may proceed with treatment after recovery and reassurance (option B is incorrect).

Tinnitus or short-term hearing loss is a rare adverse event caused by the TMS click during discharge of each magnetic pulse. To avoid this adverse effect, patients and technicians should wear hearing protection (e.g., earplugs) during treatment sessions; such measures have been shown to be effective in preventing hearing problems associated with rTMS (Rossi et al. 2009), decreasing the likelihood that this adverse event will be a contraindication to further treatment (option D is incorrect). **Chapter 30 (pp. 876–877)**

30.7   For which of the following conditions has electroconvulsive therapy (ECT) been shown to achieve better remission rates than pharmacotherapy?

A. Social anxiety disorder.
B. Major depressive disorder.
C. Obsessive-compulsive disorder.
D. Borderline personality disorder.

The correct response is option B: Major depressive disorder.

Multiple meta-analyses show the lasting and robust antidepressant effect of ECT over pharmacotherapy for unipolar and bipolar depression. ECT remains the most effective antidepressant available and has been shown to reduce mortality and decrease hospital readmission. When used to treat depression, ECT has an overall response rate of 50%–90% (option B is correct). When used in patients with treatment-resistant depression that has failed to respond to multiple antidepressant medications, ECT has a lower response rate, of 50%–70%. Remission rates after ECT for treatment-resistant depression are typically reported between 50% and 80%; however, because the therapeutic effect is highly dependent on technique, including electrode placement and dosage, remission rates can range from 20% to 80% (Lisanby 2007).

The presence of comorbid anxiety reduces the effectiveness of ECT (option A is incorrect), and ECT has not shown benefit for treatment of primary anxiety or obsessive-compulsive disorder (option C is incorrect).

Remission rates are lower for certain populations, including persons with borderline personality disorder (~20%) (option D is incorrect). **Chapter 30 (p. 867)**

30.8 A severely depressed patient whose symptoms have not responded to multiple medication trials and years of evidence-based psychotherapy asks if there are any U.S. Food and Drug Administration (FDA)–cleared stimulation treatments available. Which of the following treatments has demonstrated benefit for a patient with these characteristics but is unlikely to be covered by insurance?

A. Focused ultrasound.
B. Vagus nerve stimulation.
C. Responsive neurostimulation.
D. Repetitive transcranial magnetic stimulation.

The correct response is option B: Vagus nerve stimulation.

Vagus nerve stimulation (VNS) is an FDA-approved treatment for epilepsy and treatment-resistant unipolar and bipolar depression. A 10-week sham-controlled VNS study in patients with treatment-resistant unipolar and bipolar depression failed to show an antidepressant effect after several weeks (Rush et al. 2005), but long-term, open-label trials have demonstrated long-term antidepressant effects (Nahas et al. 2005). These findings led to FDA approval of VNS in 2005 for use in treatment-resistant depression. However, despite having received approval for this indication, VNS is not generally available to patients in the United States because insurers have determined that it is not a cost-effective intervention for treatment-resistant depression (option B is correct).

By contrast, repetitive transcranial magnetic stimulation has FDA clearance for depression and is covered by public and private insurance plans in most regions (option D is incorrect).

Both focused ultrasound and responsive neurostimulation are FDA cleared for investigational use, but not for clinical use in the treatment of depression (options A and C are incorrect). **Chapter 30 (pp. 871, 881, 886–887)**

30.9 Which of the following best explains the therapeutic mechanisms of brain stimulation therapies?

A. Effects on signaling of specific receptors.
B. Effects on functional networks of brain regions.
C. Effects on psychological processes.
D. Effects on individual brain regions.

The correct response is option B: Effects on functional networks of brain regions.

For any given intervention in psychiatry, the underlying mechanism often has an optimal "explanatory level" that lies somewhere on a spectrum extending from molecular biology at the microscopic end to societal factors at the macroscopic end. A growing body of evidence suggests that the most helpful level of explanation for understanding the mechanism of brain stimulation may be the level of functional networks of brain regions. A key discovery emerging from neuroimaging studies since the 1990s is that brain regions are organized into functional networks whose activity is correlated over time, whether during task performance or at rest. These networks have a consistent anatomy across individuals, such that surveys of large samples of healthy individuals ($N=1,000$) can reliably identify at least seven discrete functional networks (Dunlop et al. 2017) (option B is correct).

Because the brain is arranged as a set of interconnected functional networks, stimulating any given brain region also exerts an effect on the other nodes of that region's network. Thus, the best level of explanation for understanding the mechanisms of brain stimulation treatments may be that of functional brain regions rather than individual brain regions or specific molecules or receptors (options A and D are incorrect).

By contrast, cognitive-behavioral therapy may be best understood in terms of its effects on psychological mechanisms such as cognitive distortions and automatic thoughts (option C is incorrect). **Chapter 30 (pp. 888, 889 [Figure 30–8], 893)**

30.10 Hypofunctioning of which of the following functional networks has been implicated in multiple psychiatric disorders based on neuroimaging data?

A. Visual network.
B. Salience network.
C. Ventral frontoparietal network.
D. Primary somatosensory network.

The correct response is option B: Salience network.

Converging evidence from neuroimaging, stimulation, and lesion studies has identified three functional networks as playing particularly important, transdiagnostic roles across a variety of psychiatric illnesses. One of these is the *salience network*, whose core nodes include the dorsal anterior cingulate cortex (dACC) and the anterior insula. Notably, a meta-analysis of 193 structural neuroimaging studies in more than 7,000 patients across a variety of psychiatric disorders (major depressive disorder [MDD], bipolar disorder, schizophrenia, obsessive-compulsive disorder [OCD], anxiety disorders and substance use disorders) found that the most consistent sites of gray matter loss were in core salience nodes in the dACC and anterior insula (Goodkind et al. 2015). Deficits in cognitive control, reflected in hypofunctioning of the salience network, have thus been proposed as a central and transdiagnostic dimension of pathology across a variety of psychiatric disorders (option B is correct).

By contrast, some functional networks—for example, visual networks in the occipital cortex or primary somatosensory and motor networks bordering the central sulcus—perform low-level sensory or motor functions, which have not directly been implicated in psychiatric illnesses based on neuroimaging (options A and D are incorrect).

The dorsal and ventral frontoparietal networks are associated with attention and working memory, both of which are important to brain function but have not been directly implicated in psychiatric illnesses based on neuroimaging (option C is incorrect). **Chapter 30 (pp. 888–889; Figure 30–9 [p. 890])**

References

Blumberger DM, Vila-Rodriguez F, Thorpe K, et al: Effectiveness of theta burst versus high-frequency repetitive transcranial magnetic stimulation in patients with depression (THREE-D): a randomised non-inferiority trial. Lancet 391(10131):1683–1692, 2018 29726344

Brunoni AR, Moffa AH, Sampaio-Junior B, et al: Trial of electrical direct-current therapy versus escitalopram for depression. N Engl J Med 376(26):2523–2533, 2017 28657871

Carpenter LL, Janicak PG, Aaronson ST, et al: Transcranial magnetic stimulation (TMS) for major depression: a multisite, naturalistic, observational study of acute treatment outcomes in clinical practice. Depress Anxiety 29(7):587–596, 2012 22689344

Downar J, Daskalakis ZJ: New targets for rTMS in depression: a review of convergent evidence. Brain Stimulat 6(3):231–240, 2013 22975030

Dunlop K, Hanlon CA, Downar J: Noninvasive brain stimulation treatments for addiction and major depression. Ann N Y Acad Sci 1394(1):31–54, 2017 26849183

Goodkind M, Eickhoff SB, Oathes DJ, et al: Identification of a common neurobiological substrate for mental illness. JAMA Psychiatry 72(4):305–315, 2015 25651064

Greenberg BD, Rauch SL, Haber SN: Invasive circuitry-based neurotherapeutics: stereotactic ablation and deep brain stimulation for OCD. Neuropsychopharmacology 35(1):317–336, 2010 19759530

Levkovitz Y, Isserles M, Padberg F, et al: Efficacy and safety of deep transcranial magnetic stimulation for major depression: a prospective multicenter randomized controlled trial. World Psychiatry 14(1):64–73, 2015 25655160

Lisanby SH: Electroconvulsive therapy for depression. N Engl J Med 357(19):1939–1945, 2007 17989386

Magara A, Bühler R, Moser D, et al: First experience with MR-guided focused ultrasound in the treatment of Parkinson's disease. J Ther Ultrasound 2:11, 2014 25512869

Nahas Z, Marangell LB, Husain MM, et al: Two-year outcome of vagus nerve stimulation (VNS) for treatment of major depressive episodes. J Clin Psychiatry 66(9):1097–1104, 2005 16187765

O'Reardon JP, Solvason HB, Janicak PG, et al: Efficacy and safety of transcranial magnetic stimulation in the acute treatment of major depression: a multisite randomized controlled trial. Biol Psychiatry 62(11):1208–1216, 2007 17573044

Rasmussen KG, Zorumski CF: Electroconvulsive therapy in patients taking theophylline. J Clin Psychiatry 54(11):427–431, 1993 8270586

Rossi S, Hallett M, Rossini PM, et al: Safety, ethical considerations, and application guidelines for the use of transcranial magnetic stimulation in clinical practice and research. Clin Neurophysiol 120(12):2008–2039, 2009 19833552

Rush AJ, Marangell LB, Sackeim HA, et al: Vagus nerve stimulation for treatment-resistant depression: a randomized, controlled acute phase trial. Biol Psychiatry 58(5):347–354, 2005 16139580

Rush AJ, Trivedi MH, Wisniewski SR, et al; STAR*D Study Team: Bupropion-SR, sertraline, or venlafaxine-XR after failure of SSRIs for depression. N Engl J Med 354(12):1231–1242, 2006 16554525

Sackeim HA, Dillingham EM, Prudic J, et al: Effect of concomitant pharmacotherapy on electroconvulsive therapy outcomes: short-term efficacy and adverse effects. Arch Gen Psychiatry 66(7):729–737, 2009 19581564

Sienaert P, Peuskens J: Anticonvulsants during electroconvulsive therapy: review and recommendations. J ECT 23(2):120–123, 2007 17548985

Williams NR, Short EB, Hopkins T, et al: Five-year follow-up of bilateral epidural prefrontal cortical stimulation for treatment-resistant depression. Brain Stimulat 9(6):897–904, 2016 27443912

CHAPTER 31

Brief Psychotherapies

31.1   Which of the following is considered to be the key mechanism of change in short-term psychodynamic therapy?

A. Development of insight through interpretive comments.
B. Identification of patterns in defenses and interpersonal struggles through a focus on past experiences.
C. Active provision of corrective relational experiences within sessions.
D. The fostering of altered expectations in extratherapeutic relationships and experimentation with new patterns of communication.

The correct response is option C: Active provision of corrective relational experiences within sessions.

The emphasized change mechanism in short-term dynamic therapies is corrective relational experiences that the therapist actively provides within the therapy (option C is correct). In contrast, long-term psychodynamic therapy emphasizes insight as the mechanism of change and interpretation as the key mechanism for dealing with resistances (option A is incorrect). While understanding the role of the past is relevant in short-term dynamic therapy, it is not the primary focus (as it is in long-term psychodynamic therapy) (option B is incorrect). Interpersonal therapy emphasizes attempting new patterns of communication and altered expectations in extratherapeutic relationships as the mechanism of change (option D is incorrect). **Chapter 31 (pp. 902, 904, 905 [Table 31–2])**

31.2   A 31-year-old man presents to your clinic with recurrence of major depressive disorder after a recent breakup. His current symptoms include difficulty falling asleep, amotivation, social isolation, low self-esteem, and increased anxiety about meeting new people. He has been feeling lonely yet avoids going to social events. He is frequently self-critical and fears rejection. How would a provider using interpersonal therapy (IPT) conceptualize this patient's presenting problem?

A. The patient is experiencing a role transition resulting from an acute relational stressor (breakup) that exacerbates his preexisting vulnerability to avoidance and social isolation.

B. The patient has negative automatic thoughts (e.g., "no one will like me at the party") that are reinforced by cognitive distortions (e.g., catastrophizing) and driven by a self-critical core belief (e.g., "I'm unlovable").
C. The patient avoids social events and acts guardedly in an attempt to avoid rejection and abandonment, causing others to pull away from him.
D. The patient focuses excessively on his recent breakup, blinding him to his moments of success, including other fulfilling relationships.

The correct response is option A: The patient is experiencing a role transition resulting from an acute relational stressor (breakup) that exacerbates his preexisting vulnerability to avoidance and social isolation.

IPT is based on the biopsychosocial diathesis–stress model: an acute interpersonal crisis (stress), particularly in the absence of sufficient social support, will cause distress and symptoms in the area in which the person is vulnerable (diathesis). IPT targets three problem areas, one of which is role transitions, which include social transitions such as marriage and divorce—or, as in this case, a breakup (option A is correct).

Cognitive restructuring helps patients understand the relation between thoughts and feelings and the ways in which automatic thought patterns can sustain unwanted patterns of emotion and action. Cognitive therapists target cognitive distortions and link core beliefs to automatic thoughts, emotions, and behaviors (option B is incorrect).

Strategic therapies view presenting concerns as the result of attempts at solutions that unwittingly reinforce the very problems patients are attempting to address. A person concerned about rejection in relationships, for instance, might interact in guarded ways, leading others to avoid future interaction. The problem, from the vantage point of the strategic therapist, is a function of the patient's construal of the situation and the ways in which that construal is reinforced through social interaction (Quick 2008) (option C is incorrect).

In solution-focused therapy, there is an important sense that problems do not exist at all. When patients cannot reach their goals, they at some point identify that they have a problem. This reification becomes self-fulfilling: the more patients focus on their problems, the more troubled they feel and act. Equally important, such a problem focus blinds patients to the occasions in which they do, in fact, reach their goals (option D is incorrect). **Chapter 31 (pp. 903–904, 906–907, 908, 909–910)**

31.3 What would be the role of a solution-focused therapist during sessions with the patient described in question 31.2?

A. Teach the patient specific skills and coach him to use these skills during behavioral exposures.
B. Build on the patient's prior experiences of success and apply them to the current situation.

C. Collaboratively work with the patient to problem-solve ways to manage relational challenges.

D. Create powerful emotional experiences during sessions to promote change.

The correct response is option B: Build on the patient's prior experiences of success and apply them to the current situation.

A solution-focused therapist emphasizes doing more of what is already working: the therapy is not initiating new behavior and thought patterns but instead is building on existing ones (option B is correct). Behavior therapists use exposure as a core therapeutic ingredient and introduce specific skills designed to help patients control their symptoms during exposures (option A is incorrect). An interpersonal therapist acts as collaborative problem solver and focuses on relationships and communication patterns (option C is incorrect). Short-term dynamic therapists create heightened emotional contexts for change within therapy (option D is incorrect). **Chapter 31 (pp. 902–906, 910)**

31.4 Which of the following brief therapies is based on the biopsychosocial diathesis-stress model?

A. Interpersonal therapy.
B. Behavioral therapy.
C. Strategic therapy.
D. Short-term psychodynamic therapy.

The correct response is option A: Interpersonal therapy.

Interpersonal therapy is based on the psychosocial diathesis-stress model: an acute interpersonal crisis (stress), particularly in the absence of sufficient social support, will cause distress and symptoms in the area in which the person is vulnerable (diathesis) (option A is correct). Behavioral therapy views the presenting concerns of patients as learned maladaptive patterns of behavior and thought that can be unlearned (option B is incorrect). Strategic therapy views patients' presenting problems as resulting from attempts at solutions that unwittingly reinforce the very problems patients are attempting to address (option C is incorrect). Short-term psychodynamic therapy is based on the premise that patients' presenting problems result from an internalization of conflicts from earlier significant relationships (option D is incorrect). **Chapter 31 (pp. 901, 903, 905, 908)**

31.5 Which of the following brief therapies conceptualizes presenting issues as the result of interactions between patients and their contexts, rather than as intrinsic to patients?

A. Behavioral therapy.
B. Strategic therapy.
C. Short-term psychodynamic therapy.
D. Interpersonal therapy.

The correct response is option B: Strategic therapy.

Relational (i.e., short-term psychodynamic, interpersonal) and learning (i.e., behavior, cognitive) therapies begin with a common premise: the presenting concerns of patients are acquired over the life span as the result of problematic experiences such as faulty relationships or faulty learning. These therapies, in that sense, place the locus of problems within the patient (options A, C, and D are incorrect).

Contextual brief therapies (i.e., strategic, solution-focused), on the other hand, do not view problems as intrinsic to patients. Rather, problems are seen as artifacts of person–situation interactions that, once identified, can be rapidly modified (option B is correct). **Chapter 31 (p. 908)**

31.6 A 44-year-old woman presents to your clinic with ruminative anxiety, insomnia, restlessness, and low energy after having found out that her spouse is having an affair and is requesting a divorce. She has been experiencing panic attacks about twice a month since this all began. Her symptoms have improved with a selective serotonin reuptake inhibitor, but she still finds it difficult to go on dates. She says dating triggers her anxiety, and "it feels hard to trust anyone." What would the therapist's role be if this patient were undergoing behavioral therapy?

A. Use Socratic questioning to challenge the patient's belief that "no one can be trusted" and replace it with more accurate and helpful thoughts.
B. Teach the patient skills to manage her anxiety and panic, then gradually expose her to triggers to provide her with direct experiences of mastery.
C. Find the exceptions to the patient's patterns of mistrust and social isolation, then use these exceptions to help her "do more of what is already working."
D. Act as a transference object, involving him- or herself in the patient's core relationship patterns.

The correct response is option B: Teach the patient skills to manage her anxiety and panic, then gradually expose her to triggers to provide her with direct experiences of mastery.

In behavioral therapy, the therapist guides the patient in identifying specific triggers for symptom appearance and then introduces specific skills designed to help control these symptoms. The emphasized mechanism of change is rehearsal of skills and experiences of mastery during problematic situations (option B is correct).

In contrast, cognitive therapy centers on a Socratic process of guided discovery between therapist and patient that questions cognitive distortions and encourages a consideration of alternative explanations (option A is incorrect).

In solution-focused therapy, the therapist focuses on solution patterns rather than on problems. The patient is asked to identify occasions during which problems either do not occur or occur less often or less intensely, and the therapist then coaches the patient in enacting these exceptions to problem patterns—doing more of what is already working (option C is incorrect).

Finally, in short-term psychodynamic therapy, the therapist acts as a transference object. Change is catalyzed by the involvement of the therapist in the core relationship patterns, breaking the cycles of repetition by providing responses different from those anticipated by patients (option D is incorrect). **Chapter 31 (pp. 902, 905 [Table 31–2], 905–906, 907, 910)**

31.7   In which of the following types of brief psychotherapy does the therapist specifically target the patient's current relationship challenges and communication patterns?

A. Strategic therapy.
B. Solution-focused therapy.
C. Long-term psychodynamic therapy.
D. Interpersonal therapy.

The correct response is option D: Interpersonal therapy.

Like psychodynamic therapy, interpersonal therapy (IPT) sustains a focus on relationship issues and also on interpersonal communication. However, it is distinct from psychodynamic therapy in that the primary focus of IPT is on the patients' relationships and communication patterns with others who are *currently* important in their lives. The IPT therapist does not seek to understand how past events and relationships may have influenced current relationships (option D is correct; option C is incorrect).

Strategic and solution-focused therapy both emphasize the present over the past, but do not emphasize relationship challenges or communication patterns as the target of treatment. Instead, a strategic therapist would work to reframe problems in ways that lend themselves to spontaneous goal attainment (option A is incorrect). A solution-focused therapist would emphasize enacting exceptions to problem patterns and doing more of what is already working (option B is incorrect). **Chapter 31 (pp. 903, 909, 910, 912, 913)**

31.8   How would a short-term psychodynamic therapist manage a patient's resistance?

A. Actively challenge and confront the resistance.
B. Offer interpretive comments about the source of the resistance.
C. Engage with patients in a highly collaborative manner to minimize resistance.
D. Remain focused on patient's own goals to avoid resistance.

The correct response is option A: Actively challenge and confront the resistance.

Many of the brief therapies include procedures designed to elicit the understanding and cooperation of patients, such as explicit efforts at education, the use of the patient's own language in framing goals, and the collaborative formulation of treatment goals. They aim to minimize resistance to change and sustain favorable expectations for outcome.

Short-term psychodynamic therapists seek to challenge and break through patterns of defense and resistance, thereby creating a heightened emotional context for change (option A is correct). In contrast, therapists practicing traditional long-term psychodynamic therapy primarily use interpretation to deal with resistance (option B is incorrect).

The learning therapies (behavior therapy and cognitive therapy) feature the therapist in an active, directive teaching mode and the patient as a student, with the patient receiving psychosocial education in early session. Cognitive therapists engage with patients in a highly collaborative manner, minimizing resistance and sustaining the helping alliance (option C is incorrect).

Solution-focused therapists work within patient-identified goals to minimize resistance, maintain a tight solution focus, involve patients in between-session efforts to enact solution patterns, and preserve a highly active stance (Steenbarger 2018) (option D is incorrect). **Chapter 31 (pp. 902, 904, 905, 907, 910, 914)**

31.9   Which of the following statements about the existing research literature on brief therapies is *true*?

A. Short-term psychodynamic and interpersonal therapies have been formally evaluated in only a limited number of studies.
B. Study findings argue against providing maintenance sessions after a course of brief therapy.
C. Research examining the dose-effect relationship in psychotherapy indicates that approximately 20% of patients experience significant improvement within 18–26 sessions of therapy.
D. Studies suggest that patients with more chronic problems may not be appropriate for brief therapies.

The correct response is option D: Studies suggest that patients with more chronic problems may not be appropriate for brief therapies.

Chronic emotional and behavioral patterns are likely to have been overlearned and thus are more likely to require ongoing intervention than are problems of more recent origin (Steenbarger 2002); furthermore, patients with chronic and severe problem patterns frequently need more ongoing support than can be provided in short-term treatment (option D is correct).

A sizable body of studies support the effectiveness of short-term psychodynamic therapy, interpersonal therapy (IPT), and solution-focused brief therapy (Dewan et al. 2018) (option A is incorrect).

Although several studies support the long-term effectiveness of IPT and cognitive-behavioral therapies (Lambert 2013), data also suggest that highly abbreviated treatments may run an enhanced risk of patient relapse (Steenbarger 1994) and that ongoing maintenance sessions can be effective in reducing relapse rates (Lambert 2013) and improving long-term outcome (option B is incorrect).

Early investigations of the dose–effect relationship in psychotherapy found that approximately 50% of patients experienced significant improvement within 8 sessions of therapy and that 75% reached such improvement within 26 sessions (Howard et al. 1986). More recent research reviewed by Castonguay et al. (2013) found that clinically significant change occurs in half of all patients within 11–18 sessions (option C is incorrect). **Chapter 31 (pp. 914, 915, 916)**

31.10 Research findings highlight the importance of careful patient selection in the conduct of brief therapy. Which of the following patient characteristics would be predictive of a good outcome in time-limited therapy?

A. Patients with weak social supports.
B. Patients with simpler, less severe presenting problems.
C. Patients with lower interpersonal functioning.
D. Patients currently in the contemplative stage of change.

The correct response is option B: Patients with simpler, less severe presenting problems.

Reviews of the outcome literature on brief therapies (e.g., Roth and Fonagy 2006) suggest that therapeutic outcomes are more favorable for patients with less complex concerns (option B is correct). Most patients with severe presenting concerns and characterological and interpersonal problems (Lambert 2013) do not achieve clinically significant outcomes in a brief time frame.

When patients have weak or nonexistent social supports, they may look to therapy for support as well as for targeted change. In those cases, they are unlikely to embrace time limits on treatment (option A is incorrect).

Given the importance of the therapeutic alliance to change across all psychotherapies (Crits-Christoph et al. 2013), it is unlikely that patients with poor interpersonal functioning and difficulties sustaining relationships will benefit from brief intervention. Indeed, these patients may need many sessions before they can even forge a trusting relationship (option C is incorrect).

Prochaska and Norcross (2002) found that the course of therapy is different for patients who have a clear understanding and acceptance of their problems and the need for change than for patients who lack such understanding. Patients in an action phase of readiness for change are much more likely to embrace the change techniques of brief treatment than are patients in precontemplative or contemplative modes. These latter groups, in fact, may require numerous sessions of problem exploration before they even acknowledge a need for change (option D is incorrect). **Chapter 31 (pp. 916, 917)**

31.11 Which of the following brief therapies is generally the shortest in duration?

A. Behavioral therapy.
B. Interpersonal therapy.

C. Solution-focused therapy.

D. Strategic therapy.

The correct response is option D: Strategic therapy.

Strategic and solution-focused therapies are generally the briefest of the therapies and can be placed at one end of a continuum that ranges from highly abbreviated and highly structured contextual therapies to more exploratory relational treatments. Interpersonal therapy typically lasts 8–20 sessions (option B is incorrect).

Behavioral therapies include *exposure and response prevention*, which is designed to treat obsessive-compulsive disorder in a 17-session protocol, and *prolonged exposure*, which is designed to treat posttraumatic stress disorder in 8–15 sessions (option A is incorrect).

Of the two contextual therapies, strategic therapy can include single-session treatments, whereas solution-focused therapy lasts several sessions on average (option D is correct; option C is incorrect). **Chapter 31 (pp. 903, 905, 908, 910, 912, 913 [Figure 31–1])**

References

Castonguay L, Barkham M, Lutz N, et al: Practice oriented research, in Handbook of Psychotherapy and Behavior Change, 6th Edition, Edited by Lambert M, New York, Wiley, 2013, pp 85–133

Crits-Christoph P, Gibbons MBC, Mukherjee D: Psychotherapy process-outcome research, in Bergin and Garfield's Handbook of Psychotherapy and Behavior Change, 6th Edition. Edited by Lambert MJ. Hoboken, NJ, Wiley, 2013, pp 298–340

Dewan MJ, Steenbarger BN, Greenberg RP (eds): The Art and Science of Brief Psychotherapies: An Illustrated Guide, 3rd Edition. Washington, DC, American Psychiatric Publishing, 2018

Howard KI, Kopta SM, Krause MS, et al: The dose-effect relationship in psychotherapy. Am Psychol 41(2):159–164, 1986 3516036

Lambert MJ: The efficacy and effectiveness of psychotherapy, in Bergin and Garfield's Handbook of Psychotherapy and Behavior Change, 6th Edition. Edited by Lambert MJ. Hoboken, NJ, Wiley, 2013, pp 169–218

Prochaska JO, Norcross JC: Stages of change, in Psychotherapy Relationships That Work: Therapist Contributions and Responsiveness to Patients. Edited by Norcross JC. New York, Oxford University Press, 2002, pp 303–314

Quick EK: Doing What Works in Brief Psychotherapy, 2nd Edition. Burlington, MA, Elsevier, 2008

Roth A, Fonagy P: What Works for Whom? A Critical Review of Psychotherapy Research, 2nd Edition. New York, Guilford, 2006

Steenbarger BN: Duration and outcome in psychotherapy: an integrative review. Professional Psychology: Research and Practice 25(2):111–119, 1994

Steenbarger BN: Brief therapy, in Encyclopedia of Psychotherapy, Vol 1. Edited by Hersen M, Sledge W. New York, Elsevier, 2002, pp 349–358

Steenbarger BN: Solution-focused brief therapy: building strengths, achieving goals, in The Art and Science of Brief Psychotherapies: An Illustrated Guide, 3rd Edition. Edited by Dewan MJ, Steenbarger BN, Greenberg RP. Washington, DC, American Psychiatric Association Publishing, 2018, pp 199–218

CHAPTER 32

Psychodynamic Psychotherapy

32.1   The contemporary psychodynamic therapist is most likely to identify dominant issues from which of the following areas of patient focus?

A. Chief complaints.
B. Treatment satisfaction.
C. Psychiatric symptoms.
D. Early childhood experiences.

The correct response is option B: Treatment satisfaction.

In each session, the therapist identifies a *dominant issue*—an expression of conflict and defense currently active in the session—that becomes a focus for intervention. To identify a dominant issue, the therapist attends to the three channels of communication (i.e., the patient's verbal communications, the patient's nonverbal communications, and the feelings stimulated in the therapist by the patient's verbal and nonverbal communications [Caligor et al. 2018]), listening in particular for expressions of affect, descriptions of repetitive relationship patterns, communications about the therapist or about treatment, and evidence of activation of defenses (option B is correct).

Attention to transference and countertransference is a defining feature of dynamic therapy. Classical dynamic approaches to transference focused on "reliving" the past in the present, and considerable attention was directed toward exploring the relationship between childhood experience and current relational patterns. More contemporary models of transference focus not on the past as relived in the present but rather on information processing in the here and now (option D is incorrect).

In choosing between cognitive-behavioral and psychodynamic approaches, a helpful rule of thumb is that cognitive-behavioral therapy tends to focus more specifically than psychodynamic therapy on the chief complaint and symptom constellation—for example, reduction of depression, alleviation of anxiety, or improved management of parasuicidal behavior. In comparison, psychodynamic treatments tend to have a broader treatment focus, placing greater emphasis on modifying domains of personality functioning related to presenting symptoms (options A and C are incorrect). **Chapter 32 (pp. 937, 944, 947–948)**

32.2 Which of the following represents an *expressive* psychodynamic intervention?

A. Advice.
B. Psychoeducation.
C. Empathic validation.
D. Clarification.

The correct response is option D: Clarification.

Interventions used in dynamic therapies can be visualized as falling along the *supportive-expressive continuum*. Expressive interventions, also referred to as *exploratory* interventions, aim to "open things up"—to bring to the patient's awareness aspects of himself or herself that are defended against and therefore lie outside full awareness, and ultimately to help the patient make sense of these parts of the self and to take responsibility for them. The techniques used by the psychodynamic therapist that fall at the most expressive end of the continuum are referred to as *interpretive interventions*. The process of interpretation can be conceptualized as using three kinds of techniques. The most basic is clarification, followed by confrontation and interpretation proper (option D is correct).

  Supportive interventions can be seen as placing the therapist in a more active role. In some supportive interventions, the therapist is directive, suggesting certain behaviors, whereas in others, the therapist focuses more on supporting the patient emotionally—alleviating distress, reducing confusion, and providing an experience of being cared for. Supportive interventions routinely used in dynamic therapy include psychoeducation; empathic validation; directing the patient's attention to particular aspects of his or her thoughts, feelings, and behaviors that appear to be relevant to issues currently active in the therapy; and requests for elaboration or clarification (options B and C are incorrect).

  Additional techniques further along the supportive continuum that may be used in some forms of psychodynamic therapy include providing direct, concrete advice or guidance; teaching coping skills; and offering reassurance or praise (option A is incorrect). **Chapter 32 (pp. 928–929)**

32.3 The most support for the efficacy of psychodynamic therapy is established in the treatment of which of the following disorders?

A. Bulimia nervosa.
B. Delusional disorder.
C. Avoidant personality disorder.
D. Obsessive-compulsive disorder.

The correct response is option C: Avoidant personality disorder.

The efficacy of psychodynamic therapy in the treatment of personality disorders has been established for borderline personality disorder, Cluster C personality disorders (i.e., avoidant personality disorder, dependent personality disorder, and obsessive-compulsive personality disorder), and complex mental disorders (defined by Leichsenring and Rabung [2011] as personality disorders, chronic mental disorders, or multiple mental disorders) (option C is correct).

A series of controlled trials examining the efficacy of psychotherapies and pharmacotherapies for bulimia nervosa (Svaldi et al. 2019) found that cognitive-behavioral therapy (CBT) was more effective than comparable treatments such as psychodynamic psychotherapy, interpersonal therapy, weight loss treatment, and medication. Hence, CBT is regarded as the primary treatment for bulimia nervosa (option A is incorrect).

CBT can help delusion-related affective states (in delusional disorder), but there is currently no effective treatment to improve insight and to reduce delusional conviction (Peralta and Cuesta 2016) (option B is incorrect).

Freud (1973) postulated that obsessions were defensive reactions to unconscious impulses, especially sexual and aggressive impulses. Obsessions served as a way to mask these impulses and/or control them. Unfortunately, although psychodynamic therapy may help to reveal the origins of obsessions, there is little evidence that doing so changes obsessive-compulsive disorder symptoms (option D is incorrect). **Chapter 32 (pp. 948–949); see also Chapter 10 ("Schizophrenia Spectrum and Other Psychotic Disorders"; p. 265), Chapter 14 ("Obsessive-Compulsive and Related Disorders"; p. 373), and Chapter 18 ("Eating and Feeding Disorders"; p. 504)**

32.4   Which of the following potential positive outcomes of psychodynamic therapy represents a *structural* change?

A. Improved interpersonal functioning.
B. Improved capacity for mentalization.
C. Improved self-esteem.
D. Improved management of aggression.

The correct response is option B: Improved capacity for mentalization.

Empirical studies support the benefits of establishing clear goals for treatment, which may enhance both alliance and outcome Typical goals for psychodynamic therapy include improved interpersonal functioning (option A is incorrect) and capacity to sustain satisfying intimate and sexual relationships, improved occupational functioning or capacity to derive satisfaction from work, enhanced self-definition or improved self-esteem (option C is incorrect), enhanced ability to pursue long-term goals, better management of aggression (e.g., temper outbursts or inappropriate expressions of hostility, passivity, or failure of assertiveness) (option D is incorrect), and amelioration of symptoms of anxiety and depression.

In addition to descriptive treatment goals, which reflect the patient's concerns and the specific difficulties that brought the patient to treatment, the psychodynamic therapist has in mind a set of *structural* goals for the treatment, with the expectation that structural changes will lead to symptomatic improvement. Barber et al. (2013) suggested five unique, empirically supported ways in which dynamic therapy seeks to help patients: 1) fostering insight into unconscious conflict, 2) increasing the use of adaptive psychological defenses, 3) decreasing rigidity in interpersonal perceptions and behavior, 4) improving the quality of the patient's mental representations of relationships (i.e., improving the quality of object relations), and 5) increasing the patient's comprehension of his or her own and others' mental states (i.e., improving the capacity for mentalization) (option B is correct). **Chapter 32 (pp. 927, 937–938)**

32.5 Which of the following change processes has demonstrated relatively consistent clinical utility and positive outcomes?

A. Affective exploration.
B. High-frequency interpretations.
C. Minimal use of supportive interventions.
D. A focus on isolated personal themes.

The correct response is option A: Affective exploration.

Understanding how a treatment works is the first step in understanding how the treatment can be improved or how more effective treatments can be developed. In approaching these questions, it is helpful to distinguish between *change processes* introduced by the therapist and the treatment model (e.g., use of particular interventions, therapist competence in delivering the interventions) and *change mechanisms* taking place within the patient (e.g., patient self-understanding, reflective functioning) (Crits-Christoph et al. 2013). Both should be linked to positive outcome. *Common factors* are treatment elements that are provided by diverse forms of therapy—for example, therapeutic alliance, therapist empathy, use of a coherent and consistent clinical approach, patient expectation of change, and encouragement to face personal difficulties—and that overlap considerably with supportive interventions (option C is incorrect).

It is widely accepted that common factors play a role in therapeutic outcome in psychodynamic treatments. It is also clear that, at least in some settings, specific factors play a significant role in outcome. Interpersonal and affective exploration and the sparing use of accurate interpretations appear to be generally helpful (option A is correct; options B and D are incorrect). **Chapter 32 (pp. 949–951)**

32.6 Which of the following statements regarding severe personality pathology and psychodynamic psychotherapy is *true*?

A. Severe personality disorders are a contraindication to treatment with dynamic therapy.
B. Longer dynamic treatments are preferred in this population.

C. Transference work should ideally be minimized in this population.

D. Countertransference work should ideally be minimized in this population.

The correct response is option B: Longer dynamic treatments are preferred in this population.

Treatments for personality disorders are longer term, usually ranging from a minimum of 30 sessions for less severe personality pathology to weekly or twice-weekly sessions over the course of several years for more severe pathology. Another useful rule of thumb is that the more general the patient's complaints and symptoms, and the more global and severe the personality pathology, the longer the duration of treatment likely to be needed will be (option B is correct).

Patients with high-level borderline personality organization (histrionic, dependent, and avoidant personality disorders, as well as healthier narcissistic patients) do well in structured forms of dynamic therapy. Despite severity, many patients with mid-level borderline personality organization (borderline, paranoid, and schizoid personality disorders) can benefit from a variety of specialized treatments (option A is incorrect).

Ruptures of the therapeutic alliance are common and inevitable, and exploration of ruptures as they occur throughout the treatment is central to the psychotherapeutic process in the treatment of patients with low-level borderline personality organization (narcissistic personality disorder with significant antisocial features, malignant narcissistic personality disorder, and antisocial personality disorder [the latter of which is a contraindication for dynamic therapy]). Ruptures may be accompanied by strong emotional reactions on the part of the patient, often including hostility, accusations, and even paranoia and destructive acting out. Patients with more severe pathology may preferentially benefit from transference work. With this population, transferences develop rapidly and tend to be grossly distorted, highly affectively charged, and extreme and are often negative and intrusive—both demanding of clinical attention and providing a central vehicle for exploration and change (option C is incorrect).

As a general rule, as personality pathology becomes more severe, attending to countertransference becomes increasingly central to clinical work (option D is incorrect). **Chapter 32 (pp. 929, 933, 935 [Table 32–4], 943–944, 946, 947, 949)**

References

Barber JP, Muran C, McCarthy KS, et al: Research on dynamic therapies, in Bergin and Garfield's Handbook of Psychotherapy and Behavior Change, 6th Edition. Edited by Lambert MJ. Hoboken, NJ, Wiley, 2013, pp 443–494

Caligor E, Kernberg OF, Clarkin JF, et al: Psychodynamic Therapy for Personality Pathology: Treating Self and Interpersonal Functioning. Arlington, VA, American Psychiatric Association Publishing, 2018

Crits-Christoph P, Connolly Gibbons M, Mukherjee D: Psychotherapy process-outcome research, in Bergin and Garfield's Handbook of Psychotherapy and Behavior Change, 6th Edition. Edited by Lambert MJ. Hoboken, NJ, Wiley, 2013, pp 298–340

Freud S: Three Case Histories: The "Wolf Man," the "Rat Man," and the Psychotic Doctor Schreber (1909). Translated by Rieff P. New York, Macmillan, 1973

Leichsenring F, Rabung S: Long-term psychodynamic psychotherapy in complex mental disorders: update of a meta-analysis. Br J Psychiatry 199(1):15–22, 2011 21719877

Peralta V, Cuesta MJ: Delusional disorder and schizophrenia: a comparative study across multiple domains. Psychol Med 46(13):2829–2839, 2016 27468631

Svaldi J, Schmitz F, Baur J, et al: Efficacy of psychotherapies and pharmacotherapies for bulimia nervosa. Psychol Med 49(6):898–910, 2019 30514412

CHAPTER 33

Cognitive-Behavioral Therapy

33.1 Which of the following patient interventions is a primary focus of cognitive-behavioral therapy (CBT) (as opposed to psychodynamic psychotherapy or interpersonal therapy)?

A. Cognitive appraisal and emotional responses to external events.
B. Relationship with the therapist.
C. Wishes, dreams, and fantasies.
D. Interpersonal communication patterns.

The correct response is option A: Cognitive appraisal and emotional responses to external events.

The CBT Model (Wright et al. 2017; Figure 33–1) posits a close relationship between cognition and emotion. The general thrust of CBT is that emotional responses are largely dependent on cognitive appraisals of the significance of environmental cues (option A is correct). For example, sadness is likely when a person perceives an event (or memory of an event) in a negative way (e.g., as a loss, a defeat, or a rejection), and anger is common when a person judges that there are threats to oneself or one's loved ones. The cognitive model also incorporates the effects of emotion on cognitive processing. Heightened emotion can stimulate and intensify cognitive distortions. Therapeutic procedures in CBT involve interventions at all points in the model diagrammed in Figure 33–1. However, most of the effort is directed at stimulating either cognitive or behavioral change.

The psychodynamic treatments (see Chapter 32, "Psychodynamic Psychotherapy"), on the other hand, are distinguished on the basis of 1) a focus on affect and emotional expression; 2) identification of recurring patterns of behavior, feelings, experiences, and relationships; 3) a focus on interpersonal relationships; 4) exploration of the therapeutic relationship (option B is incorrect); 5) exploration of the patient's tendency to defend against and avoid certain issues; and 6) exploration of wishes, dreams, and fantasies (option C is incorrect).

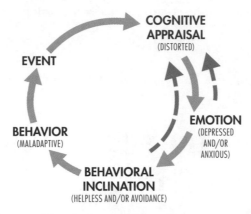

FIGURE 33–1. Basic cognitive-behavioral model.

Source. Reprinted from Wright JH, Brown GK, Thase ME, Basco MR: *Learning Cognitive-Behavior Therapy: An Illustrated Guide,* 2nd Edition (Core Competencies in Psychotherapy Series; Glen O. Gabbard, series ed). Arlington, VA, American Psychiatric Association Publishing, 2017, p. 4. Copyright © 2017, American Psychiatric Association Publishing. Used with permission.

Interpersonal therapy (IPT; see Chapter 31, "Brief Psychotherapies"), a brief psychotherapy, sustains a focus on relationship issues and also on interpersonal communication (option D is incorrect). The primary focus of IPT is on the patients' relationships and communication patterns with others who are currently import-ant in their lives. **Chapter 33 (pp. 957–958); see also Chapter 31 ("Brief Psycho-therapies"; p. 903) and Chapter 32 ("Psychodynamic Psychotherapy"; p. 925)**

33.2   Which of the following types of pathological information processing is character-istic of both anxiety disorders and depressive disorder?

A. Fears of harm or danger.
B. Impaired performance on tasks requiring effort or abstract thinking.
C. Demoralization.
D. Overestimates of risk in situations.

The correct response is option C: Demoralization.

The role of cognitive functioning in depressive and anxiety disorders has been studied extensively. Table 33–1 shows pathological information processing that occurs primarily in depressive disorders, anxiety disorders, or both. Predominant in depression are hopelessness, low self-esteem, negative view of environment, automatic thoughts with negative themes, misattributions, overestimates of neg-ative feedback, enhanced recall of negative memories, and impaired performance on cognitive tasks requiring effort or abstract thinking (option B is incorrect).

Predominant in anxiety are fears of harm or danger (option A is incorrect); high sensitivity to information about potential threat; automatic thoughts associ-ated with danger, risk, uncontrollability, or incapacity; overestimates of risk in sit-

TABLE 33–1. Pathological information processing in depression and anxiety disorders

Predominant in depression	Predominant in anxiety disorders	Common to both depression and anxiety disorders
Hopelessness	Fears of harm or danger	Demoralization
Low self-esteem	High sensitivity to information	Self-absorption
Negative view of environment	about potential threat	Heightened automatic information processing
Automatic thoughts with negative themes	Automatic thoughts associated with danger, risk, uncontrollability, incapacity	Maladaptive schemas
Misattributions	Overestimates of risk in situations	Reduced cognitive capacity for problem solving
Overestimates of negative feedback	Enhanced recall of memories for threatening situations	
Enhanced recall of negative memories		
Impaired performance on cognitive tasks requiring effort, abstract thinking		

uations (option D is incorrect); and enhanced recall of memories for threatening situations.

Shared between the two disorders are demoralization (option C is correct), self-absorption, heightened automatic information processing, maladaptive schemas, and reduced cognitive capacity for problem solving. **Chapter 33 (pp. 960–961; Table 33–3 [p. 961])**

33.3 Which of the following is one of the most frequently used techniques for identifying and modifying problematic cognitions in cognitive-behavioral therapy (CBT)?

A. Confrontation.
B. Direct guidance.
C. Socratic questioning.
D. Empathic validation.

The correct response is option C: Socratic questioning.

One of the most frequently used procedures in CBT is Socratic questioning. Socratic questioning usually involves a series of inductive questions that are likely to reveal dysfunctional thought patterns (option C is correct).

The use of expressive interventions—also referred to as *exploratory* interventions and including clarification, confrontation, and interpretation proper—distinguishes psychodynamic therapies from other forms of treatment, including CBT. Exploratory interventions aim to "open things up"—to bring to the patient's awareness aspects of himself or herself that are defended against and therefore lie outside full awareness, and ultimately to help the patient make sense of these parts of the self and to take responsibility for them. For this exploration, psychodynamic therapists use *interpretation*, a process involving three kinds of techniques: clarification, confrontation, and interpretation proper (option A is incorrect).

Supportive interventions routinely used in psychodynamic therapy include psychoeducation; empathic validation; directing the patient's attention to particular aspects of his or her thoughts, feelings, and behaviors that appear to be relevant to issues currently active in the therapy; and requests for elaboration or clarification (options B and D are incorrect). **Chapter 33 (p. 970); see also Chapter 32 ("Psychodynamic Psychotherapy"; pp. 928–929)**

33.4   Which of the following is one of the main behavioral techniques employed in cognitive-behavioral therapy (CBT) for anxiety disorders?

A. Examining the evidence.
B. Exposure.
C. Thought recording.
D. Cognitive rehearsal.

The correct response is option B: Exposure.

Exposure techniques are a central part of cognitive-behavioral approaches to anxiety disorders. Typically, a hierarchy of feared stimuli is developed with the patient. The hierarchy should contain several different stimuli that cause varying degrees of distress. After the hierarchy is established, the therapist and patient work collaboratively to set goals for gradual exposure, starting with the items that are ranked lower on the distress scale (option B is correct).

Examining the evidence, thought recording, and cognitive rehearsal are cognitive CBT techniques, not behavioral ones (options A, C, and D are incorrect). Other cognitive methods used in CBT include Socratic questioning (guided discovery), use of mood shifts to demonstrate automatic thoughts, in vivo imagery exercises, role-play, generating alternatives, decatastrophizing, and reattribution. **Chapter 33 (pp. 970 [Table 33–8], 977–978)**

33.5   Research evidence supports use of cognitive-behavioral therapy (CBT) as a primary (first-line) intervention for which of the following disorders?

A. Schizophrenia.
B. Eating disorders.
C. Bipolar disorders.
D. Depression with psychotic features.

The correct response is option B: Eating disorders.

CBT can be considered a primary treatment for 1) disorders in which it has been proven to be effective in controlled research (e.g., unipolar depression [nonpsychotic], anxiety disorders, eating disorders, psychophysiological disorders) and 2) other conditions for which a clearly detailed treatment method has been developed (e.g., personality disorders, substance abuse) and some evidence supports CBT's effectiveness (option B is correct).

CBT should be considered as an adjunctive therapy for disorders such as major depressive disorder with psychotic features, bipolar disorder, and schizophrenia—disorders for which there is clear evidence for the effectiveness of pharmacotherapy but limited or no research examining the effectiveness of CBT alone compared with pharmacotherapy (options A, C, and D are incorrect). **Chapter 33 (p. 981)**

Reference

Wright JH, Brown GK, Thase ME, Basco MR: Learning Cognitive-Behavior Therapy: An Illustrated Guide, 2nd Edition (Core Competencies in Psychotherapy Series; Gabbard GO, series ed). Arlington, VA, American Psychiatric Association Publishing, 2017

CHAPTER 34

Supportive Psychotherapy

34.1   Which of the following statements best describes the organizing goals of supportive psychotherapy?

A. To provide severely impaired patients with interventions aimed at improving ego functions, day-to-day coping, and self-esteem.
B. To change the patient's underlying personality structure.
C. To develop a supportive relationship between the therapist and the patient.
D. To utilize specifically definable techniques or interventions that are unique within the fields of psychiatry and psychology.

The correct response is option A: To provide severely impaired patients with interventions aimed at improving ego functions, day-to-day coping, and self-esteem.

Supportive psychotherapy is an extensively practiced form of individual psychotherapy that focuses on ameliorating symptoms, improving self-esteem, fostering resilience, and strengthening adaptive skills. Supportive psychotherapy is helpful for the most impaired patients, who require direct interventions aimed at improving ego functions, day-to-day coping, and self-esteem (option A is correct).

Supportive psychotherapy is not merely a supportive relationship between the therapist and the patient (option C is incorrect); rather, it is highly intentional therapeutic work that emphasizes relational and interpersonal issues and the self within the reality of the present everyday world as opposed to conflict and instinctual issues and a focus on the past.

Supportive therapy does not seek to change the patient's underlying personality structure; instead, supportive psychotherapy is oriented toward coping, adaptation, and well-being (option B is incorrect).

Supportive psychotherapy includes specifically definable techniques or interventions that draw from across the fields of psychiatry and psychology (option D is incorrect). **Chapter 34 (pp. 999–1001)**

34.2 For which of the following diagnoses would supportive psychotherapy be contra-indicated?

A. Acute bereavement.
B. Late-stage dementia.
C. Substance use disorder.
D. Pancreatic cancer.

The correct response is option B: Late-stage dementia.

Supportive psychotherapy has value in the care of very impaired individuals, in the care of less impaired individuals in acute situational distress, in the care of medically ill patients, in the context of grief, and as an adjuvant strategy in the care of individuals living with addiction. Supportive psychotherapy is contraindicated only when psychotherapy itself is contraindicated, such as in patients with delirium, drug intoxication, late-stage dementia, or malingering (option B is correct), or when providing supportive psychotherapy would deprive the patient of a more appropriate form of care. In the care of patients with substance use disorders, supportive psychotherapy may play an invaluable adjuvant role, helping individuals to develop coping strategies to control or reduce substance use and diminish anxiety and dysphoria (option C is incorrect).

For many medical conditions, supportive psychotherapy is the only psychotherapeutic treatment that should be recommended. Early studies showed that supportive psychotherapy could be successfully used in patients with breast cancer, in HIV-positive patients with depression, in patients with pancreatic cancer (option D is incorrect), in cancer patients with depression, in patients with chronic pain, in patients with HIV-related neuropathic pain, and in patients with somatization disorder (Winston et al. 2012). Supportive psychotherapy is also helpful in caring for a person after an acute loss of a loved one (option A is incorrect). **Chapter 34 (pp. 1001–1002)**

34.3 Which of the following patients would be most likely to have a good outcome from supportive psychotherapy?

A. A patient with new-onset delirium secondary to electrolyte abnormalities.
B. A patient with an adjustment disorder after the loss of a loved one.
C. A patient with unremitting panic disorder and agoraphobia.
D. A patient with obsessive-compulsive disorder and contamination phobias.

The correct response is option B: A patient with an adjustment disorder after the loss of a loved one.

In considering whether supportive psychotherapy is appropriate, it is important to note that for some conditions, treatments other than supportive psychotherapy have been shown to be more effective. For example, panic disorder (Barlow and Craske 1989) and obsessive-compulsive disorder (Foa and Franklin 2002) have been shown to have better outcomes with cognitive-behavioral therapy than with supportive psychotherapy (options C and D are incorrect).

Supportive psychotherapy is contraindicated when psychotherapy itself is contraindicated, such as in patients with delirium, drug intoxication, late-stage dementia, or malingering (option A is incorrect).

Supportive psychotherapy has value in the context of grief and is helpful in caring for a person after an acute loss of a loved one (option B is correct). **Chapter 34 (pp. 1001–1003)**

34.4   Which of the following is one of the key strategies of supportive psychotherapy?

A. Promoting patient self-esteem.
B. Working primarily on conflict and instinctual issues with a focus on the past.
C. Self-disclosing to the patient in the interest of the therapist.
D. Questioning and directly confronting patient defenses.

The correct response is option A: Promoting patient self-esteem.

Supportive psychotherapy is highly intentional therapeutic work that emphasizes relational and interpersonal issues and the self within the reality of the present everyday world as opposed to conflict and instinctual issues and a focus on the past. Although the therapist should understand many of the patient's dynamic issues and unconscious conflicts, these generally are not explored in supportive psychotherapy (option B is incorrect).

Improvement in self-esteem is an important goal of supportive psychotherapy. The therapist's positive regard, approval, acceptance, interest, respect, and genuineness help to promote the patient's self-esteem (option A is correct).

In regard to the therapeutic relationship, intentional revelations by the therapist about himself or herself should have a therapeutic rationale—that is, they should be in the interest of the patient (Roberts 2016). Self-disclosure does have transference implications, and if self-disclosure is in the therapist's interest and takes the form of bragging, complaining, seductiveness, and so on, then it is a boundary violation and exploitative (option C is incorrect).

In supportive psychotherapy, defenses are questioned or confronted only when they are maladaptive and interfere with functioning. In practice, the clinician does not work directly with a defense, but rather works on the attitude or behavior it expresses (option D is incorrect). **Chapter 34 (pp. 999, 1003–1004)**

34.5   Which of the following statements accurately describes the difference between a structural case formulation and a dynamic case formulation?

A. A *structural case formulation* attempts to capture the relatively fixed characteristics of an individual's personality, which are understood within a functional context; a *dynamic case formulation* focuses on conflicting wishes, needs, or feelings and on their meanings.

B. A *structural case formulation* focuses on conflicting wishes, needs, or feelings and on their meanings; a *dynamic case formulation* involves exploration of early development and life events that may help to explain an individual's current situation.

C. A *structural case formulation* addresses an individual's underlying psychological structure and the content of his or her thoughts; a *dynamic case formulation* attempts to capture the relatively fixed characteristics of an individual's personality, which are understood within a functional context.

D. A *structural case formulation* involves exploration of early development and life events that may help to explain an individual's current situation; a *dynamic case formulation* addresses an individual's underlying psychological structure and the content of his or her thoughts.

The correct response is option A: A *structural case formulation* attempts to capture the relatively fixed characteristics of an individual's personality, which are understood within a functional context; a *dynamic case formulation* focuses on conflicting wishes, needs, or feelings and on their meanings.

The case formulation is an explanation of the patient's symptoms and psychosocial functioning and depends on an accurate and thorough assessment of the patient. There are many approaches to case formulation. A structural case formulation attempts to capture the relatively fixed characteristics of an individual's personality, which are understood within a functional context. The dynamic approach concerns mental and emotional tensions that may be conscious or unconscious. This approach focuses on conflicting wishes, needs, or feelings and on their meanings (option A is correct).

The genetic approach to case formulation involves exploration of early development and life events that may help to explain an individual's current situation (options B and D are incorrect).

The cognitive-behavioral approach addresses an individual's underlying psychological structure and the content of his or her thoughts (option C is incorrect).

Overall, the structural and cognitive-behavioral formulations are the most important in supportive psychotherapy, because mapping out current areas of difficulty and ameliorating them are more important than understanding the genetic basis or dynamic cause of the difficulty. **Chapter 34 (pp. 1005–1006)**

34.6 Which of the following best describes the communication style used in supportive psychotherapy?

A. There is a give-and-take exchange between patient and therapist.
B. Therapists typically ask patients challenging questions.
C. Patients are permitted extended periods of silence to reflect on their experiences.
D. Therapists often start questions with "Why."

The correct response is option A: There is a give-and-take exchange between patient and therapist.

The style of communication in supportive psychotherapy tends to be more conversational than in expressive psychotherapy. Silences are avoided because they can raise the individual's level of anxiety (option C is incorrect). There is a give-and-take exchange (option A is correct), and challenging questions are not asked (option B is correct). Questions beginning with "Why" are avoided because they can increase anxiety and threaten self-esteem (option D is incorrect). **Chapter 34 (p. 1009)**

34.7   Which of the following quoted therapist statements is an example of *clarification* in supportive psychotherapy?

   A. "Most people with your condition improve."
   B. "It's good that you can be so considerate of other people."
   C. "Could it be that you got into the argument with them to avoid asking them for money?"
   D. "It sounds like a lot of things are troubling you and you are feeling overwhelmed."

The correct response is option D: "It sounds like a lot of things are troubling you and you are feeling overwhelmed."

Supportive psychotherapists use clearly defined interventions designed to achieve the goals of maintaining or improving the patient's self-esteem, functioning, and adaptation to the environment (Table 34–1). *Clarification* encompasses summarizing, paraphrasing, or organizing without elaboration or inference. Clarification frames communication so that both parties agree on what is being discussed. Summarizing and restating help organize the patient's thinking and provide structure (option D is correct).

Option A is an example of *reassurance*. Words spoken in an attempt to reassure a patient must not be empty or without basis. For example, many patients ask their therapist if they will get better. A response of "Yes, you will get better" may be misleading and false. A more appropriate response would be "Most people with your condition improve" (option A is incorrect).

Option B is an example of *praise*, which is considered a useful technique for promoting self-esteem and supporting more adaptive behaviors (option B is incorrect).

Option C is an example of *empathic confrontation*, which addresses a patient's defensive behavior by bringing to the patient's attention a pattern of behaviors, ideas, or feelings he or she has not recognized or has avoided (option C is incorrect). **Chapter 34 (pp. 1009–1011; Table 34–4 [p. 1010])**

TABLE 34–1. Therapeutic interventions used in supportive psychotherapy

Conversational style of communication

Praise, reassurance, and encouragement

Advice

Rationalizing and reframing

Rehearsal or anticipatory guidance

Empathic confrontation, clarification, and interpretation

Processing, elaborative processing, generation, interleaving, and critical reflection

34.8 Historically, the components of the therapeutic relationship have been considered to be the transference–countertransference configuration, the real relationship, and the therapeutic alliance. Which of the following statements best describes the roles of transference and the real relationship in supportive psychotherapy?

A. In supportive psychotherapy, the therapist explores positive feelings and thoughts in the transference.
B. The real relationship is not a focus in supportive psychotherapy.
C. In supportive psychotherapy, the therapist must investigate negative transference reactions.
D. Supportive psychotherapy places more emphasis on the transference than on the real relationship.

The correct response is option C: In supportive psychotherapy, the therapist must investigate negative transference reactions.

At the supportive end of the psychotherapy continuum, transference can be used to guide therapeutic interventions. Positive transference reactions generally are not explored but rather are simply accepted (option A is incorrect). Negative transference reactions always must be investigated, however, because they may compromise treatment (Winston and Winston 2002) (option C is correct).

The real relationship underlies all psychotherapy; it is paramount and is based on overt mutuality in the conduct of therapy (option B is incorrect). Expressive therapy places more emphasis on the transference, whereas supportive psychotherapy focuses more on the real relationship (options B and D are incorrect). **Chapter 34 (pp. 1012–1013; Table 34–5 [p. 1013])**

34.9 Which of the following is a therapeutic intervention used in supportive psychotherapy?

A. Critical reflection.
B. Interpretation focused on the patient's past relationships.
C. Contradiction.
D. Exploration and interpretation of transference phenomena.

The correct response is option A: Critical reflection.

Supportive psychotherapy uses many ideas and techniques derived from cognitive-behavioral therapy and learning theory (see Table 34–1). *Critical reflection* (Mezirow 1998) is an important technique of learning theory. It is the process by which a person questions and then replaces or reframes an assumption. It is the process through which alternative perspectives are formed on ideas, actions, and forms of reasoning previously taken for granted. Supportive psychotherapy approaches use reframing and critical reflection to attempt to provide patients with alternative ways of thinking about the world, relating to others, and solving problems (option A is correct).

An *interpretation* is an explanation that brings meaning to the patient's behavior or thinking. Generally, it makes the individual aware of something that was not previously conscious. Interpretation can be used to link thoughts, feelings, and behaviors toward people in the patient's current life to people from the past and/or to the therapist; however, in supportive psychotherapy, interpretation generally emphasizes present rather than past relationships (option B is incorrect).

Processing (deWinstanley and Bjork 2002), an important technique used to facilitate learning in supportive psychotherapy, involves interpretation that is focused and accurate, accompanied by thorough elaboration. Information that can be interpreted (linked) through associations with preexisting knowledge will be easier to learn than information that is not interpreted. It is important to note that interpretation as a technique of learning theory is not the same as the classic technique of interpretation in dynamic psychotherapy (option D is incorrect); instead, it is more of a linkage to preexisting knowledge.

Rationalizing and reframing are important CBT techniques that provide the patient with an alternative way of looking at an event that was previously perceived as painful or negative. The challenge in using rationalization and reframing is to avoid sounding fatuous or arguing with and contradicting a patient (option C is incorrect). **Chapter 34 (pp. 1009–1011)**

34.10 Which of the following statements accurately describes the role of the therapeutic alliance in supportive psychotherapy?

A. The therapeutic alliance tends to be more stable on the supportive psychotherapy side of the continuum.
B. The therapeutic alliance is a static process between patient and therapist.
C. The therapeutic alliance is a component of the transference.
D. Patients with limited capacity to form a therapeutic alliance should not receive supportive psychotherapy.

The correct response is option A: The therapeutic alliance tends to be more stable on the supportive psychotherapy side of the continuum.

The stability of the therapeutic alliance appears to be related to the psychotherapy continuum. The alliance tends to be more stable on the supportive psychotherapy side of the continuum because it is not threatened by challenging confrontations or interpretations that may heighten patient anxiety (Hellerstein et al. 1998) (option A is correct).

The therapeutic alliance is a component of the real relationship (option C is incorrect) and forms an essential part of the foundation on which all psychotherapy stands. Zetzel (1956) first used the term *therapeutic alliance* for the "unobjectionable positive transference" that was seen as an essential element in the success of psychotherapy. She believed that the capacity to form an alliance is based on an individual's early experiences with the primary caregiver. In the absence of this capacity, the task of the therapist in early treatment is to provide a supportive relationship to foster the development of a therapeutic alliance (option D is incorrect).

Bordin (1979) operationalized the therapeutic alliance concept as the degree of agreement between patient and therapist concerning the tasks and goals of psychotherapy and the quality of the bond between them. He conceptualized the alliance as evolving and changing as the result of a dynamic interactive process occurring between patient and therapist (option B is incorrect). **Chapter 34 (pp. 1014, 1015)**

References

Barlow D, Craske M: Mastery of Your Anxiety and Panic. Albany, Center for Stress and Anxiety Disorders, State University of New York, 1989

Bordin ES: The generalizability of the psychoanalytic concept of the working alliance. Psychotherapy: Theory, Research and Practice 16(3):252–260, 1979

deWinstanley PA, Bjork RA: Successful lecturing: presenting information in ways that engage effective processing, in Applying the Science of Learning to University Teaching and Beyond (New Directions for Teaching and Learning, No 89). Edited by Halpern DF, Hakel MD. San Francisco, CA, Jossey-Bass, 2002, pp 19–31

Foa EB, Franklin ME: Psychotherapies for obsessive compulsive disorder: a review, in Obsessive Compulsive Disorder, 2nd Edition. Edited by Maj M, Sartorius N, Okasha A, et al. Chichester, UK, Wiley, 2002, pp 93–115

Hellerstein DJ, Rosenthal RN, Pinsker H, et al: A randomized prospective study comparing supportive and dynamic therapies: outcome and alliance. J Psychother Pract Res 7(4):261–271, 1998 9752637

Mezirow J: On critical reflection. Adult Education Quarterly 48:185–198, 1998

Roberts LW: A Clinical Guide to Psychiatric Ethics. Arlington, VA, American Psychiatric Association Publishing, 2016

Winston A, Winston B: Handbook of Integrated Short-Term Psychotherapy. Washington, DC, American Psychiatric Publishing, 2002

Winston A, Rosenthal RN, Pinsker H: Introduction to Supportive Psychotherapy. Washington, DC, American Psychiatric Publishing, 2004

Winston A, Rosenthal RN, Pinsker H: Learning Supportive Psychotherapy: An Illustrated Guide. Washington, DC, American Psychiatric Publishing, 2012

Zetzel E: Current concepts of transference. Int J Psychoanal 37(4–5):369–375, 1956 13366506

CHAPTER 35

Mentalizing
in Psychotherapy

35.1   Which of the following statements best characterizes implicit mentalizing (as opposed to explicit mentalizing)?

A. Implicit mentalizing is relatively automatic, procedural, and nonconscious.
B. Implicit mentalizing usually takes the form of a narrative.
C. Implicit mentalizing can be as simple as putting feelings into words.
D. Implicit mentalizing can be used to learn from past mistakes in the service of interacting more effectively in the future.

The correct response is option A: Implicit mentalizing is relatively automatic, procedural, and nonconscious.

Implicit mentalizing is relatively automatic, procedural, and nonconscious, such as in turn-taking in conversation, adapting voice tone and posture to others' emotional states, and taking others' knowledge into account automatically (option A is correct).

In contrast, *explicit* mentalizing is relatively controlled, predominantly taking the form of narrative (option B is incorrect).

The narratives in explicit mentalizing vary in complexity, ranging from putting feelings into words to creating elaborate autobiographical narratives (option C is incorrect).

Explicit mentalizing permits mental time travel: people mentalize not only about the present but also about the past and the future. Thus, as in psychotherapy, individuals use explicit mentalizing to learn from past mistakes in the service of interacting more effectively in the future (option D is incorrect). **Chapter 35 (pp. 1020–1021)**

35.2   Which of the following is a characteristic of *external* mentalizing (as opposed to internal mentalizing)?

A. Intellectualizing.
B. Feeling emotions.

C. Responsiveness to observable aspects of behavior.
D. Requiring inference and imagination to understand the mental states conjoined with external behavior.

The correct response is option C: Responsiveness to observable aspects of behavior.

External mentalizing entails responsiveness to external, observable aspects of behavior—most prominently facial expressions but also voice tone and posture (option C is correct). In contrast, *internal* mentalizing requires inference and imagination in the service of understanding the mental states conjoined with external behavior (i.e., desires, feelings, beliefs, and relationship proclivities) (option D is incorrect).

Another facet of mentalizing entails the opposing dimensions of *cognitive* and *affective* mentalizing. Extreme imbalance in either direction poses challenges for psychotherapy. For example, relying on cognition, intellectualizing patients might be adept at generating explicit reasons for their own or others' behavior, but such insight—devoid of any real emotional meaning—does not promote change (option A is incorrect).

Conversely, relying on feelings, patients who are more prone to being flooded with affect (e.g., as in borderline personality disorder) are using implicit processes conducive to emotional contagion and impaired self–other differentiation (option B is incorrect).

For patients at both ends of this spectrum, *mentalizing emotion*—thinking and feeling about thinking and feeling—is a crucial therapeutic goal. **Chapter 35 (pp. 1020–1021)**

35.3 Which of the following is considered a hallmark of skillful mentalizing?

A. Focusing primarily on assumptions about others.
B. Mentalizing with high confidence in the accuracy of one's perceptions and interpretations of others.
C. Linking external behavior with internal mental states.
D. Mentalizing with the goal of benignly controlling others' thoughts or actions.

The correct response is option C: Linking external behavior with internal mental states.

To a great degree, skillful mentalizing entails flexible integration of the multiple facets of mentalizing: balancing focus on self and others, integrating cognitive and affective mentalizing, and being able to link external behavior with internal mental states (option C is correct).

Focusing primarily on assumptions about others, mentalizing with high confidence in the accuracy of one's perceptions and interpretations of others, and mentalizing with the goal of benignly controlling others' thoughts or actions are not features of skillful mentalizing (options A, B, and D are incorrect). **Chapter 35 (Table 35–2 [p. 1022])**

35.4   Mentalizing overlaps in some respects with *mindfulness*, a concept that has received considerable attention in recent years. Which of the following characteristics is exclusive to *mentalizing* and is not a focus of mindfulness?

A. Reflection and interpretation.
B. Problem-centered attention.
C. Attention to mental states in oneself or others.
D. A nonjudgmental attitude of acceptance, compassion, and curiosity.

The correct response is option A: Reflection and interpretation.

The distinction between mentalizing and mindfulness bears particular attention because the two concepts are easily confused and conflated. Moreover, mindfulness has become a popular concept and is likely to be far more familiar to clinicians and patients, who may question the difference when they hear about mentalizing. *Mindfulness* refers to present-centered attention (option B is incorrect), which can include attention to mental states in self or others (option C is incorrect).

In contrast, *mentalizing* also includes reflection and interpretation, typically in the form of narrative (option A is correct).

Mindful attentiveness to mental states is a necessary condition for skillful mentalizing. Mindfulness and mentalizing overlap in two key respects: 1) both emphasize the need to distinguish between mental states and the reality they represent, and 2) both advocate a nonjudgmental, open-minded attitude of curiosity and inquisitiveness about mental states in oneself and others (option D is incorrect). **Chapter 35 (pp. 1021–1022)**

35.5   Which of the following actions is characteristic of *mentalizing* (as opposed to *prementalizing* or *nonmentalizing* modes of experience)?

A. Living in a mental state unmoored from reality.
B. Expressing mental states in goal-directed action.
C. Equating one's own mental states with reality.
D. Reflecting on the meaning of mental states.

The correct response is option D: Reflecting on the meaning of mental states.

The theory of mentalizing proposes a developmentally and neuroscientifically based conceptualization of the processes that are activated when mentalizing fails. These processes are called *prementalizing*, or *nonmentalizing*, modes of experience, and they are associated with the interpersonal or intrasubjective dysfunction most commonly associated with personality disorders but also with many experiences of mental disorders. Prementalizing modes of experience include psychic equivalence, pretend mode, and teleological mode (Allen et al. 2008). *Psychic equivalence* involves equating one's own mental contents with reality and failing to distinguish mental representations from the external reality that they represent (option C is incorrect). *Pretend mode* describes a state in which mental contents are too divorced from reality, taking on a feeling of unreality, often due to a lack of anchoring in emotion or sense of self (e.g., as in dissociative states) (option A is incorrect). *Teleological mode* refers to the expression of mental states through goal-directed action rather than through narrative communication (option B is incorrect).

Reflecting on the meaning of mental states is a defining characteristic of mentalizing and does not relate to prementalizing modes of experience (option D is correct). **Chapter 35 (p. 1023 [Table 35–4])**

35.6   In mentalization-based therapy for a patient in a state of *psychic equivalence*, which of the following would be the best initial approach for the therapist?

A. Point out logical inconsistencies in the patient's perspective.
B. Encourage the patient to imagine him- or herself as another person.
C. Attempt to see the situation through the eyes of the patient.
D. Introduce alternative perspectives to the patient.

The correct response is option C: Attempt to see the situation through the eyes of the patient.

For a patient in a state of psychic equivalence, the initial approach of a mentalization-based therapist would be to attempt to see the situation through the eyes of the patient (option C is correct).

Once the patient has had the experience of feeling understood and recognized, the therapist might be able to introduce alternative perspectives (option D is incorrect) that might involve a shift in view. Trying to force another person to mentalize is inherently nonmentalizing (option B is incorrect), and likewise, simply pointing out inconsistencies in a person's perspective will not beget mentalization (option A is incorrect). **Chapter 35 (pp. 1032–1033)**

35.7   Which of the following statements about the mentalizing approach is *true*?

A. Mentalizing is highly structured.
B. Mentalizing should be based on an explicit formulation.
C. Mentalizing is prescriptive.
D. Mentalizing is inherently freewheeling.

The correct response is option B: Mentalizing should be based on an explicit formulation.

The mentalizing approach is neither highly structured nor prescriptive (options A and C are incorrect). However, it is not freewheeling either (option D is incorrect). Sound treatment must be based on an explicit formulation that guides the treatment—ideally, a written formulation provided to the patient based on a collaborative process of understanding (Allen et al. 2008) (option B is correct). **Chapter 35 (p. 1035)**

35.8   Which of the following statements best describes the relation of mentalizing to other therapeutic modalities?

A. Mentalizing is inherently limited in its scope of application.
B. Mentalizing is an integrative approach to psychotherapy.
C. Mentalizing is a new and groundbreaking therapeutic approach.
D. Because of its highly specialized techniques, mentalizing is compatible with only a few other therapies.

The correct response is option B: Mentalizing is an integrative approach to psychotherapy.

Mentalizing is what psychotherapists do—with Oldham's (2008) caveat: *when they are doing their job*. Mentalizing represents an integrative approach to psychotherapy (option B is correct).

Mentalizing is transtheoretical, transdiagnostic, and applicable to multiple treatment modalities (option A is incorrect).

Mentalizing is both a specialized brand of therapy and a common factor in psychotherapy (option C is incorrect).

Mentalizing is consistent with the expansive applications of other therapeutic approaches, including psychoanalysis, interpersonal psychotherapy, cognitive therapy, and mindfulness practice (option D is incorrect). **Chapter 35 (pp. 1034, 1035, 1036)**

35.9   To which of the following patient problems would mentalizing-based treatment (MBT) be most applicable?

A. Deficits in social cognition in individuals with borderline personality disorder (BPD).
B. Psychotic disorders.
C. Problems in communication in individuals with autism spectrum disorder (ASD).
D. Impulsivity in individuals with attention-deficit/hyperactivity disorder (ADHD).

The correct response is option A: Deficits in social cognition in individuals with borderline personality disorder (BPD).

MBT was originally developed for the treatment of BPD. The core symptoms of BPD—emotional dysregulation, impulsivity, self-destructive behavior, and unstable relationships—are embedded in highly insecure (i.e., preoccupied and disorganized) attachment relationships and severe mentalizing impairments. More specifically, patients with BPD show marked impairments in the explicit, internal, and cognitive facets of mentalizing: they are reactive to external behavioral cues (e.g., a grimace or a yawn), they have difficulty linking such cues appropriately to internal mental states, and they are subject to implicit mentalizing and emotional contagion concomitant with impaired capacity for explicit, reflective thinking (Fonagy and Luyten 2009). MBT was designed to provide a mentalizing-rich and trustworthy interpersonal environment in which these core deficits in social cognition could be rectified (option A is correct).

Other psychiatric disorders may improve with a mentalizing focus in psychotherapy; however, psychotic disorders, communication deficits in ASD, and impulsivity in ADHD are not appropriate targets for mentalization-based psychotherapy (options B, C, and D are incorrect). **Chapter 35 (pp. 1028, 1037)**

35.10 Which of the following is an outcome of trauma during the formation of attachment relationships?

A. Infant distress when separated from parent in the Strange Situation, followed by quick recovery when reunited with parent.
B. Secure attachment as measured in the Strange Situation.
C. Increased capacity for mentalization in adulthood.
D. Intergenerational transmission of impaired mentalizing capacity.

The correct response is option D: Intergenerational transmission of impaired mentalizing capacity.

In their research examining the relationship between parental mentalizing (elicited with the Adult Attachment Interview) and subsequent infant attachment security (assessed via Ainsworth's Strange Situation), Fonagy et al. (1991) found that parents' mentalizing capacity in relation to their own attachment history predicted their infants' attachment security in relation to them. Although securely attached infants were more or less distressed by the separation, at the point of reunion they sought contact and comfort from the parent, and then, reassured, returned to play. At the opposite extreme from infants of parents with secure attachment in childhood, infants of parents with unresolved–disorganized attachment (the most profound form of attachment insecurity in the Adult Attachment Interview) were at higher risk for showing the most severe form of insecure attachment in the Strange Situation—namely, disorganized attachment. Infant disorganized attachment behavior is anomalous in showing extreme conflict (e.g., screaming in protest when the parent leaves the room and then running away when the parent returns) as well as manifesting frankly confused or disoriented behavior (e.g., wandering around the room as if lost, or entering into a dissociative, trancelike state). Liable to have their own traumatic attachment history evoked in response to their infant's attachment needs or distress, profoundly insecure parents become frightening or frightened and unable to mentalize; in turn, their infants are liable to feel frightened and unable to seek solace in the relationship. This chain of effects illustrates how trauma in attachment relationships contributes to the intergenerational transmission of impaired mentalizing capacities (option D is correct).

Infants who have experienced trauma are more likely to develop an *insecure* attachment to their caregivers and in the Strange Situation show distress both when separated from their parents and when reunited with them (option A is incorrect). Trauma in attachment formation would not lead to *secure* attachment as measured in the Strange Situation (option B is incorrect). Trauma is associated with a *diminished* capacity for mentalization in adulthood (option C is incorrect). **Chapter 35 (pp. 1023–1024)**

35.11 Randomized controlled trials examining the effectiveness of mentalization-based therapy (MBT) for treating borderline personality disorder (BPD) have reported which of the following findings?

   A. Increased difficulty in interpersonal functioning.
   B. Increased emergency room visits.
   C. Decreased impulsivity and suicide attempts.
   D. Increased inpatient psychiatric admissions.

The correct response is option C: Decreased impulsivity and suicide attempts.

Bateman and Fonagy conducted a series of randomized controlled trials to examine the effectiveness of MBT among patients with BPD in a day-hospital setting, with BPD patients receiving treatment as usual in the community serving as the comparison group. The day-hospital program was investigated in a series of outcome studies, culminating in an 8-year follow-up study (Bateman and Fonagy 2008), the longest follow-up of treatment for BPD conducted to date. In comparison with treatment as usual, MBT was associated with decreased suicide attempts, emergency department visits, inpatient admissions, medication and outpatient treatment use, and impulsivity (option C is correct; options B and D are incorrect).

   Far fewer patients in the MBT group than in the comparison group met criteria for BPD at follow-up (13% vs. 87%). Moreover, in addition to symptomatic improvement, patients in the MBT group showed greater improvement in interpersonal and occupational functioning (Bateman and Fonagy 2008) (option A is incorrect). **Chapter 35 (p. 1033)**

References

Allen JG, Fonagy P, Bateman A: Mentalizing in Clinical Practice. Washington, DC, American Psychiatric Publishing, 2008
Bateman A, Fonagy P: 8-Year follow-up of patients treated for borderline personality disorder: mentalization-based treatment versus treatment as usual. Am J Psychiatry 165(5):631–638, 2008 18347003
Fonagy P, Luyten P: A developmental, mentalization-based approach to the understanding and treatment of borderline personality disorder. Dev Psychopathol 21(4):1355–1381, 2009 19825272
Fonagy P, Steele H, Steele M: Maternal representations of attachment during pregnancy predict the organization of infant-mother attachment at one year of age. Child Dev 62(5):891–905, 1991 1756665
Oldham JM: Epilogue, in Mentalizing in Clinical Practice. Edited by Allen JG, Fonagy P. Washington, DC, American Psychiatric Publishing, 2008, pp 341–346

CHAPTER 36

Hybrid Practitioners and Digital Treatments

36.1 Which of the following patient-referral options is available to a psychiatrist working in a traditional practice setting?

A. Arrange an in-person office consultation at a specialist psychiatry clinic.
B. Arrange an asynchronous telepsychiatry consultation for clinic or home.
C. Arrange a synchronous telepsychiatry consultation for clinic or home.
D. Arrange for a patient to be seen by a psychiatrist in the primary care clinic.

The correct response is option A: Arrange an in-person office consultation at a specialist psychiatry clinic.

Yellowlees and Shore (2017) have described hybrid providers as "clinicians who interact with patients both in person and online, so that their doctor–patient relationships cross both environments. The addition of interactions via videoconferencing, e-mail, text messaging, and telephony leads to improved access and interactions at times and places not possible when care is restricted to the in-person venue" (p. 254). The effect of the transition to providing hybrid care is also significant for the systems and providers that psychiatrists interact with. For example, primary care physicians traditionally, when referring a patient to a psychiatrist, had only three options:

1. Arrange an in-person office consultation at a specialist psychiatry clinic (option A is correct).
2. Telephone for a curbside consultation.
3. Instruct the patient to go to the emergency department.

In a hybrid practice environment, many more options are available. For example, when a University of California–Davis (UCD) primary provider wishes to obtain psychiatric advice, or to attend regular educational sessions offered by a UCD psychiatrist, he or she may use the following additional options:

1. Schedule a psychiatric review through the care coordination team.
2. Submit an e-consultation request via the electronic medical record.
3. Arrange an asynchronous telepsychiatry consultation for clinic or home (option B is incorrect).
4. Arrange a synchronous telepsychiatry consultation for clinic or home (option C is incorrect).
5. Arrange for a patient to be seen by a psychiatrist in the primary care clinic (option D is incorrect).

Chapter 36 (pp. 1046, 1048–1049)

36.2 Which of the following is reduced in online psychotherapy?

A. Anxiety.
B. Safety in the virtual space.
C. Sense of self-control.
D. Option to engage.

The correct response is option A: Anxiety.

Telepsychotherapy can be less anxiety provoking, because patients have the option to be "seen" from their homes or other familiar settings. Similarly, therapists have the option of seeing patients from a setting that is more comfortable for them—such as from home. Kocsis and Yellowlees (2018) noted that this geographic relocation may help both parties to feel more relaxed or "settled" and could foster the development of psychotherapeutic intimacy (option A is correct).

The concept of a "virtual space" in telepsychotherapy, representing a combination of the increased physical and psychological distance that arises by virtue of the teleconferencing medium, provides more safety to allow an increased sharing of intimacy (option B is incorrect).

Likewise, in telepsychotherapy, the patient experiences a greater sense of physical and psychological control of the session and the therapist is less likely to be successful with a paternalistic approach (option C is incorrect).

Finally, patients with high levels of anxiety or hypervigilance—such as phobic patients, patients on the autism spectrum, and traumatized patients—may more readily engage in telepsychotherapy than in traditional in-person psychotherapy (option D is incorrect). **Chapter 36 (pp. 1049–1050)**

36.3 A primary care clinic keeps track of patients who are maintained on antipsychotics. This patient roster is reviewed at regular intervals by a psychiatrist to ensure that appropriate metabolic screening is being completed. This arrangement is an example of which of the following clinical services?

A. E-consultations.
B. Direct consultation.

C. Evidence-based clinical reviews.

D. Patient registries.

The correct response is option D: Patient registries.

In patient registries, lists of patients with specific disorders, such as depression or bipolar disorder, are reviewed by psychiatrists with expertise in those disorders to make sure that best practices are being followed—for instance, by checking that all patients taking lithium are receiving annual renal and thyroid function tests, or that all patients with depression are being offered therapeutic dosages of antidepressants and appropriate psychotherapies (option D is correct).

E-consultations essentially represent an enhanced form of curbside consultations in which psychiatrists can respond to certain primary provider consultation questions via electronic medical record messaging, rendering an opinion or treatment suggestions without face-to-face patient evaluation when appropriate (option A is incorrect).

Direct consultation, in contrast, represents the traditional form of consultation in which a patient is referred by another medical provider for an in-person psychiatric evaluation to answer evaluation or treatment questions (option B is incorrect).

In evidence-based clinical reviews, a multidisciplinary (including psychiatrists) team reviews panels of patients, or individual patients, often through use of routine screening of patients with validated tools such as the Patient Health Questionnaire–9, the Generalized Anxiety Disorder–7, and the Alcohol Use Disorders Identification Test (option C is incorrect). **Chapter 36 (pp. 1045–1046)**

36.4   Which of the following technology-based approaches has been reported to be potentially more effective than in-person treatment of children with attention-deficit/hyperactivity disorder and patients with posttraumatic stress disorder?

A. Telephony.

B. E-mail or secure messaging.

C. Videoconferencing.

D. Web-based applications.

The correct response is option C: Videoconferencing.

Telephony has long been used with patients, especially to deal with emergent issues, although all practitioners will be aware of the pains involved in playing "phone tag" with patients. Interactive voice response systems have been used for several years to collect information and to monitor patients, and the increasing combination of traditional telephony approaches with those possible on smart devices is radically changing the way that telephony is thought about (option A is incorrect).

E-mail or secure messaging occurs either in real time (synchronous) or in delayed time (asynchronous) and is especially useful for communication between or after sessions and for monitoring treatment. With the use of enterprise electronic medical record (EMR) systems, psychiatrists will increasingly communicate with their patients via secure messaging within the EMRs, and e-mail communication with patients will also be carried out via smartphones and similar devices. E-mail has already been transforming administrative communication around patient care for decades (option B is incorrect).

Web-based applications are currently being widely deployed for clinical purposes, with a focus on psychoeducation and patient support, as well as monitoring and data collection. Many web sites incorporate synchronous and asynchronous communication capacities, allowing them to be used as an adjunct to treatment, taking the place of, for instance, paper charts or tools, or as the portal through which treatment occurs, such as with online cognitive-behavioral programs, which are becoming increasingly common, with an emerging evidence base confirming their utility. A review of YouTube.com will rapidly show how much psychiatric educational material is available for patients (option D is incorrect).

Live interactive videoconferencing has rapidly developed as a field over the past three decades. The American Telemedicine Association has reported that more than a million individual patients were treated with telepsychiatry in the United States in 2016 (Yellowlees and Shore 2017), with the Department of Veterans Affairs being the largest national provider of such services (National Academy of Sciences 2017). Videoconferencing has moved past a tipping point of use and is now commonly used by psychiatrists around the United States, with many commercial virtual telepsychiatry companies emerging and patients routinely asking their psychiatrists if they can be seen at home on video. Several studies and reviews have been published identifying areas where treatment with videoconferencing seems to be more effective than in-person treatment, such as in children with attention-deficit/hyperactivity disorder (Myers et al. 2015) and in patients with posttraumatic stress disorder (Azarang et al. 2019) (option C is correct). **Chapter 36 (pp. 1042–1043)**

36.5   Which of the following emergent technologies is used in mobile phones to detect the position of the device and estimate the activity of the user?

A. Virtual reality.
B. Virtual worlds.
C. GPS.
D. Social networking apps.

The correct response is option C: GPS.

The typical smartphone is equipped with accelerometers to detect the position of the smartphone and estimate the activity of the user; with Wi-Fi and *GPS (Global Positioning System)* to locate the user; and with software that can capture the user's interactions (option C is correct).

Virtual reality involves the use of virtual gaming systems that use technology (wraparound three-dimensional goggles; body location sensors to direct movement, touch, smell, and other sensory components) to immerse the user in a computer-generated environment (option A is incorrect).

Virtual worlds are massive online multiplayer systems (e.g., Second Life) that allow individuals to interact with both virtual environments and other individuals for psychoeducation and treatment purposes (option B is incorrect).

Both individual practitioners and health care organizations are exploring methods to leverage *social networking apps* for engaging and educating patients as well as for potentially monitoring (both actively and passively) patients' activities to assess location, social engagement, and so forth (option D is incorrect). **Chapter 36 (pp. 1044–1045)**

36.6 A patient wears wraparound three-dimensional goggles and body sensors while being immersed in a computer-generated environment for pain management. This scenario is an example of which of the following emergent technologies?

A. Virtual reality.
B. Virtual worlds.
C. GPS.
D. Social networking apps.

The correct response is option A: Virtual reality.

Virtual reality involves the use of virtual gaming systems that use technology (wraparound three-dimensional goggles; body location sensors to direct movement, touch, smell, and other sensory components) to immerse the user in a computer-generated environment (option A is correct).

Virtual worlds are massive online multiplayer systems (e.g., Second Life) that allow individuals to interact with both virtual environments and other individuals for psychoeducation and treatment purposes (option B is incorrect).

Both individual practitioners and health care organizations are exploring methods to leverage *social networking apps* for engaging and educating patients as well as for potentially monitoring (both actively and passively) patients' activities to assess location, social engagement, and so forth (option D is incorrect).

The typical smartphone is equipped with accelerometers to detect the position of the smartphone and estimate the activity of the user; with Wi-Fi and *GPS (Global Positioning System)* to locate the user; and with software that can capture the user's interactions (option C is incorrect). **Chapter 36 (pp. 1044–1045)**

36.7 Which of the following technologies is routinely used by psychiatrists for clinical, administrative, and reimbursement purposes?

A. Videoconferencing.
B. Web-based applications.
C. Mobile devices.
D. Electronic medical records.

The correct response is option D: Electronic medical records.

Electronic medical records are now used routinely by psychiatrists for clinical, administrative, and reimbursement purposes (option D is correct).

The American Telemedicine Association has reported that more than a million individual patients were treated with telepsychiatry in the United States in 2016 (Yellowlees and Shore 2017), but videoconferencing is not described to include administrative or reimbursement purposes (option A is incorrect).

Web-based applications are currently being widely deployed for clinical purposes, with a focus on psychoeducation and patient support, as well as monitoring and data collection (option B is incorrect).

Mobile telephones encompass all of the time-honored uses of telephone systems along with texting and applications (apps) with monitoring, recording, and note-taking capacities, and are typically equipped with accelerometers to detect the position of the smartphone and estimate the activity of the user; with Wi-Fi and GPS (Global Positioning System) to locate the user; and with software that can capture the user's interactions (option C is incorrect). **Chapter 36 (pp. 1042–1044)**

36.8 Asynchronous telepsychiatry consultations, while possibly involving no direct patient contact, may allow psychiatrists to potentially provide care for many more patients. In which of the following populations might psychiatrists find the largest number of potential patients for telepsychiatry?

A. Primary care patients.
B. Psychotic patients.
C. Highly anxious patients.
D. Patients on the autism spectrum.

The correct response is option A: Primary care patients.

Psychiatrists can potentially provide care for many more patients if they work both in-person and online, doing a combination of synchronous and asynchronous electronic consultations (using e-mail, messaging, videoconferencing, and telephony), while also remaining in closer and more regular contact with patients (Yellowlees and Shore 2017). Although all of the patient groups identified in the options above would benefit from improved access to mental health care, the primary care population, which encompasses all individuals who receive care in the health care system, would yield the largest number of potential patients (option A is correct).

Psychotic patients seem to feel more at ease when the provider is not in the room, and the increased physical and psychological distance afforded with videoconferencing may reduce anxiety in this population (Sharp et al. 2011) (option B is incorrect).

Highly anxious patients can use a video-based modality to access a therapeutic relationship in a way that feels safe for them (Fortney et al. (2015) (option C is incorrect).

Higher-functioning patients on the autism spectrum enjoy using computers and find a sense of community online, such that they may feel more comfortable with this modality for receiving psychiatric care (Boada and Parellada 2017) (option D is incorrect). **Chapter 36 (pp. 1050–1051)**

36.9 Which of the following scenarios would constitute the only absolute contraindication to seeing a patient via videoconferencing?

A. The patient is engaging in behavior dangerous to him- or herself or others at the time of the interview.
B. The patient has paranoid ruminations about televisions or radios.
C. The patient suffers from severe anxiety that prevents him or her from leaving home.
D. The patient has a significant trauma history involving an "authority figure."

The correct response is option A: The patient is engaging in behavior dangerous to him- or herself or others at the time of the interview.

After years of telemedicine use by many psychiatrists in their practices, the consensus is clear that any type of patient with a psychiatric disorder may be seen via videoconferencing (Bashshur et al. 2016). The only absolute contraindications to a psychiatric interview or intervention via telepsychiatry are when a patient refuses to attend, as some do, or when a patient is actively acting out and engaging in behavior dangerous to him- or herself or others at the time of the interview (option A is correct).

By virtue of their illness, psychotic patients often seem to feel very unsafe, and despite some having paranoid thoughts about televisions and radios, these patients seem to feel more at ease when the provider is not in the room. The increased physical and psychological distance afforded with videoconferencing may reduce anxiety in this population (Sharp et al. 2011) (option B is incorrect).

Psychotherapy via video may be particularly helpful for anxious patients who have difficulty leaving their homes (Morland et al. 2015). With a video-based modality, patients who might otherwise delay or forgo treatment can access a therapeutic relationship in a way that feels safe for them, as Fortney et al. (2015) have demonstrated (option C is incorrect).

Patients with significant childhood or adult abuse histories may have an especially difficult time feeling safe around the "authority figure" of the doctor or therapist in a closed office setting, and an online approach may help to build the important initial rapport and sense of safety (option D is incorrect). **Chapter 36 (pp. 1050–1051)**

36.10 Which of the following types of clinical services uses "less intensive and less expensive interventions at the outset and gradually adds more intensive services if patients fail to improve"?

A. Evidence-based clinical reviews.
B. Patient registries.
C. Stepped models of care.
D. Online provider to online provider consultations.

The correct response is option C: Stepped models of care.

Integrated behavioral health care is a comprehensive approach to care that involves a team of primary care and behavioral health clinicians working together with patients and families. It uses a systematic and cost-effective approach to provide patient-centered care for a defined population through an integrated primary care medical home (Katon and Unützer 2011).

A crucial step in expanding mental health care services to where patients are, which is mainly in the primary care setting, is to improve the flow of clinical work across primary care and specialty care settings. This workflow objective is best achieved by implementing efficient, provider-compatible, administratively simple electronic synchronous and asynchronous solutions to integrate behavioral health care into the primary care setting via a stepped-care model. *Stepped models of care* use less intensive and less expensive interventions at the outset and gradually add more intensive services if patients fail to improve (Hilty et al. 2013), delivering the right level of triage and treatment based on patients' needs (option C is correct).

Evidence-based clinical reviews are a multidisciplinary (including psychiatrists) team that reviews panels of patients, or individual patients, often involving routine screening of patients with tools such as the Patient Health Questionnaire–9, Generalized Anxiety Disorder–7, and Alcohol Use Disorders Identification Test, where feedback and treatment planning suggestions are then returned to the patients' primary care physicians electronically through electronic medical records (EMRs), messaging, or similar systems (Raney et al. 2014) (option A is incorrect).

Patient registries are registries of patients with specific disorders (e.g., depression, bipolar disorder) that are reviewed by psychiatrists with expertise in those disorders to make sure that best practices are being followed—for instance, by checking that all patients taking lithium are receiving annual renal and thyroid function tests, or that all patients with depression are being offered therapeutic dosages of antidepressants and appropriate psychotherapies (option B is incorrect).

Online provider to online provider consultations (e-consultations) and responding to primary provider questions via EMR messaging are becoming increasingly common and essentially represent an enhanced form of curbside consultation. In these communications, the psychiatrist receives a formal referral or set of questions from a primary care provider, perhaps with some algorithmically developed questions; ideally reviews the patient's notes in a shared EMR; and then responds with an opinion and treatment suggestions for the provider to consider (option D is incorrect). **Chapter 36 (pp. 1045–1046)**

References

Azarang A, Pakyurek M, Giroux C, et al: Information technologies: an augmentation to post-traumatic stress disorder treatment among trauma survivors. Telemed J E Health 25(4):263–271, 2019 30004318

Bashshur RL, Shannon GW, Bashshur N, et al: The empirical evidence for telemedicine interventions in mental disorders. Telemed J E Health 22(2):87–113, 2016 26624248

Boada L, Parellada M: Seeing the doctor without fear: www.doctortea.org for the desensitization for medical visits in autism spectrum disorders. Rev Psiquiatr Salud Ment 10(1):28–32, 2017 27964853

Fortney JC, Pyne JM, Kimbrell TA, et al: Telemedicine-based collaborative care for posttraumatic stress disorder: a randomized clinical trial. JAMA Psychiatry 72(1):58–67, 2015 25409287

Hilty DM, Ferrer DC, Parish MB, et al: The effectiveness of telemental health: a 2013 review. Telemed J E Health 19(6):444–454, 2013 23697504

Katon W, Unützer J: Consultation psychiatry in the medical home and accountable care organizations: achieving the triple aim. Gen Hosp Psychiatry 33(4):305–310, 2011 21762825

Kocsis BJ, Yellowlees P: Telepsychotherapy and the therapeutic relationship: principles, advantages, and case examples. Telemed J E Health 24(5):329–334, 2018 28836902

Morland LA, Poizner JM, Williams KE, et al: Home-based clinical video teleconferencing care: clinical considerations and future directions. Int Rev Psychiatry 27(6):504–512, 2015 26619273

Myers K, Vander Stoep A, Zhou C, et al: Effectiveness of a telehealth service delivery model for treating attention-deficit/hyperactivity disorder: a community-based randomized controlled trial. J Am Acad Child Adolesc Psychiatry 54(4):263–274, 2015 25791143

Myers K, Nelson E, Hilty DM, et al: American Telemental Association practice guidelines for telemental health with children and adolescents. Telemed J Health 23(10):779–804, 2017 28930496

National Academy of Sciences: Evaluation of the Department of Veterans Affairs Mental Health Services. Washington, DC, National Academies Press, 2017

Raney L, Pollack D, Parks J, et al: The American Psychiatric Association response to the "joint principles: integrating behavioral health care into the patient-centered medical home." Fam Syst Health 32(2):147–148, 2014 24955687

Sharp IR, Kobak KA, Osman DA: The use of videoconferencing with patients with psychosis: a review of the literature. Ann Gen Psychiatry 10(1):14, 2011 21501496

Yellowlees PM, Shore J (eds): Telepsychiatry and Health Technologies: A Guide for Mental Health Professionals. Arlington, VA, American Psychiatric Association Publishing, 2017

CHAPTER 37

Complementary and Integrative Psychiatry

37.1 A 30-year-old woman presents to your office to discuss pharmacological options for treatment of major depressive disorder (MDD). After discussion of the benefits, side effects, and alternatives to antidepressant medications, she asks if there are any vitamins or nutrients she could take instead. Which of the following nutrients has the strongest evidence of effectiveness as monotherapy for MDD?

A. Vitamin D_3.
B. L-methylfolate.
C. Vitamin B_{12}.
D. S-adenosylmethionine (SAMe).

The correct response is option D: S-adenosylmethionine (SAMe).

A meta-analysis by the U.S. Department of Health and Human Services Agency for Healthcare Research and Quality (Sharma et al. 2017), which included 28 double-blind, randomized controlled trials, concluded that SAMe monotherapy was more effective than placebo and as effective as conventional antidepressants for treating MDD (option D is correct). Studies do not support the use of folate or B_{12} as monotherapies for MDD (options B and C are incorrect). Current evidence does not support a role for vitamin D in the treatment or prevention of depression (option A is incorrect). **Chapter 37 (pp. 1058–1059)**

37.2 A 70-year-old man diagnosed with major depressive disorder (MDD) with a seasonal pattern is still feeling depressed despite taking sertraline 200 mg/day for the past 3 months, over the winter. He follows a strict vegan diet. Although he would prefer to stop the sertraline, he is willing to continue taking it if advised. He asks whether there are any vitamins or nutrients he can take to supplement his treatment. Which of the following would be the best next step in managing this patient's depression?

A. Recommend that he take a daily multivitamin tablet containing vitamin B_{12} and folic acid.
B. Check levels of vitamin B_{12}, folate, and 25-hydroxyvitamin D.
C. Recommend that he take vitamin D_3 at a dosage of 2,000 IU/day.
D. Recommend that he discontinue the sertraline and start L-methylfolate.

The correct response is option B: Check levels of vitamin B_{12}, folate, and 25-hydroxyvitamin D.

This patient has several risk factors for vitamin D and vitamin B_{12} insufficiency, including low sunlight exposure over the winter months, advanced age, and a strict vegan diet. Although supplementation with vitamin D can be justified for "general health" in patients with confirmed vitamin D insufficiency, two systematic reviews found that studies on vitamin D for MDD were inconclusive, and current evidence does not support a role for vitamin D in the treatment or prevention of depression (option C is incorrect).

Evidence that supplementation with folate or B_{12} can beneficially augment antidepressant treatment is stronger for patients with insufficiencies of these vitamins; hence, it is best to check levels of these nutrients before starting supplementation (option B is correct; option A is incorrect). Although adjunctive L-methylfolate may be an effective treatment strategy for patients with MDD who have a partial response or no response to selective serotonin reuptake inhibitors, studies do not support the use of folate as monotherapy for MDD (option D is incorrect). **Chapter 37 (pp. 1058–1059)**

37.3 Which of the following statements regarding vitamin B_{12} is *true*?

A. Adverse effects of vitamin B_{12} have been noted at dosages of 8 mg/day.
B. The ability to absorb vitamin B_{12} remains strong throughout the life span.
C. Supplementation with vitamin B_{12} may help preserve cognitive function in geriatric patients.
D. There is evidence that vitamin B_{12} can augment antidepressant treatment regardless of whether there is a deficiency.

The correct response is option C: Supplementation with vitamin B_{12} may help preserve cognitive function in geriatric patients.

Vitamin B_{12} supplementation may help preserve cognitive function in geriatric patients (option C is correct). No adverse effects or safe upper limit of B_{12} dose or level has been identified (option A is incorrect). Up to 30% of elderly persons may have difficulty absorbing B_{12} from food because of low levels of stomach acid (weakening of the stomach lining or the use of antacids), which may contribute to the vitamin insufficiency (option B is incorrect). Evidence that supplementation with folate or B_{12} can beneficially augment antidepressant treatment is stronger for patients with insufficiencies of these vitamins (Almeida et al. 2015) (option D is incorrect). **Chapter 37 (p. 1058)**

37.4 Which of the following statements about omega-3 fatty acids is *true*?

A. α-Linoleic acid (ALA) is the omega-3 fatty acid best used by the body.
B. Fishy aftertaste can be avoided by freezing capsules before consuming.
C. Dosages above 3 g/day are optimal.
D. Docosahexaenoic acid (DHA) appears to have the main antidepressant effect.

The correct response is option B: Fishy aftertaste can be avoided by freezing capsules before consuming.

The omega-3 fatty acids best utilized by the body are eicosapentaenoic acid (EPA; 20:5) and docosahexaenoic acid (DHA; 22:6). Flaxseed and hemp oils contain the omega-3 fatty acid linoleic acid (ALA), which the body must convert to EPA or DHA. In approximately 15% of people, this conversion is impaired (option A is incorrect).

Most complaints of side effects, such as gastrointestinal upset and fishy aftertaste ("fish burps" or "seal burps"), can be avoided by freezing capsules before consuming or by ingesting them with food (option B is correct).

Daily dosages of 1–3 g (EPA+DHA) are safe without physician supervision. Dosages greater than 3 g/day may affect platelet function and increase bleeding times (option C is incorrect).

EPA rather than DHA appears to have the main antidepressant effect, because most of the significant positive studies in depression used at least 60% EPA (option D is incorrect). **Chapter 37 (pp. 1061–1062)**

37.5 A 75-year-old woman with a history of mild cognitive impairment and depression comes to your office stating that since she started taking a supplement, she has noticed improved mood and memory function, but has also noted foul-smelling urine and constipation. Which of the following supplements is the patient most likely taking?

A. Acetyl-L-carnitine.
B. Omega-3 fatty acids.
C. Kava (kava-kava, *Piper methysticum*).
D. St. John's wort (*Hypericum perforatum*).

The correct response is option A: Acetyl-L-carnitine.

Acetyl-L-carnitine (ALC) was found to have significant advantages compared with placebo in mild cognitive impairment and Alzheimer's disease, and a few studies have shown its superiority to placebo for dysthymia, major depressive disorder, and geriatric depression. The most common side effects include diarrhea, foul-smelling urine, constipation, and dyspepsia (option A is correct). Common side effects of *omega-3 fatty acids* include increased bleeding times, gastrointestinal upset, and a fishy aftertaste (option B is incorrect). Long-term heavy use of *kava* can lead to facial swelling, scaly rash, dyspnea, and low albumin levels (option C is incorrect). Side effects of *St. John's wort* include phototoxic rash, nausea, heartburn, and loose stools; at higher doses, this agent can cause sexual dysfunction, teeth clenching, and restless legs syndrome (option D is incorrect). **Chapter 37 (pp. 1061–1062, 1065, 1067)**

37.6 A 37-year-old man returns to your office with increased difficulty maintaining an erection and decreased sexual performance since starting a selective serotonin reuptake inhibitor (SSRI) for anxiety. He also takes a benzodiazepine. Which adaptogenic herb is safe for this patient and may be used to mitigate symptoms of sexual dysfunction?

A. St. John's wort (*Hypericum perforatum*).
B. Maca (*Lepidium meyenii*).
C. American ginseng (*Panax quinquefolius*, Xi Yang Shen).
D. Kava (kava-kava, *Piper methysticum*).

The correct response is option B: Maca (*Lepidium meyenii*).

Maca is a Peruvian herb that grows at high altitudes in the Andes and is used to enhance sexual function, fertility, alertness, mental focus, mood, and physical resilience. A double-blind, randomized pilot study found that maca (3 g/day) significantly reduced SSRI-induced sexual dysfunction (Dording et al. 2008). At recommended doses, maca causes minimal side effects, although at excess doses it may cause overactivation. In clinical practice, maca can be a useful adjunctive treatment for asthenia, sexual dysfunction, or infertility (option B is correct).

St. John's wort (*Hypericum perforatum*) is an herb used for treatment of mild to moderate depression and somatic symptom disorder and at higher doses may cause side effects similar to those of SSRIs, including sexual dysfunction, bruxism (teeth clenching), and restless legs syndrome (option A is incorrect).

American ginseng administered as a single dose may improve cognition and has few side effects. Although animal and in vitro studies suggest that ginseng may have some estrogenic activity, the clinical significance of such activity in humans is unclear (option C is incorrect).

Kava (kava-kava, *Piper methysticum*) has been studied in the treatment of anxiety; however, taking kava with alcohol, benzodiazepines, or muscle relaxants may result in coma and thus would be contraindicated in this patient taking a benzodiazepine. Additionally, the use of kava is not recommended until more information is available on safety, efficacy, and quality (option D is incorrect). **Chapter 37 (pp. 1064–1065, 1067)**

37.7 A 29-year-old woman with schizophrenia and HIV (for which she is currently taking antiretroviral medication) asks if there are any natural treatments that she could add to her current antipsychotic regimen to help with her symptoms of psychosis, which include hallucinations and social withdrawal. Which of the following interventions may be helpful for this patient's symptoms?

A. Mindfulness.
B. Cannabis sativa.

C. Schizandra (*Schisandra chinensis*).

D. St. John's wort (*Hypericum perforatum*).

The correct response is option C: Schizandra (*Schisandra chinensis*).

In studies of *Schisandra* for schizophrenia, several trials reported remission of catatonic stupor, decreased hallucinations, and increased sociability (Panossian and Amsterdam 2017). Older studies with less rigorous methodology suggested that *Schisandra* may have a place in treatment of schizophrenia for amelioration of catatonia, negative symptoms, fatigue, and side effects of first-generation antipsychotics and other sedating medications (option C is correct).

Patients with psychosis are not good candidates for meditation or mindfulness because psychotic thoughts may emerge during unstructured meditation (option A is incorrect).

Cannabis sativa use has been reported in treatment of nausea, anorexia, headaches, neuropathic pain, glaucoma, seizures, and muscle spasms in patients with multiple sclerosis. However, one of the main adverse effects associated with cannabis is psychosis, and thus it is not an advisable therapy for a patient with a primary psychotic disorder (option B is incorrect).

Finally, while most phytomedicines do not interfere with the cytochrome P450 (CYP) enzyme system, St. John's wort (*Hypericum perforatum*) has significant induction of CYP3A4. Given this, St. John's wort may interfere with antiretroviral treatment in this patient and thus would be contraindicated (option D is incorrect). **Chapter 37 (pp. 1063–1067, 1071)**

37.8   A 60-year-old man presents with depression. He has a history of hypertension and diabetes, and had a successful renal transplant several years ago. He takes maintenance immunosuppressive therapy consisting of cyclosporine, azathioprine, and prednisone. He is also takes an anticoagulant as he has paroxysmal atrial fibrillation. He does not want to add to his already long list of medications, and asks you about "natural products." Which of the following herbs is most likely to be safe and effective in treating this patient's depression?

A. St. John's wort (*Hypericum perforatum*).

B. Kava.

C. Arctic root (*Rhodiola rosea*).

D. Ginkgo biloba.

The correct response is option C: Arctic root (*Rhodiola rosea*).

Among herbs used in psychiatric practice, most have no clinically significant interactions with drugs when used at therapeutic doses. The exceptions are St. John's wort (*Hypericum perforatum*), ginkgo, and kava. Caution is required when combining herbs that interact with drugs having a narrow therapeutic window (i.e., a small difference between therapeutic and toxic levels or between therapeutic and subtherapeutic levels) or with drugs having the potential to cause serious adverse effects at levels outside the therapeutic range, such as warfarin, cyclosporine, or digoxin. In humans, significant interactions have been reported between St. John's wort and immunosuppressants via induction of cytochrome P450 (CYP) 3A4, so St. John's wort could be unsafe in this patient taking cyclosporine (option A is incorrect).

The use of kava is not recommended until more information is available on safety, efficacy, and quality (option B is incorrect).

A 6-week double-blind randomized controlled trial of *R. rosea* (SHR-5) in mild to moderate depression showed significant antidepressant effects compared with placebo (Darbinyan et al. 2007). It is considered safe, and adverse effects are rare (option C is correct).

Inhibition of platelet activating factor by ginkgolide B suggests that ginkgo can have additive effects with drugs that affect platelet function and/or coagulation, such as nonsteroidal anti-inflammatory drugs (e.g., aspirin, ibuprofen, selective cyclooxygenase 2 [COX-2] inhibitors) and anticoagulants (e.g., warfarin) (option D is incorrect). **Chapter 37 (pp. 1062–1063, 1065–1067)**

37.9   A 36-year-old pregnant woman presents with several weeks of low mood, poor sleep, decreased motivation, and decreased concentration. She has no history of manic symptoms. She does not want to take a conventional antidepressant, and is interested in taking an alternative treatment for her symptoms. Which of the following may be as effective as an antidepressant and would be safe for this patient?

A. s-adenosylmethionine (SAMe).
B. Ashwagandha (*Withania somnifera*).
C. Saffron (*Crocus sativus*).
D. St. John's wort (*Hypericum perforatum*).

The correct response is option A: s-Adenosylmethionine (SAMe).

Ashwagandha (*Withania somnifera*) may improve GABA-ergic signaling dysfunctions that may occur in anxiety and insomnia; however, it may precipitate miscarriage (option B is incorrect).

Saffron (*Crocus sativus*) has been documented in randomized controlled trials to have benefits in mild to moderate depression; however, doses of 10 g of saffron have been used to induce abortion and thus use in pregnancy is not recommended (option C is incorrect).

Some research on St. John's wort (*Hypericum perforatum*) supports its use for mild to moderate depression; however, safety in pregnancy has not been established (option D is incorrect).

When used as monotherapy, SAMe has been shown to be more effective than placebo and as effective as conventional antidepressants for treating major depressive disorder. It may be given at dosages of 80–1,200 mg/day for mild to moderate depression or for antidepressant augmentation, and at dosages up to 2,400 mg/day as tolerated for treatment-resistant illness. Additionally, SAMe is thought to be safe in pregnancy, given that SAMe treatment for cholestasis in pregnancy caused no adverse effects on neonates and healthy infants have higher cerebrospinal fluid levels of SAMe than do adults (option A is correct). **Chapter 37 (pp. 1059–1060, 1065–1067)**

37.10 Which of the following complementary and alternative treatments is considered to be a safe and possibly effective treatment for bipolar disorder?

A. Ashwagandha (*Withania somnifera*).
B. s-adenosylmethionine (SAMe).
C. Arctic root (*Rhodiola rosea*).
D. St. John's wort (*Hypericum perforatum*).

The correct response is option A: Ashwagandha (*Withania somnifera*).

Ashwagandha (*Withania somnifera*) is an adaptogenic herb that may improve GABAergic signaling dysfunctions and has been described as a safe and possibly effective agent in bipolar disorder (option A is correct).

SAMe may be used to augment antidepressants; however, it can be stimulating and may initially exacerbate anxiety and in bipolar disorder can induce hypomanic or manic symptoms (option B is incorrect).

Arctic root (*Rhodiola rosea*) has been used in the treatment of asthenia neuroses, schizophrenia, and mild to moderate depression. Sensitive individuals may experience excessive stimulation such as anxiety, irritability, or insomnia. The stimulatory effect can exacerbate agitation and irritability in bipolar disorder, hence may be unsafe in this patient population (option C is incorrect).

A clear temporal association exists between St. John's wort use and induction of hypomania or mania. As with conventional antidepressants, caution is advised in people with a personal or family history of bipolar disorder (option D is incorrect). **Chapter 37 (pp. 1059, 1063, 1065)**

37.11 Which of the following effects can be produced by slow-breathing practices?

A. Decreased heart rate variability.
B. Decreased underactivity in prefrontal emotion regulatory centers.
C. Decreased levels of GABA (γ-aminobutyric acid).
D. Reduced overactivity in the amygdala.

The correct response is option D: Reduced overactivity in the amygdala.

Evidence shows that slow-breathing practices (through vagal afferents) can reduce overactivity in the amygdala (option D is correct), increase underactivity in prefrontal emotion regulatory centers (option B is incorrect), modulate hypothalamic-pituitary-adrenal axis function, increase levels of the inhibitory neurotransmitter GABA (option C is incorrect), stimulate oxytocin release, and improve cognitive function. For most adults, gentle breathing at 4.5 to 6 cycles per minute significantly increases heart rate variability, leading to a calm state (option A is incorrect). **Chapter 37 (p. 1071)**

37.12 An 81-year-old man with arthritis and a pacemaker presents with several years of gradually worsening memory, and a declining ability to care for himself. He is evaluated and subsequently diagnosed with major neurocognitive disorder. Which of the following interventions would be safe for this patient and has shown benefit for maintaining a stable clinical dementia rating over 5 months?

A. Qigong.
B. Yoga.
C. Cranial electrotherapy stimulation.
D. Vitamin E.

The correct response is option A: Qigong.

Comparative studies suggest that participation in qigong/tai chi may be more effective than conventional exercise for reducing anxiety, increasing frontal electroencephalogram theta-wave activity, and maintaining a stable clinical dementia rating over 5 months (Abbott et al. 2017) (option A is correct).

In this elderly patient with arthritis, qigong may be preferred to yoga because participants are not required to lie down or contort into difficult positions in qigong (option B is incorrect).

Cranial electrotherapy stimulation is contraindicated because this patient has a pacemaker (option C is incorrect).

Vitamin E is known to act as an antioxidant to scavenge toxic free radicals, and it has been studied extensively in the treatment of mild cognitive impairment (MCI) and Alzheimer's dementia. However, evidence for its benefit in MCI or Alzheimer's disease is lacking, with the exception of a study that reported that vitamin E may slow functional decline in Alzheimer's disease (Dysken et al. 2014). Because long-term vitamin E supplementation was found to be associated with a small increased risk of cardiovascular events in a large trial involving older patients with vascular disease or diabetes mellitus (Lonn et al. 2005), vitamin E has become less popular as a treatment approach (option D is incorrect). **Chapter 37 (pp. 1071–1073); see also Chapter 25 ("Neurocognitive Disorders"; p. 702)**

References

Abbott R, Chang DD, Eyre H, et al: Mind-body practices tai chi and qigong in the treatment and prevention of psychiatric disorders, in Complementary and Integrative Treatments in Psychiatric Practice. Edited by Gerbarg PL, Muskin PR, Brown RP. Arlington, VA, American Psychiatric Association Publishing, 2017, pp 261–280

Almeida OP, Ford AH, Flicker L: Systematic review and meta-analysis of randomized placebo-controlled trials of folate and vitamin B12 for depression. Int Psychogeriatr 27(5):727–737, 2015 25644193

Dysken MW, Guarino PD, Vertrees JE, et al: Vitamin E and memantine in Alzheimer's disease: clinical trial methods and baseline data. Alzheimers Dement 10(1):36–44, 2014 23583234

Darbinyan V, Aslanyan G, Amroyan E, et al: Clinical trial of Rhodiola rosea L. extract SHR-5 in the treatment of mild to moderate depression. Nord J Psychiatry 61(5):343–348, 2007 [Erratum in: Nord J Psychiatry 61(6):503, 2007] 17990195

Dording CM, Fisher L, Papakostas G, et al: A double-blind, randomized, pilot dose-finding study of maca root (L. meyenii) for the management of SSRI-induced sexual dysfunction. CNS Neurosci Ther 14(3):182–191, 2008 18801111

Lonn E, Bosch J, Yusuf S, et al; HOPE and HOPE-TOO Trial Investigators: Effects of long-term vitamin E supplementation on cardiovascular events and cancer: a randomized controlled trial. JAMA 293(11):1338–1347, 2005 15769967

Panossian A, Amsterdam JD: Adaptogens in psychiatric practice, in Complementary and Integrative Treatments in Psychiatric Practice. Edited by Gerbarg PL, Muskin PR, Brown RP. Arlington, VA, American Psychiatric Association Publishing, 2017, pp 113–134

Sharma A, Gerbarg P, Bottiglieri T, et al: S-Adenosylmethionine (SAMe) for neuropsychiatric disorders: a clinician-oriented review of research. J Clin Psychiatry 78(6):e656–e667, 2017 28682528

CHAPTER 38

Integrated
and Collaborative Care

38.1 A 79-year-old woman with high cholesterol, diabetes complicated by retinopathy, peripheral arterial disease, and schizoaffective disorder lives in a rural area without public transportation and with limited numbers of mental health providers. Which of the following integrated treatment modalities would help this patient receive the care she needs?

A. Colocated care.
B. Collaborative care.
C. Telepsychiatry.
D. Medical care for psychiatric patients.

The correct response is option C: Telepsychiatry.

Integrated care delivery encompasses several models, including colocation of a psychiatrist within a general medical setting (colocated care), collaborative care, telepsychiatry, and provision of general medical services to psychiatric patients with chronic severe mental illnesses (Table 38–1). The target population for *telepsychiatry* is providers or patients at distant sites or unable to come in person (option C is correct). The target population for *colocated care* is patients referred by primary care providers (option A is incorrect). The target population for *collaborative care* is a clinic or health system patient population (option B is incorrect). The target population for *medical care for psychiatric patients* is psychiatric patients, especially in community mental health (option D is incorrect). **Chapter 38 (Table 38–1 [p. 1083])**

38.2 Which of the following collaborative care principles refers to an approach focused on a defined population, such as all individuals served by a particular primary care clinic, medical center, or health care system?

A. Population-based care.
B. Evidence-based care.
C. Measurement-based treatment to target.
D. Accountability.

TABLE 38–1. Models of integrated care

	Colocated care	Collaborative care	Telepsychiatry	Medical care for psychiatric patients
Target population	Patients referred by primary care providers	Clinic or health system patient population	Providers or patients at distant sites or unable to come in person	Psychiatric patients, especially in community mental health
Personnel	Consulting psychiatrist or behavioral health specialist	Team of patient, primary care provider, care manager, psychiatrist	Psychiatrist or other mental health specialist	General medical provider
Methods	Direct (in-person) consultation	Population-based screening; team provides patient-centered and evidence-based interventions, outcome measurement, stepped care	Direct or indirect consultation by telephone or videoconferencing	Preventive and primary medical care delivered within psychiatric treatment setting
Advantages	Improved access, patient satisfaction, provider interactions, outcomes for referred patients	Improved access, care quality, population outcomes, cost-effectiveness	Improved access for smaller/rural areas, patients who are unable to come to appointments	Improved access to medical care
Limitations	Limited capacity; treats only referred patients	Requires changes in practice; varying reimbursement	Requires specialized equipment; varying reimbursement	Need for medical providers in mental health setting or psychiatrists providing medical care

The correct response is option A: Population-based care.

In *population-based care*, the focus is on a defined population, such as all individuals served by a particular primary care clinic, medical center, or health care system (option A is correct).

Evidence-based care refers to the principle that treatments delivered in collaborative care are based on the best available evidence (option B is incorrect).

In the *measurement-based treatment to target* approach, the collaborative care team establishes a patient-centered treatment goal for each person who is identified as having a mental health condition. Patients are then systematically tracked with the help of outcome measures, such as symptom rating scales, and timely treatment adjustments are made until the predefined goal is achieved (option C is incorrect).

Accountability refers to the principle that the psychiatric consultants within collaborative care teams take responsibility both for the treatment outcomes of patients in their identified population who are active in treatment and for continuous improvement in the overall quality of care provided by their team (option D is incorrect). **Chapter 38 (pp. 1084–1085)**

38.3 Which of the following is an appropriate method for tracking progress toward a measurable treatment goal in the collaborative care model?

A. Recording an increase in a patient's fluoxetine dosage from 20 mg/day to 60 mg/day.
B. Recording a patient's "no-show" rate over a 3-month period.
C. Reassessing a patient's symptom ratings on the Patient Health Questionnaire–9 (PHQ-9) during each appointment.
D. Reviewing utilization of new coping skills with a patient.

The correct response is option C: Reassessing a patient's symptom ratings on the Patient Health Questionnaire–9 (PHQ-9) during each appointment.

In the collaborative care model, the team establishes a patient-centered treatment goal for each person who is identified as having a mental health condition. Patients are then systematically tracked with the help of relevant outcome measures, such as symptom rating scales (e.g., the PHQ-9 for depression [Kroenke et al. 2001]) (option C is correct).

Reviewing a patient's "no-show" rate over several months is one of the responsibilities of the care manager or behavioral health care provider. A significant "no show" rate could be due to many factors but is not necessarily an appropriate measure of treatment response (option B is incorrect). Recording antidepressant dosage adjustments is an important aspect of patient care but is not in itself a patient-centered treatment goal (option A is incorrect). A patient's utilization of new coping skills does not necessarily indicate that the patient's mood has responded to treatment (option D is incorrect). **Chapter 38 (p. 1085)**

38.4 In the collaborative care model, which of the following roles is primarily the responsibility of the psychiatrist?

A. Serving as the first contact for the patient.
B. Managing the details of patient care.
C. Providing brief, evidence-based psychotherapies.
D. Providing indirect consultation and recommendations for patients who are not improving.

The correct response is option D: Providing indirect consultation and recommendations for patients who are not improving.

In the collaborative care model, mental health care providers work together with primary care providers and the patient as a team. A collaborative care team consists of the patient and at least a primary care provider, a care manager or behavioral health care provider, and a psychiatric consultant. Each team member has a clear role in order to coordinate care most effectively (Ratzliff et al. 2016):
    The psychiatric consultant in collaborative care spends most of his or her time *providing indirect consultations* (option D is correct).
    The *first contact for the patient* in the collaborative care model is the primary care provider (option A is incorrect).
    The *care manager* or *behavioral health care provider* has two main roles in the collaborative care model. The first is to *manage patient care*, which includes engaging the patient in treatment, seeing the patient every 2 weeks, performing systematic initial and follow-up assessments, coordinating the care being provided to the patient, adding the patient to the registry, maintaining and updating the registry, tracking the treatment response of the patient with behavioral health measures, and regularly reviewing the caseload with the psychiatric consultant, usually on a weekly basis. The second major function of the care manager is to *provide brief, evidence-based psychotherapies*, such as behavioral activation, problem-solving therapy, cognitive-behavioral therapy, interpersonal therapy, and motivational interviewing (options B and C are incorrect). **Chapter 38 (pp. 1087–1088)**

38.5 Which of the following options describes an appropriate role for the psychiatrist in the collaborative care model?

A. Teaching the team how to identify hypomania in geriatric patients.
B. Spending 3 days per week providing short-term interpersonal therapy to patients in an outpatient setting.
C. Routinely working alongside the primary care provider during appointments to examine severely ill patients.
D. Exclusively providing direct, in-person patient care.

The correct response is option A: Teaching the team how to identify hypomania in geriatric patients.

In the collaborative care model, the psychiatric consultant performs primarily indirect consultation, reviewing care managers' caseloads and providing recommendations for additional assessment and treatment for patients whose symptoms are not improving. In a minority of cases (usually reserved for situations in which the psychiatric provider needs to see the patient to clarify the diagnosis or reassess the treatment approach for treatment-refractory symptoms), the psychiatric consultant sees the patient directly, either in person or by teleconferencing (option D is incorrect).

In addition to clinical consultation duties, the psychiatrist has several other important responsibilities, including providing education and training for other team members (option A is correct) and taking on a leadership role to support the team and the collaborative care model (Raney 2015).

Provision of brief, evidence-based psychotherapies is a major function of the care manager, not of the psychiatric consultant (option B is incorrect). Similarly, examination of patients is typically performed only by the primary care provider (option C is incorrect). **Chapter 38 (pp. 1082, 1087–1089)**

38.6   In the United States, approximately what percentage of people with psychiatric disorders see any mental health specialist?

A. 21%.
B. 2%.
C. 30%.
D. 65%.

The correct response is option A: 21%.

Mental disorders are responsible for significant morbidity and mortality, accounting for about 25% of disability worldwide (Murray et al. 2012). However, in the United States, only 12% of people with psychiatric disorders see a psychiatrist, and only 21% see any mental health specialist (Wang et al. 2005) (option A is correct; options B, C, and D are incorrect). **Chapter 38 (p. 1081)**

38.7   Which of the following is a population-based model that uses systematic mental health screening of the clinic or health system population to identify patients for further diagnostic evaluation and evidence-based treatment?

A. Collaborative care model.
B. Colocated care model.
C. Telepsychiatry model.
D. Medical care for psychiatric patients model.

The correct response is option A: Collaborative care model.

Collaborative care is a population-based model that uses systematic mental health screening of a clinic or health system population to identify patients for further diagnostic evaluation and treatment (see Table 38–1). In this model, a team—consisting of the patient, a primary care provider, a care manager, and a psychiatrist—provides patient-centered and evidence-based interventions, outcome measurement, and stepped care based on patient response (option A is correct).

In the *colocated care* model, a consulting psychiatrist or behavioral health specialist working within a general medical clinic provides on-site consultation and direct care to patients referred by clinic providers (option B is incorrect).

In the *telepsychiatry* model, a psychiatrist or other mental health care specialist provides direct or indirect consultation via telephone or videoconferencing (option C is incorrect).

In the *medical care for psychiatric patients* model, a general medical care practitioner or a psychiatrist trained in screening for and first-line treatment of common medical conditions delivers preventive and primary medical care to patients within the psychiatric treatment setting (option D is incorrect). **Chapter 38 (pp. 1082, 1083 [Table 38–1])**

38.8 Which of the following terms refers to an approach that brings together mental health care and primary medical care to increase access to care and to improve mental health and medical outcomes for patients in a cost-effective manner?

A. Telepsychiatry.
B. Collaborative care.
C. Colocated care.
D. Integrated care.

The correct response is option D: Integrated care.

Integrated behavioral health care has been defined as "the care that results from a practice team of primary care and [mental] health clinicians, working together with patients and families, using a systematic and cost-effective approach to provide patient-centered care for a defined population" (Peek and The National Integration Academy Council 2013, p. 2). Studies of integrated care have confirmed the effectiveness of this approach in addressing the triple aim of improving access to care, improving quality and outcomes of care, and reducing total health care costs (Katon and Unützer 2011) (option D is correct).

Specific models of integrated care include colocation of a psychiatrist within a primary care setting, collaborative care, telepsychiatry, and delivery of preventive and general medical care to psychiatric patients (options A, B, and C are incorrect). **Chapter 38 (pp. 1081–1082, 1092)**

38.9 Which of the following care models delivers treatment through a team consisting of the patient, a primary care provider, a care manager, and a psychiatric consultant?

A. Collaborative care model.
B. Telepsychiatry model.
C. Medical care for psychiatric patients model.
D. Colocated care model.

The correct response is option A: Collaborative care model.

The *collaborative care model* uses systematic mental health screening of a clinic or health system population to identify patients for further diagnostic evaluation and treatment (see Table 38–1). The collaborative care team consists of the patient and at least a primary care provider, a care manager or behavioral health care provider, and a psychiatric consultant (option A is correct). In the *telepsychiatry* model, direct or indirect consultation via telephone or videoconferencing is provided by a psychiatrist or other mental health care specialist (option B is incorrect). In the *medical care for psychiatric patients* model, preventive and primary medical care is delivered to patients in the psychiatric treatment setting by a general medical care practitioner or a psychiatrist trained in screening for and first-line treatment of common medical conditions (option C is incorrect).

In the *colocated care* model, on-site consultation and direct care to referred patients is provided by a consulting psychiatrist or behavioral health specialist working within a general medical clinic (option D is incorrect). **Chapter 38 (pp. 1083 [Table 38–1], 1087)**

38.10 In the collaborative care model, which of the following practitioners is responsible for delivering evidence-based brief psychotherapy interventions to patients?

A. Care manager or behavioral health care provider.
B. Primary care provider.
C. Psychiatric consultant.
D. Any member of the team may be assigned responsibility for providing brief psychotherapy to patients.

The correct response is option A: Care manager or behavioral health care provider.

In the collaborative care model, the care manager (typically a licensed social worker, a registered nurse, or a psychologist) works closely with the primary care provider and psychiatric consultant to provide mental health care to patients. Care managers have two main roles. The first is *care management*, which includes engaging the patient in treatment, seeing the patient every 2 weeks, performing systematic initial and follow-up assessments, coordinating the care being provided to the patient, adding the patient to the registry, maintaining and updating the registry, tracking the treatment response of the patient with behavioral health measures, and regularly reviewing the caseload with the psychiatric consultant, usually on a weekly basis. The second major function of the care manager is to *provide brief, evidence-based psychotherapies*, such as behavioral activation, problem-solving therapy, cognitive-behavioral therapy, interpersonal therapy, and motivational interviewing (option A is correct; option D is incorrect).

The primary care provider retains the overall responsibility of overseeing all aspects of care provided to the patient. He or she has several important roles, including identifying patients who need behavioral health treatment, doing the initial assessment, starting appropriate first-line treatment, introducing the collaborative care model to the patient, and referring the patient to the care manager for further assessment and treatment. The primary care provider works with the rest of the team to develop shared treatment goals, monitor treatment response, and encourage the patient to engage in collaborative care. The primary care provider prescribes medications, orders laboratory tests, and adjusts treatment in consultation with the care manager and psychiatric consultant (option B is incorrect).

The psychiatric consultant is responsible for performing primarily indirect consultation, reviewing care managers' caseloads and providing recommendations for additional assessment and treatment for patients whose symptoms are not improving (option C is incorrect). **Chapter 38 (pp. 1082, 1087–1088)**

38.11 Each of the various models of care delivery has advantages and limitations. Which of the following options describes a limitation of the *colocated care model*?

A. The requirement for specialized equipment.
B. The need for medical care providers to work within the mental health care setting.
C. The restriction that only patients who are specifically referred can be treated.
D. The requirement for many changes in the way providers usually practice.

The correct response is option C: The restriction that only patients who are specifically referred can be treated.

Whereas all of main models of integrated care are associated with the advantage of providing patients with improved access to care, each model has one or two specific disadvantages (see Table 38–1). The *telepsychiatry* model is most specifically limited by its requirement for specialized equipment (option A is incorrect). Models focused on improving *medical care for psychiatric patients* are most limited by the need to place medical care providers in mental health care settings (and vice versa) (option B is incorrect). The *colocated care* model is most limited by both capacity and the fact that it only allows for treatment of referred patients (option C is correct). Requiring changes in the way providers practice is a limitation of the *collaborative care* model (option D is incorrect). **Chapter 38 (Table 38–1 [p. 1083])**

38.12 A 24-year-old man with a medical history significant for schizophrenia is being followed by his primary care provider (PCP) at a collaborative care clinic. Over the past 4 months, the patient has had two separate episodes of increased paranoia, auditory hallucinations, and disorganized thinking that impaired his ability to maintain safety in the community. These episodes required treatment in an inpatient psychiatric unit. The PCP notes that the patient was most recently discharged on paliperidone 6 mg daily, quetiapine 150 mg at night, trazodone 100 mg at night, alprazolam 1 mg twice daily as needed for anxiety, benztropine 1 mg twice daily, and valproic acid 1,000 mg at night. Which of the following would be the most appropriate next step for the PCP?

A. Have the consulting psychiatrist schedule a series of in-person visits to examine the patient and provide treatment recommendations.
B. Have the care manager refer the patient to a specialty mental health care service and continue following the patient until care is established.
C. Schedule a "curbside consult" with the psychiatrist to discuss adjustment of the patient's current medication regimen.
D. Ask the care manager to increase the frequency of visits for psychodynamic therapy.

The correct response is option B: Have the care manager refer the patient to a specialty mental health care service and continue following the patient until care is established.

In the collaborative care model, the primary care provider has several important roles, including identifying patients who need behavioral health treatment, starting appropriate first-line treatment, and referring the patient to the care manager for further assessment and treatment. The care manager is in charge of tracking the treatment response of the patient with behavioral health measures and regularly reviewing the caseload with the psychiatric consultant, usually on a weekly basis; it would be inappropriate in this situation to respond to the increased needs of this patient by only asking the case manager to increase the frequency of visits (option D is incorrect).

Typically, patients are in active treatment for 3–6 months, after which two outcomes are possible: either the patient achieves remission or the patient needs referral to specialized mental health care services for longer-term, more intensive treatment. If a patient does not improve despite multiple treatment adjustments or requires a level of care that cannot be provided within the collaborative care model, the care manager facilitates referrals to specialty mental health care services and follows up until the patient has established care there (option B is correct).

In the collaborative care model, the psychiatric consultant performs primarily indirect consultation, reviewing care managers' caseloads and providing recommendations for additional assessment and treatment for patients whose symptoms are not improving. Indirect consultations include caseload reviews with the care manager and "curbside consults." This scenario displays a level of complexity that would be inappropriate for a curbside consult (option C is incorrect).

Direct consultations are usually reserved for situations in which the psychiatric provider needs to see the patient to clarify the diagnosis or reassess the treatment approach in treatment-refractory cases (option A is incorrect). **Chapter 38 (pp. 1087–1088, 1089)**

38.13 In which model of care would the psychiatric consultant most often provide indirect consultation to the patient without seeing the patient?

A. Collaborative care model.
B. Telepsychiatry model.

C. Medical care for psychiatric patients model.

D. Colocated care model.

The correct response is option A: Collaborative care model.

In other integrated care models, particularly colocated care and some telepsychiatry services, the psychiatrist provides direct consultation, seeing the patient in person or by teleconferencing, doing an assessment, and providing treatment recommendations to the primary care provider (options B, C, and D are incorrect). In contrast, the psychiatric consultant in collaborative care spends most of his or her time providing indirect consultations. Indirect consultations include caseload reviews with the care manager and "curbside consults." For weekly caseload reviews, the psychiatric consultant reviews the registry (i.e., the comprehensive list of patients who are in active treatment) with the care manager and develops treatment recommendations without seeing the patient; this is done by gathering information from the care manager, from the assessment conducted by the primary care provider, and from behavioral health measures such as symptom rating scales. In the collaborative care model, direct consultations are usually reserved for situations in which the psychiatric provider needs to see the patient to clarify the diagnosis or reassess the treatment approach in treatment-refractory cases (option A is correct). **Chapter 38 (p. 1089)**

References

Katon W, Unützer J: Consultation psychiatry in the medical home and accountable care organizations: achieving the triple aim. Gen Hosp Psychiatry 33(4):305–310, 2011 21762825

Kroenke K, Spitzer RL, Williams JB: The PHQ-9: validity of a brief depression severity measure. J Gen Intern Med 16(9):606–613, 2001 11556941

Murray CJL, Vos T, Lozano R, et al: Disability-adjusted life years (DALYs) for 291 diseases and injuries in 21 regions, 1990–2010: a systematic analysis for the Global Burden of Disease Study 2010. Lancet 380(9859):2197–2223, 2012 23245608

Peek CJ, The National Integration Academy Council: Lexicon for Behavioral Health and Primary Care Integration: Concepts and Definitions Developed by Expert Consensus (AHRQ Publ No 13-IP001-EF). Rockville, MD, Agency for Healthcare Research and Quality, 2013. Available at: http://integrationacademy.ahrq.gov/sites/default/files/Lexicon.pdf. Accessed September 3, 2017.

Raney LE: Integrating primary care and behavioral health: the role of the psychiatrist in the Collaborative Care Model. Am J Psychiatry 172(8):721–728, 2015 26234599

Ratzliff A, Cerimele J, Katon W, et al: Working as a team to provide Collaborative Care, in Integrated Care: Creating Effective Mental and Primary Health Care Teams. Edited by Ratzliff A, Unützer J, Katon W, et al. Hoboken, NJ, Wiley, 2016, pp 1–23

Wang PS, Lane M, Olfson M, et al: Twelve-month use of mental health services in the United States: results from the National Comorbidity Survey Replication. Arch Gen Psychiatry 62(6):629–640, 2005 15939840

CHAPTER 39

Standardized Assessment and Measurement-Based Care

39.1   Which of the following options correctly defines the term *measurement-based care*?

    A. The process of making decisions by formulating, testing, and refining hypotheses based on clinical information that is often incomplete or inconsistent, often in the context of very brief clinical encounters.

    B. The ongoing administration of validated measures throughout the course of treatment to track patient progress, and the use of those data to inform clinicians' and patients' decisions about clinical interventions.

    C. The use of validated brief tools to enable improved detection and more accurate diagnosis of mental disorders in primary care.

    D. The use of tests of behavior that assess people by rating their performance on standardized tasks.

The correct response is option B: The ongoing administration of validated measures throughout the course of treatment to track patient progress, and the use of those data to inform clinicians' and patients' decisions about clinical interventions.

Measurement-based care (MBC) refers to the ongoing administration of validated measures throughout the course of treatment to track patient progress, and the use of those data to inform clinicians' and patients' decisions about clinical interventions (Scott and Lewis 2015) (option B is correct).

The assessment process requires the clinician to make decisions by formulating, testing, and refining hypotheses based on clinical information that is often incomplete or inconsistent, often in the context of very brief clinical encounters (option A is incorrect). Evidence has been mounting for decades that in such contexts, subjective clinical judgment does not yield diagnoses that are as accurate or comprehensive as standardized diagnostic measures. Consequently, evidence-based assessment is now recognized as a key component of evidence-based care.

Several studies indicate that use of validated brief screening tools enables improved detection and more accurate diagnosis of mental disorders in primary care (Bufka and Campl 2010) (option C is incorrect).

Standardized assessment involving tests of behavior that assess people by rating their performance on standardized tasks (Groth-Marnat and Wright 2016) is the approach used in neuropsychiatric assessment (option D is incorrect). **Chapter 39 (pp. 1095–1098)**

39.2   What type of measure is the Alcohol Use Disorders Identification Test—Consumption (AUDIT-C)?

A. Broad symptom measure.
B. Scale of functioning or quality of life.
C. Screening tool.
D. Comprehensive self-report assessment battery.

The correct response is option C: Screening tool.

The measures used for initial treatment planning or monitoring progress should match the clinical purpose of the assessment and the clinical focus of the treatment (Table 39–1). *Screening tools* such as the AUDIT-C and the two-item Patient Health Questionnaire (PHQ-2) are used to identify individuals who should be referred for further assessment (option C is correct). *Broad symptom measures* such as the 45-item Outcome Questionnaire (OQ-45) and the Brief Symptom Inventory can be used in treatment planning and assessment of progress (option A is incorrect). *Scales of functioning or quality of life* are also used for treatment planning and assessment of progress; examples include the 24-item Behavior and Symptom Identification Scale (BASIS-24) and the Medical Outcomes Study 36-item Short Form (SF-36) (option B is incorrect). *Comprehensive self-report assessment batteries* such as the Minnesota Multiphasic Personality Inventory (MMPI) and the Millon Clinical Multiaxial Inventory (MCMI) are used for formulation of complex cases, personality assessment, or differential diagnosis (option D is incorrect). **Chapter 39 (Table 39–1 [p. 1101])**

39.3   A college student sees a psychiatrist for academic difficulties after minimal improvement with the help of an academic tutor. After assessment, the psychiatrist gives a diagnosis of attention-deficit/hyperactivity disorder (ADHD) and rules out other psychiatric disorders. After 3 months on a stimulant with improvements in attention, the student reports ongoing difficulty with testing performance and executive functioning tasks. What type of assessment would be most appropriate as a next step in differential diagnosis and treatment planning?

A. A comprehensive neuropsychiatric assessment using standardized measures.
B. A self-assessment personality questionnaire such as the Minnesota Multiphasic Personality Inventory.
C. A structured clinical interview such as the Mini International Neuropsychiatric Interview.
D. A projective personality test such as the Rorschach.

TABLE 39–1. Purposes and uses of standardized measures

Type of measure	Purpose	Which patients	Who administers and interprets it	Examples
Screening tools	Identification of persons who should be referred for further assessment	Everyone	Primary care staff or mental health professionals	PHQ-2, AUDIT-C
Broad symptom measures	Treatment planning; assessment of progress	Patients in mental health treatment	Mental health professionals	OQ-45, Brief Symptom Inventory
Specific symptom measures	Treatment planning; assessment of progress	Patients in mental health treatment	Mental health professionals	PHQ-9, GAD-7
Scales of functioning or quality of life	Treatment planning; assessment of progress	Patients in mental health treatment	Mental health professionals	BASIS-24, SF-36
Ratings of quality of therapeutic alliance or patient satisfaction	Assessment of progress	Patients in mental health treatment	Mental health professionals	Working Alliance Inventory
Comprehensive self-report assessment batteries	Formulation of complex cases; personality assessment; differential diagnosis	Complex cases that pose assessment challenges	Assessment experts (typically psychologists)	MMPI, MCMI
Medication adherence and side effects	Assessment of medication compliance and physical side effects	Individuals using psychotropic medication	Psychiatrists	Morisky Medication Adherence Scale; UKU Side Effect Rating Scale
Neuropsychiatric assessments	Assessment of cognitive deficits and strengths relative to established norms	Individuals who may have cognitive impairment	Neuropsychologists	WAIS, Halstead-Reitan

Note. AUDIT-C=Alcohol Use Disorders Identification Test—Consumption; BASIS-24=24-item Behavior and Symptom Identification Scale; GAD-7=Generalized Anxiety Disorder seven-item scale; MCMI=Millon Clinical Multiaxial Inventory; MMPI=Minnesota Multiphasic Personality Inventory; OQ-45=45-item Outcome Questionnaire; PHQ-2=two-item Patient Health Questionnaire; PHQ-9=nine-item Patient Health Questionnaire; SF-36=Medical Outcomes Study 36-item Short Form; UKU=Udvalg fur Kliniske Undersøgelser; WAIS=Wechsler Adult Intelligence Scale.

The correct response is option A: A comprehensive neuropsychiatric assessment using standardized measures.

Referral for comprehensive neuropsychiatric assessment using standardized measures can enable detection of cognitive deficits and strengths that might not otherwise be immediately apparent (Roebuck-Spencer et al. 2017). Neuropsychiatric tests assess domains such as attention and concentration, memory, language, visuospatial abilities, and problem solving (Groth-Marnat and Wright 2016). Results of such assessments can inform recovery and treatment and can identify existing strengths that can be leveraged to improve functioning (option A is correct).

The Mini International Neuropsychiatric Interview (Groth-Marnat and Wright 2016) is a structured clinical interview that requires substantial training and often takes a long time to administer, so it is used more often in research studies than in clinical practice (option C is incorrect).

The Minnesota Multiphasic Personality Inventory (MMPI), is a self-assessment questionnaire that assesses personality disorders as well as other symptoms (Groth-Marnat and Wright 2016) (option B is incorrect).

Clinical psychology training programs are placing increasing emphasis on use of validated self-report batteries rather than projective personality tests such as the Rorschach (Stedman et al. 2018) (option D is incorrect). **Chapter 39 (p. 1098)**

39.4   Which of the following statements describes a test that has high *validity*?

A. A test that yields consistent scores when administered to the same person under similar circumstances.
B. A test for which two interviewers assessing the same person arrive at similar results.
C. A test that measures the trait it is intended to measure.
D. A test that shows the same result on two different occasions.

The correct response is option C: A test that measures the trait it is intended to measure.

Validity refers to the extent to which a test measures the trait it is intended to measure (Groth-Marnat and Wright 2016; Tarescavage and Ben-Porath 2014) (option C is correct).

Reliability is the degree to which a measure yields consistent scores when administered to the same person under similar circumstances (Groth-Marnat and Wright 2016) (option A is incorrect).

Ways of assessing reliability include *test-retest reliability* (administering the test on two different occasions and comparing results) (option D is incorrect) and *interrater reliability* (comparing results from two interviewers or observers assessing the same person) (Groth-Marnat and Wright 2016) (option B is incorrect). **Chapter 39 (pp. 1098–1099)**

39.5   For which of the following clinical purposes is a *structured interview* most useful?

A. Enabling detection of cognitive deficits and strengths that might not otherwise be immediately apparent.
B. Identification of people who may potentially have a psychiatric disorder who should be referred for further assessment.
C. Identification of stigmatizing problems such as substance use.
D. Informing treatment planning and differential diagnosis in complicated cases.

The correct response is option D: Informing treatment planning and differential diagnosis in complicated cases.

Structured interviews can be extremely useful in informing treatment planning and differential diagnosis in complicated cases (option D is correct).

Referral of individuals for comprehensive neuropsychiatric assessment using standardized measures can enable detection of cognitive deficits and strengths that might not otherwise be immediately apparent (Roebuck-Spencer et al. 2017) (option A is incorrect).

Screening tools are intended to identify people who may potentially have a psychiatric disorder who should be referred for further assessment (option B is incorrect).

Several studies suggest that people are more likely to disclose stigmatizing problems such as substance use in an online survey or paper questionnaires than in a clinical interview (Del Boca and Darkes 2003) (option C is incorrect). **Chapter 39 (pp. 1096–1098)**

39.6   Which of the following standardized measures is designed to be administered by professionals in the primary care setting?

A. Morisky Medication Adherence Scale.
B. 24-Item Behavior and Symptom Identification Scale (BASIS-24).
C. Two-item Patient Health Questionnaire (PHQ-2).
D. Halstead-Reitan.

The correct response is option C: Two-item Patient Health Questionnaire (PHQ-2).

Staff resources are an important consideration in the choice of assessment measures (see Table 39–1).The PHQ-2 is designed to be administered and interpreted by primary care staff (option C is correct). The Morisky Medication Adherence Scale (Morisky et al. 1986) is designed to be administered and interpreted by psychiatrists (option A is incorrect). The BASIS-24 is designed to be administered and interpreted by mental health professionals (option B is incorrect). The Halstead-Reitan is designed to be administered and interpreted by neuropsychologists (option D is incorrect). **Chapter 39 (Table 39–1 [p. 1101])**

39.7   A 65-year-old man with depression has been your patient for 6 months and has tolerated a selective serotonin reuptake inhibitor (SSRI). As you review symptoms with the patient, you notice that he shows marked improvements in many of his depressive symptoms. When you comment on this, he says dejectedly, "I'm glad your checklist thinks I'm better." Which of the following standardized measures would be most appropriate as a next step?

A. Nine-item Patient Health Questionnaire (PHQ-9).
B. Generalized Anxiety Disorder seven-item scale (GAD-7).
C. 32-Item Behavior and Symptom Identification Scale (BASIS-32).
D. Alcohol Use Disorders Identification Test—Consumption (AUDIT-C).

The correct response is option C: 32-Item Behavior and Symptom Identification Scale (BASIS-32).

Although symptom severity is normally thought of as the primary target of measurement-based care, the choice of outcome measure can change over time as the goals of treatment shift (see Table 39–1). For example, patients' goals for improvement often go beyond simple symptom reduction to include a return to their usual self, with an improvement in functioning and a heightened sense of well-being. Validated assessment measures such as the BASIS-32 and the Medical Outcomes Study 36-item Short Form (SF-36) assess overall functioning and quality of life (Tarescavage and Ben-Porath 2014) (option C is correct).

The PHQ-9 is a specific symptom measure and thus is not likely to yield additional information at this time (option A is incorrect).

The GAD-7 is a symptom measure for generalized anxiety disorder, which does not appear to be a relevant clinical issue for this patient (option B is incorrect).

The AUDIT-C is a screening tool for alcohol use disorder; there is no evidence from the vignette that this is clinically suspected (option D is incorrect). **Chapter 39 (p. 1100; Table 39–1 [p. 1101])**

39.8   Which of the following is considered a best practice for measurement-based care (MBC)?

A. Introduce MBC as a tool for increasing patients' control over their own treatment.
B. Streamline assessment protocols by limiting patient feedback.
C. Rely on standardized outcome data rather than resorting to collaborative decision making.
D. Provide concrete evidence to patients when they disagree with an assessment.

The correct response is option A: Introduce MBC as a tool for increasing patients' control over their own treatment.

Best practices for measurement-based care include introducing MBC as a tool for increasing patients' control over their own treatment (option A is correct).

People are individuals; no one treatment works for everyone. Provide some feedback every time patients complete an assessment to reinforce the idea that the assessment is a clinical tool to improve their care, not simply paperwork (option B is incorrect).

Standardized outcome data should enhance clinical judgment and collaborative decision making, not replace it (option C is incorrect).

Do not argue if a patient disagrees with what the measure is indicating. Explore the discrepancy with the patient's experience and validate his or her emotional reactions (option D is incorrect). **Chapter 39 (Table 39–2 [p. 1104])**

39.9   Which of the following statements best describes the function of actigraphy?

A. Recording of outcome data prior to appointments.
B. Detection of behavioral changes and disruptions in sleep that patients may not be aware of at the time.
C. Detection of changes in mood, thought process, and suicidality from social media postings and other patient writings.
D. Detection of mood or psychosis episodes on mobile phones prior to patients' or providers' awareness of a pending episode.

The correct response is option B: Detection of behavioral changes and disruptions in sleep that patients may not be aware of at the time.

Future advances in technology may greatly expand the type of outcome data that can be collected (Hallgren et al. 2017). Emerging technology allows for passive data collection from patients, if implemented with proper safeguards and patient consent (see Chapter 7, "Ethical Considerations in Psychiatry"). Actigraphy can detect behavioral changes and disruptions in sleep that patients may not be aware of at the time (option B is correct).

Web-based and mobile technology can already be used by patients to record outcome data prior to appointments so that results are available at the time of their appointment (option A is incorrect).

Voice analysis technology on mobile phones has the potential to monitor conversations and detect mood or psychosis episodes prior to patients' or providers' awareness of a pending episode (option D is incorrect).

Natural language processing tools have the potential to detect changes in mood, thought processes, and suicidality from postings and other patient writings (option C is incorrect). **Chapter 39 (p. 1107)**

39.10   Which of the following changes is likely to result from implementation of Electronic Medical Record–embedded Measurement-Based Care (EMR-embedded MBC)?

A. Increased time spent in session to collect data.
B. Expanded need for additional data entry.
C. Improved overall quality of mental health care.
D. Reduced time waste during patient–provider discussions.

The correct response is option C: Improved overall quality of mental health care.

The full benefits of MBC are realized when interventions and outcomes are recorded in an EMR or an MBC platform in a manner that allows for easy extraction and analyses across a patient population. In addition to assisting in improving individual patient outcomes, EMR-embedded MBC has the potential to improve the overall quality of mental health care (option C is correct).

EMR-embedded MBC allows for progress to be tracked easily over time and to be graphically presented in a manner that facilitates patient–provider discussions (option D is incorrect).

EMR embedding also expands the possibilities for collection of MBC data to include kiosks, mobile devices, and web-based applications, thereby decreasing the time spent in session to collect the data (option A is incorrect).

Well-designed mental health care EMR systems minimize the need for additional data entry and maintain ease of use (option B is incorrect). **Chapter 39 (p. 1106)**

References

Bufka LF, Campl N: Brief measures for screening and measuring mental health outcomes, in Assessment and Treatment Planning for Psychological Disorders, 2nd Edition. Edited by Antony MM, Barlow DH. New York, Guilford, 2010, pp 62–94

Del Boca FK, Darkes J: The validity of self-reports of alcohol consumption: state of the science and challenges for research. Addiction 98(suppl 2):1–12, 2003 14984237

Groth-Marnat G, Wright AJ: Handbook of Psychological Assessment, 6th Edition. Hoboken, NJ, John Wiley and Sons, 2016

Hallgren KA, Bauer AM, Atkins DC: Digital technology and clinical decision making in depression treatment: current findings and future opportunities. Depress Anxiety 34(6):494–501, 2017 28453916

Morisky DE, Green LW, Levine DM: Concurrent and predictive validity of a self-reported measure of medication adherence. Med Care 24(1):67–74, 1986 3945130

Roebuck-Spencer TM, Glen T, Puente AE, et al: Cognitive screening tests versus comprehensive neuropsychological test batteries: a National Academy of Neuropsychology education paper. Arch Clin Neuropsychol 32(4):491–498, 2017 28334244

Scott K, Lewis CC: Using measurement-based care to enhance any treatment. Cognit Behav Pract 22(1):49–59, 2015 27330267

Stedman JM, McGeary CA, Essery J: Current patterns of training in personality assessment during internship. J Clin Psychol 74(3):398–406, 2018 28685823

Tarescavage AM, Ben-Porath YS: Psychotherapeutic outcomes measures: a critical review for practitioners. J Clin Psychol 70(9):808–830, 2014 24652811

CHAPTER 40

Women

40.1 How do the presentations of women diagnosed with schizophrenia differ from those of men diagnosed with schizophrenia?

A. Women tend to have worse premorbid functioning.
B. Women are less likely to have a family history of schizophrenia.
C. Women are diagnosed earlier.
D. Women tend to have more mood symptoms.

The correct response is option D: Women tend to have more mood symptoms.

Compared with men, women have better premorbid functioning (option A is incorrect), are diagnosed later (option C is incorrect), and are more likely to have a family history of schizophrenia (option B is incorrect); have less substance abuse and are less likely to commit suicide; have more mood symptoms (option D is correct), more positive symptoms, and fewer negative symptoms; and have better language proficiency and better social functioning. **Chapter 40 (p. 1114 [Table 40–1])**

40.2 In what phase of the menstrual cycle do the symptoms of premenstrual dysphoric disorder (PMDD) begin?

A. Early luteal phase.
B. Late luteal phase.
C. Early follicular phase.
D. Late follicular phase.

The correct response is option B: Late luteal phase.

PMDD comprises recurrent physical and emotional symptoms that begin in the late luteal phase of the menstrual cycle (option B is correct; options A, C, and D are incorrect) and remit within several days following the onset of menstruation. In addition to experiencing physical symptoms (i.e., bloating, breast tenderness, cramping, and headaches) women with PMDD have emotional symptoms that may include depression, irritability, anxiety, and insomnia. **Chapter 40 (pp. 1116–1117)**

40.3　A 32-year-old woman is attempting to conceive, but wants to continue her anti-depressant medications for depression and anxiety. Which of the following medications would pose the greatest risk of congenital malformation?

A. Paroxetine.
B. Fluoxetine.
C. Escitalopram.
D. Sertraline.

The correct response is option A: Paroxetine.

Paroxetine may increase risk of congenital anomalies, particularly ventricular-septal defects, and should be avoided if possible (option A is incorrect). Studies have found that paroxetine may be associated with cardiac defects (especially right-ventricle defects) in 1–2 per 100 infants; however, a large-scale cohort study of close to 950,000 women found no significant association between cardiac malformations and first-trimester antidepressant use, including paroxetine (Huybrechts et al. 2014). Nonetheless, the recommendation is to avoid paroxetine.

As a group, selective serotonin reuptake inhibitors other than paroxetine do not appear to increase risk for major congenital malformations (options B, C, and D are incorrect). Numerous peer-reviewed studies on the use of selective serotonin reuptake inhibitors (SSRIs) during pregnancy have found no significantly increased risk of birth defects beyond the general population risk of 3% (Huybrechts et al. 2014; Margulis et al. 2013; Nordeng et al. 2012); however, several studies have suggested possible teratogenicity with in utero exposure to SSRIs (Jimenez-Solem et al. 2012; Malm et al. 2011). Nevertheless, studies finding increased risks have been compromised by reliance on prescription data, lack of control for underlying psychiatric condition, low numbers of exposed subjects, low background absolute risk for uncommon defects, and inadequate control for substance and alcohol use or abuse. **Chapter 40 (pp. 1121, 1124 [Table 40–4])**

40.4　A patient who was started on sertraline 100 mg/day during the third trimester of her first pregnancy delivers a full-term baby. The newborn is found to be irritable and jittery, with poor muscle tone and a weak cry. Which of the following is the most likely diagnosis for this infant?

A. Cardiac malformation.
B. Persistent pulmonary hypertension of the newborn.
C. Neonatal adaptation syndrome.
D. Small-for-gestational-age infant.

The correct response is option C: Neonatal adaptation syndrome.

Third-trimester exposure to selective serotonin reuptake inhibitors (SSRIs) is associated with an approximately 25% risk of perinatal symptoms—including irritability, jitteriness, poor muscle tone, weak or absent cry, respiratory distress, hypoglycemia, and seizures—that sometimes require admission to special care nurseries (Salisbury et al. 2016). These symptoms—collectively termed *neonatal adaptation syndrome* (option C is correct)—are usually mild, transient, and self-limited. It appears that neonatal symptoms do not differ between babies of women who discontinue SSRIs in the third trimester of pregnancy and babies of women who continued their antidepressant through delivery.

As a group, SSRIs other than paroxetine do not appear to increase risk for major congenital malformations. Although some studies have found that paroxetine may be associated with cardiac defects (especially right-ventricle defects) in 1–2 per 100 infants, a large-scale cohort study of close to 950,000 women found no significant association between cardiac malformations and first-trimester antidepressant use, including paroxetine (Huybrechts et al. 2014) (option A is incorrect).

Exposure to SSRIs in late pregnancy has been reported to increase the risk of persistent pulmonary hypertension of the newborn (PPHN), a rare illness affecting fewer than 2 per 1,000 live births at baseline (option B is incorrect).

While some studies have suggested that SSRIs may be associated with an increased risk of shorter gestation, small-for-gestational-age babies, and admission to special care nurseries, other studies, a large systematic review, and a meta-analysis of pregnancy and delivery outcomes after prenatal exposure to antidepressants (Ross et al. 2013) found statistically but not clinically significant decreases in length of gestation (3 days fewer), birth weight (75 grams lower), and Apgar scores (less than half a point on the 1- and 5-minute scores). Thus, although gestation length, birth weight, and fetal growth may be somewhat decreased with prenatal antidepressant exposure, the differences appear to be small, and Apgar scores, which measure the condition of neonates on delivery, are not clinically significantly different (option D is incorrect). **Chapter 40 (pp. 1121–1122)**

40.5 A 25-year-old woman with bipolar disorder who was recently hospitalized for a severe manic episode and stabilized on valproate is interested in trying to conceive. What is the best initial recommendation for her mood stabilizer?

A. Discontinue valproate.
B. Continue valproate.
C. Cross-taper to carbamazepine.
D. Cross-taper to lithium.

The correct response is option D: Cross-taper to lithium.

For women with mild to moderate bipolar disorder, an attempt should be made to withhold mood stabilizers during the first trimester (option A is incorrect, given the patient's recent severe manic episode requiring hospitalization). For women with moderate to severe bipolar disorder, mood stabilizers and other psychiatric medications should be continued as needed to maintain euthymia throughout pregnancy. Because all mood stabilizers carry some teratogenic risk and potential for peripartum toxicity, choice of treatment should be made after a careful case-by-case analysis of the safest regimen to maintain maternal mood stability and fetal safety.

Lithium, despite its risk of cardiovascular teratogenicity, is probably a reasonable choice for the pregnant bipolar patient. Lithium is preferable to carbamazepine and valproate because of its lower risk of teratogenicity (option D is correct; options B and C are incorrect). **Chapter 40 (pp. 1123–1126, 1126 [Table 40–5])**

40.6   Which of the following substances, when used by a mother during pregnancy, can cause a lifelong disabling condition in the offspring?

A. Alcohol.
B. Marijuana.
C. Cocaine.
D. Opioids.

The correct response is option A: Alcohol.

Fetal alcohol syndrome, a lifelong disabling condition that results from in utero exposure to alcohol (option A is correct), occurs in as many as 1.5 in 1,000 live births in the United States. Isolated abnormalities (fetal alcohol effects) occur more often than the full syndrome. In utero exposure to alcohol increases the risk of fetal brain developmental deficits, microcephaly, abnormal facial features, and a number of psychiatric sequelae. No safe quantity of prenatal alcohol consumption has been established.

The effects of cannabis on the developing fetus are largely unknown but may include increased risk of stillbirth, fetal growth restriction, preterm birth, and adverse neurodevelopmental outcomes (Metz and Stickrath 2015) (option B is incorrect).

Antenatal cocaine use is associated with miscarriage, preterm labor, abruptio placentae, and other obstetrical complications secondary to cocaine's vasoconstrictive effects. Exposed neonates may experience a withdrawal syndrome lasting several months (option C is incorrect).

Pregnant women who are dependent on opioids tend to have inconsistent prenatal care, and antenatal opioid use has been associated with miscarriage, stillbirth, poor fetal growth, preterm labor, and sudden infant death syndrome. Exposed neonates are at risk for a neonatal abstinence syndrome characterized by irritability, poor feeding, respiratory difficulties, and tremulousness (option D is incorrect). **Chapter 40 (pp. 1131–1132)**

40.7   You are following a 23-year-old woman with a history of major depressive disorder who gave birth 4 months ago. Her husband calls you with some concerns. He says that over the past few months, she has become increasingly isolative and irritable, taking poor care of herself and sleeping only 3–4 hours each night, and he has noticed that she has recently begun speaking to herself and making less sense. What is your initial recommendation?

A. Send a prescription for an antipsychotic and say you will follow up tomorrow.
B. Assess the patient over the phone and then schedule an office visit for the coming week.

C. Instruct the husband to bring the patient to your office tomorrow.

D. Tell the husband to bring the patient to the emergency room immediately for a full medical and psychiatric evaluation.

The correct response is option D: Tell the husband to bring the patient to the emergency room immediately for a full medical and psychiatric evaluation.

Postpartum psychosis is a psychiatric emergency and requires a full evaluation, including a medical rule-out and stabilization in an inpatient setting (option D is correct). Postpartum psychosis occurs in 0.25–0.6 of every 1,000 births. The condition is characterized by mood lability, agitation, confusion, thought disorganization, hallucinations, and disturbed sleep. Because postpartum psychosis carries with it the risk of suicide, infant neglect, and infanticide, patients should be hospitalized (options B and C are incorrect). The initial evaluation includes a medical assessment to rule out pathophysiological causes such as postpartum thyroiditis, Sheehan's syndrome, pregnancy-related autoimmune disorders, N-methyl-D-aspartate-encephalitis, HIV-related infection, and intoxication or withdrawal states. Acute pharmacological treatment includes a benzodiazepine, an antipsychotic, and a mood stabilizer (with lithium as the preferred agent) (option A is incorrect, given the primary need for hospitalization, although the patient will likely require an antipsychotic medication). **Chapter 40 (p. 1136)**

40.8   Which of the following is the most common postpartum psychopathology?

A. Postpartum "blues."

B. Postpartum depression.

C. Postpartum anxiety.

D. Postpartum psychosis.

The correct response is option A: Postpartum "blues."

For many women, the period following delivery is a time of heightened risk for emotional instability. Conditions involving disordered mood following childbirth include postpartum blues, postpartum depression and anxiety, and postpartum psychosis. Postpartum "blues" is very common, occurring in up to 85% of births (option A is correct). Postpartum depression occurs in approximately 15% of births; however, estimates vary widely across studies, depending on the population being studied, the definition used, and the mode of assessment employed (option B is incorrect). Postpartum anxiety has an overall prevalence of 8.5% (broken down as 3.6% for generalized anxiety disorder, 1.7% for panic disorder, and 2.5% for obsessive-compulsive disorder) (option C is incorrect). Postpartum psychosis affects fewer than 1 in 1,000 births, although the prevalence is higher among women with a history of bipolar disorder or previous postpartum psychosis (option D is incorrect). **Chapter 40 (pp. 1132–1133, 1134–1135 [Table 40–9])**

References

Aleman A, Kahn RS, Selten JP: Sex differences in the risk of schizophrenia: evidence from meta-analysis. Arch Gen Psychiatry 60(6):565–571, 2003 12796219

Huybrechts KF, Palmsten K, Avorn J, et al: Antidepressant use in pregnancy and the risk of cardiac defects. N Engl J Med 370(25):2397–2407, 2014 24941178

Jimenez-Solem E, Andersen JT, Petersen M, et al: Exposure to selective serotonin reuptake inhibitors and the risk of congenital malformations: a nationwide cohort study. BMJ Open 2(3):e001148, 2012 22710132

Malm H, Artama M, Gissler M, et al: Selective serotonin reuptake inhibitors and risk for major congenital anomalies. Obstet Gynecol 118(1):111–120, 2011 21646927

Margulis AV, Abou-Ali A, Strazzeri MM, et al: Use of selective serotonin reuptake inhibitors in pregnancy and cardiac malformations: a propensity-score matched cohort in CPRD. Pharmacoepidemiol Drug Saf 22(9):942–951, 2013 23733623

Metz TD, Stickrath EH: Marijuana use in pregnancy and lactation: a review of the evidence. Am J Obstet Gynecol 213(6):761–778, 2015 25986032

Nordeng H, van Gelder MM, Spigset O: Pregnancy outcome after exposure to antidepressants and the role of maternal depression: results from the Norwegian Mother and Child Cohort Study. J Clin Psychopharmacol 32(2):186–194, 2012 22367660

Ross LE, Grigoriadis S, Mamisashvili L, et al: Selected pregnancy and delivery outcomes after exposure to antidepressant medication: a systematic review and meta-analysis. JAMA Psychiatry 70(4):436–443, 2013 23446732

Salisbury AL, O'Grady KE, Battle CL, et al: The roles of maternal depression, serotonin reuptake inhibitor treatment, and concomitant benzodiazepine use on infant neurobehavioral functioning over the first postnatal month. Am J Psychiatry 173(2):147–157, 2016 26514656

C H A P T E R   4 1

Children and Adolescents

41.1 A 12-year-old boy with a history of Tourette's disorder is brought by his parents to your office for evaluation of attention-deficit/hyperactivity disorder (ADHD) after scoring positive for ADHD on the Vanderbilt ADHD Diagnostic Rating Scales. He is not currently on any medications. The parents say that his tics are present throughout the day and feel that they inhibit his ability to focus on tasks such as schoolwork and household chores. Which of the following treatment strategies showed the greatest benefit for chronic tic disorders comorbid with ADHD in a randomized controlled trial?

A. Treatment of Tourette syndrome with aripiprazole.
B. Treatment of ADHD with clonidine.
C. Treatment of both disorders (ADHD and comorbid Tourette syndrome) with clonidine and methylphenidate.
D. Treatment of ADHD with methylphenidate.

The correct response is option C: Treatment of both disorders (ADHD and comorbid Tourette syndrome) with clonidine and methylphenidate.

Evidence supports the efficacy of risperidone and aripiprazole in reducing tic severity in children and adolescents with Tourette's disorder; however, patients with Tourette's disorder who have comorbid ADHD are often far more disabled by the ADHD than by the tics. Stimulant treatment is effective in these cases (option A is incorrect). A randomized controlled trial in children with both ADHD and a chronic tic disorder (Tourette's Syndrome Study Group 2002) found significant improvements in all three treatment groups (clonidine, methylphenidate, and the combination). The greatest benefit compared with placebo was seen in the combination medication group (option C is correct; options B and D are incorrect). **Chapter 41 (pp. 1153, 1155–1156, 1165)**

41.2 A 16-year-old boy with a history of attention-deficit/hyperactivity disorder and epilepsy has received trials of multiple stimulants, but none have adequately controlled his symptoms. His parents therefore would like to switch him to the non-stimulant medication atomoxetine, given its more favorable risk–benefit profile. Which of the following statements correctly describes a U.S. Food and Drug Administration (FDA) bolded warning regarding atomoxetine?

A. Atomoxetine has been reported to prolong QTc and lead to arrhythmias.
B. Atomoxetine has been known to cause significant effects on growth (height and weight).
C. Atomoxetine has been shown to lower the seizure threshold.
D. Atomoxetine has been associated with severe liver injury in extremely rare cases.

The correct response is option D: Atomoxetine has been associated with severe liver injury in extremely rare cases.

Atomoxetine carries two FDA bolded warnings: one for extremely rare severe liver injury and one (based on limited evidence) for increased hostility and aggression or suicidal ideation (option D is correct). The risk for suicidal ideation has been examined in depth and, in comparison with placebo, was found to be not significant (Bangs et al. 2014).

Atomoxetine does not increase tics, lower the seizure threshold, or cause QTc prolongation (options A and C are incorrect).

There is no evidence that atomoxetine has any significant effect on height and weight (option B is incorrect). **Chapter 41 (pp. 1158–1159)**

41.3 Which of the following is the best first-line medication choice for treating pediatric mania?

A. Olanzapine.
B. Risperidone.
C. Lamotrigine.
D. Oxcarbazepine.

The correct response is option B: Risperidone.

For pediatric mania, risperidone appears to be more effective than either lithium or divalproex (Geller et al. 2012) (option B is correct).

Quetiapine, aripiprazole, and olanzapine all have demonstrated efficacy as well, although olanzapine should be avoided as a first-line agent because of its metabolic effects (option A is incorrect).

Oxcarbazepine has not been found to be effective in multicenter trials and is not generally considered to be useful in children with bipolar disorder (option D is incorrect).

No placebo-controlled trials of lamotrigine monotherapy have been conducted for psychiatric conditions in the pediatric population, and there is no support for lamotrigine's use as an add-on treatment for pediatric bipolar I disorder. It is, however, used with some frequency for bipolar depression and bipolar II disorder in adolescents (option C is incorrect). **Chapter 41 (pp. 1163–1164)**

41.4 Which of the following is a first-line medication choice for treating adolescent depression?

A. Bupropion.
B. Venlafaxine.
C. Clomipramine.
D. Sertraline.

The correct response is option D: Sertraline.

The guidelines from the Texas Children's Medication Algorithm Project (Hughes et al. 2007) recommend fluoxetine, sertraline, and citalopram as first-line medication choices for the treatment of pediatric major depressive disorder (MDD) (option D is correct).

Bupropion has been demonstrated to be effective in treatment of pediatric attention-deficit/hyperactivity disorder (ADHD) in controlled trials and is a third-line treatment for that disorder. Its use as an antidepressant is generally limited to adolescents who have had one or more failed trials of a selective serotonin reuptake inhibitor (SSRI) and have low energy and difficulty concentrating as symptoms of depression, or who have comorbid ADHD (option A is incorrect).

Use of venlafaxine is generally limited to adolescents with MDD who have had one or more failed trials of an SSRI. In the Treatment of Resistant Depression in Adolescents (TORDIA) study, after one failed trial of an SSRI, switching to another SSRI was as effective as switching to venlafaxine, and venlafaxine produced more side effects (Brent et al. 2008) (option B is incorrect).

Until the introduction of the SSRIs, tricyclic antidepressants (TCAs) were used in the pharmacological treatment of a variety of disorders in children and adolescents. However, the paucity of clinical studies demonstrating the efficacy of TCAs in pediatric depression, the cardiac side effects of this class of medication, and the availability of alternative medications have resulted in a shift away from using TCAs in children, except for clomipramine, which is used to treat obsessive-compulsive disorder that has not responded to an SSRI (option C is incorrect). **Chapter 41 (pp. 1161, 1162)**

41.5 "PRIDE skills" are a component of parent–child interaction therapy. What does the acronym *PRIDE* stand for?

A. Playing with the child, Reflecting on appropriate talk, Imitating appropriate play, Describing appropriate behavior, and being Enthusiastic.
B. Playing with the child, Reflecting on appropriate talk, Imitating appropriate play, Describing appropriate behavior, and being Engaging.
C. Praising the child's appropriate behavior, Reflecting on appropriate talk, Imitating appropriate play, Describing appropriate behavior, and being Enthusiastic.
D. Praising the child's appropriate behavior, Reflecting on appropriate talk, Imitating appropriate play, Describing appropriate behavior, and being Engaging.

The correct response is option C: Praising the child's appropriate behavior, Reflecting on appropriate talk, Imitating appropriate play, Describing appropriate behavior, and being Enthusiastic.

Parent–child interaction therapy has been shown to be effective in reducing disruptive behaviors in children up to 7 years old. It is based on both social learning theory and attachment theory. The two phases of treatment are child-directed interaction and parent-directed interaction. In the first phase, the parents practice PRIDE skills, which include Praising the child's appropriate behavior, Reflecting on appropriate talk, Imitating appropriate play, Describing appropriate behavior, and being Enthusiastic (option C is correct; options A, B, and D are incorrect). The parent in this stage is also encouraged to avoid the use of commands, questions, or criticisms and to ignore minor misconduct but to stop play for aggressive misconduct. **Chapter 41 (p. 1174)**

41.6   A depressed 17-year-old adolescent is struggling with new relationships and roles as he is transitioning to adult life. Which of the following therapy modalities would be most relevant for this patient?

A. Supportive therapy.
B. Interpersonal psychotherapy.
C. Cognitive-behavioral therapy.
D. Dialectical behavior therapy.

The correct response is option B: Interpersonal psychotherapy.

Interpersonal psychotherapy may be successfully adapted for depressed adolescents and has demonstrated efficacy in several controlled studies. This treatment focuses on improving interpersonal relationships in the lives of depressed adolescents through role clarification and enhanced communication. Such treatment may be especially effective when an older adolescent is struggling with changing roles and changing relationships in the period of transition to adult life (option B is correct).

   In supportive therapy, the therapist provides support to the patient until a stressor resolves, a developmental crisis has passed, or the patient or environment changes sufficiently so that other adults can take on the supportive role. There is a real relationship with the therapist, who facilitates verbal expression of feelings and provides understanding and judicious advice (option A is incorrect).

   Cognitive-behavioral therapy (CBT) techniques adapted for children and adolescents have been shown in controlled trials to be efficacious in the treatment of anxiety disorders. Results in the treatment of depression are somewhat less consistent, but CBT is considered to be an important treatment option for depressed adolescents. The depression treatments involve techniques such as examining and changing cognitive distortions regarding the world and relationships, social problem solving, behavioral activation, and goal-setting (option C is incorrect).

   Dialectical behavior therapy (DBT) has been modified for treatment of adolescents, especially those with suicidal or self-injurious behaviors, and involves a combination of individual, group, and family treatment. Key components are development of coping skills and self-soothing techniques to help such patients modulate unstable affective states and reduce impulsive destructive behaviors.

Family members must be actively involved in the treatment to improve their own coping skills and learn how to help their teen put his or her coping skills to good use. The availability of a therapist on call is an important feature of this treatment to address crises (option D is incorrect). **Chapter 41 (pp. 1171–1172)**

41.7   An 8-year-old boy has a history of attention-deficit/hyperactivity disorder (ADHD) and comorbid anxiety. He complains of insomnia, which has worsened since the start of school 2 weeks ago. The boy's parents have him get ready for bed at 9 P.M.; however, he is unable to fall asleep until midnight, despite having to wake up at 6 A.M. for school. Which of the following interventions should be *avoided* in the initial treatment of this child's insomnia?

A. Melatonin.
B. Benzodiazepines.
C. Sleep hygiene.
D. Clonidine.

The correct response is option B: Benzodiazepines.

Benzodiazepines are best avoided in the treatment of acute pediatric agitation or anxiety because of their propensity to cause disinhibition reactions, which can manifest as psychomotor agitation, aggression, hostility, irritability, or anxiety (option B is correct).

Although pharmacological treatment can be appropriate, particularly in the short term, behavioral interventions and improvement of sleep hygiene are the best initial treatments for insomnia in children (option C is incorrect).

Melatonin can be used either to shift the sleep phase forward (as a chronobiotic) or to induce sleep (as a hypnotic). As a chronobiotic, it is best administered 3–5 hours before bedtime, but as a hypnotic it should be given 30 minutes beforehand (option A is incorrect).

Clonidine is commonly used for insomnia, particularly in pediatric patients with comorbid ADHD (option D is incorrect). **Chapter 41 (p. 1168)**

References

Bangs ME, Wietecha LA, Wang S, et al: Meta-analysis of suicide-related behavior or ideation in child, adolescent, and adult patients treated with atomoxetine. J Child Adolesc Psychopharmacol 24(8):426–434, 2014 25019647

Brent D, Emslie G, Clarke G, et al: Switching to another SSRI or to venlafaxine with or without cognitive behavioral therapy for adolescents with SSRI-resistant depression: the TORDIA randomized controlled trial. JAMA 299(8):901–913, 2008 18314433

Geller B, Luby JL, Joshi P, et al: A randomized controlled trial of risperidone, lithium, or divalproex sodium for initial treatment of bipolar I disorder, manic or mixed phase, in children and adolescents. Arch Gen Psychiatry 69(5):515–528, 2012 22213771

Hughes CW, Emslie GJ, Crimson ML, et al: Texas Children's Medication Algorithm Project: update from Texas Consensus Conference Panel on Medication Treatment of Childhood Major Depressive Disorder. J Am Acad Child Adolesc Psychiatry 46(6):667–686, 2007 17513980

Tourette's Syndrome Study Group: Treatment of ADHD in children with tics: a randomized controlled trial. Neurology 58(4):527–536, 2002 11865128

CHAPTER 42

Lesbian, Gay, Bisexual, and Transgender Patients

42.1 What is the DSM-5 diagnosis given to an individual experiencing clinically significant distress or impairment due to a marked incongruence between their experienced gender and their assigned gender?

A. Gender incongruence.
B. Transsexualism.
C. Gender dysphoria.
D. Gender identity disorder.

The correct response is option C: Gender dysphoria.

The diagnosis of "trans-sexualism" first appeared in the International Classification of Diseases, 9th Revision (ICD-9; World Health Organization 1977). The DSM-III (American Psychiatric Association 1980) authors felt that there was a large enough database to support the inclusion of transsexualism. The diagnosis of transsexualism led to growing psychiatric recognition of a patient population that could benefit from gender reassignment rather than forced conformity with the sex assigned at birth (option B is incorrect).

In DSM-IV (American Psychiatric Association 1994), transsexualism was replaced by "gender identity disorder (GID) in adolescents and adults" (option D is incorrect).

In anticipation of DSM-5 (American Psychiatric Association 2013), transgender activists appealed to the American Psychiatric Association, requesting that the diagnosis of GID be removed in order to lessen the stigma that they faced (Drescher 2010). GID was replaced by "gender dysphoria" in DSM-5 (option C is correct).

In 2018, the World Health Organization replaced "gender identity disorders" with "gender incongruence" in ICD-11 and moved the diagnosis to a new chapter on "conditions related to sexual health" (World Health Organization 2018) (option A is incorrect). **Chapter 42 (p. 1188)**

42.2   To which of the following does the term *cisgender* refer?

A. Gender role.
B. Sexual orientation.
C. Gender expression.
D. Gender identity.

The correct response is option D: Gender identity.

Gender identity is defined as a person's self-identification as male, female, or other gender (e.g., genderqueer). *Cisgender* is a term used to describe an individual whose gender identity aligns with their assigned sex at birth (option D is correct).

Gender role is defined as the presentation and behaviors deemed acceptable or appropriate for one's assigned sex, as determined by cultural norms (option A is incorrect).

Gender expression is defined as how individuals demonstrate their gender to others via manner of dress, behaviors, and appearance (option C is incorrect).

Sexual orientation (the sex to which one is attracted) is a variable independent from gender identity (whether one feels like a man or a woman) (option B is incorrect). **Chapter 42 (pp. 1209–1211)**

42.3   Epidemiological research indicates that sexual minority youth show which of the following trends in comparison with their heterosexual peers?

A. Lower rates of substance use disorders.
B. Lower rates of alcohol use and smoking.
C. Lower rates of depression and suicide attempts.
D. Higher rates of bullying and victimization.

The correct response is option D: Higher rates of bullying and victimization.

Bullying can be a problem for any gender-nonconforming child. A compelling longitudinal study of 10,655 individuals used data from the Growing Up Today Study to assess depressive symptoms from ages 12 to 30 years, prevalence of bullying victimization, and gender nonconformity before age 11 years (Roberts et al. 2013). The investigators compared depressive symptoms by gender nonconformity and explored the relationship between gender nonconformity and depressive symptoms by bullying and childhood abuse. The investigators found that individuals who reported gender nonconformity in childhood had an elevated risk of depressive symptoms, and that experiences of childhood abuse and bullying accounted for approximately one-half of the increased depression symptoms among individuals who were gender nonconforming (option D is correct).

Sexual minority individuals who had been victims of discrimination have also been found to be at greater risk for substance use disorders (Lee et al. 2016) (option A is incorrect). Smoking and alcohol consumption may be higher among lesbian, gay, and bisexual (LGB) youth than among heterosexual youth (Institute of

Medicine 2011) (option B is incorrect). LGB youth are at increased risk for suicidal ideation and attempts as well as depression (option C is incorrect). **Chapter 42 (pp. 1190, 1194–1196; Table 42–1 [p. 1195])**

42.4 During the course of a comprehensive sexual history, a 24-year-old male patient reports having experienced same-sex attraction since adolescence and engaging exclusively in sexual relationships with men. After this disclosure, he requests professional help in order to change his sexual orientation. This request reflects which of the following phenomena?

A. Gender dysphoria.
B. Outing.
C. Internalized homophobia.
D. Ego-dystonic homosexuality.

The correct response is option C: Internalized homophobia.

Internalized homophobia refers to the self-hatred lesbian, gay, and bisexual (LGB) individuals may feel toward themselves as a product of antihomosexual and transphobic attitudes of the dominant culture (option C is correct).

Some may have sought to change their sexual orientation through conversion therapy (Drescher 2001). Clinicians should keep in mind that efforts to change an individual's sexual or gender identity are potentially harmful. As of February 2019, 14 U.S. states, the Canadian province of Ontario, and many local municipalities have banned conversion therapies for lesbian, gay, bisexual, and transgender (LGBT) minors younger than 18 years (Drescher et al. 2016). In DSM-5, gender identity disorder was changed to gender dysphoria. To meet criteria for the diagnosis, a person must have "a marked incongruence between their experienced/expressed gender and their assigned gender, of at least 6 months' duration" (DSM-5, p. 452) (option A is incorrect).

Outing is a colloquial term for an unwanted revelation by a third party of an individual's sexual orientation or gender identity to others (option B is incorrect).

In DSM-III (American Psychiatric Association 1980), sexual orientation disturbance was replaced with "ego-dystonic homosexuality," but this diagnosis was inconsistent with the growing evidence-based approach of the new diagnostic system and was removed from DSM-III-R (American Psychiatric Association 1987). It was obvious to psychiatrists at this time that neither sexual orientation disturbance nor ego-dystonic homosexuality met the definition of a disorder (Drescher 2015) (option D is incorrect). **Chapter 42 (pp. 1187, 1193, 1197, 1210–1211); see also Chapter 22 ("Gender Dysphoria"; p. 600)**

References

American Psychiatric Association: Diagnostic and Statistical Manual of Mental Disorders, 3rd Edition. Washington, DC, American Psychiatric Association, 1980
American Psychiatric Association: Diagnostic and Statistical Manual of Mental Disorders, 3rd Edition Revised. Washington, DC, American Psychiatric Association, 1987

American Psychiatric Association: Diagnostic and Statistical Manual of Mental Disorders, 4th Edition. Washington, DC, American Psychiatric Association, 1994

American Psychiatric Association: Diagnostic and Statistical Manual of Mental Disorders, 5th Edition. Arlington, VA, American Psychiatric Association, 2013

Drescher J: Psychoanalytic Therapy and the Gay Man. New York, Routledge, 2001

Drescher J: Queer diagnoses: parallels and contrasts in the history of homosexuality, gender variance, and the diagnostic and statistical manual. Arch Sex Behav 39(2):427–460, 2010 19838785

Drescher J: Out of DSM: depathologizing homosexuality. Behav Sci 5(4):565–575, 2015 26690228

Drescher J, Schwartz A, Casoy F, et al: The growing regulation of conversion therapy. J Med Regul 102(2):7–12, 2016 27754500

Institute of Medicine: The Health of Lesbian, Gay, Bisexual and Transgender People: Building a Foundation for Better Understanding. Washington, DC, National Academies Press, 2011

Lee JH, Gamarel KE, Bryant KJ, et al: Discrimination, mental health, and substance use disorders among sexual minority populations. LGBT Health 3(4):258–265, 2016 27383512

Roberts AL, Rosario M, Slopen N, et al: Childhood gender nonconformity, bullying victimization, and depressive symptoms across adolescence and early adulthood: an 11-year longitudinal study. J Am Acad Child Adolesc Psychiatry 52(2):143–152, 2013 23357441

World Health Organization: International Classification of Diseases, 9th Revision. Geneva, Switzerland, World Health Organization, 1977

World Health Organization: Classifying disease to map the way we live and die. June 18, 2018. Available at: https://www.who.int/health-topics/international-classification-of-diseases. Accessed January 11, 2019.

CHAPTER 43

Older Adults

43.1   A resident on her consultation-liaison psychiatry rotation receives a request for assistance in managing acute-onset agitation in a 79-year-old patient who received hip replacement surgery 5 days ago. The patient has no prior psychiatric history and up until the surgery has been living alone and fully functional. Upon entering the room, the resident observes a disheveled elderly woman who does not know where she is. When asked the date, the patient recites her birth date. She is unable to recite the months of the year in reverse, and nursing staff report that the patient spoke of visiting with a deceased family member earlier today. Nurses report that the patient was oriented to person, place, and time earlier in the day and until now has been calm and cooperative, with few needs other than pain control (for which she has been given scheduled morphine doses around the clock). Which of the following is the most likely diagnosis?

A. Neurocognitive disorder due to Alzheimer's disease.
B. Delirium.
C. Vascular neurocognitive disorder.
D. Very-late-onset schizophrenia.

The correct response is option B: Delirium.

Acute confusion, or delirium, is a transient neurocognitive disorder (NCD) characterized by acute onset and global impairment of cognitive function. The hallmark of delirium is impaired attention. Many persons with delirium remain oriented to person, place, and time but demonstrate impairment on tests of sustained attention such as digit span and months of the year in reverse (option B is correct).

Once delirium has been ruled out, the initial cognitive diagnostic task is to differentiate among usual neurocognitive function (cognitive aging), mild NCD, and major NCD. The second step is to assign an etiological category, such as NCD due to Alzheimer's disease, vascular NCD, or frontotemporal NCD (Blazer et al. 2015). Late-life memory loss is typically accompanied by a more or less sustained decline in cognitive function from a previously obtained intellectual level, usually with an insidious onset. State of consciousness is usually not altered until very late in the memory loss syndrome, which is in contrast with acute confusion (delirium) (options A and C are incorrect).

Very-late-onset-schizophrenia is characterized by marked paranoid delusions in older adults who nevertheless maintain their functioning in the community for months or even years (option D is incorrect). **Chapter 43 (pp. 1213, 1215, 1226); see also Chapter 25 ("Neurocognitive Disorders"; p. 688)**

43.2   Which of the following options is the most appropriate first step in managing behavioral disturbances associated with delirium?

A. Implementation of restraints and mittens.
B. Administration of haloperidol 0.5 mg PO.
C. Administration of lorazepam 0.5 mg IV.
D. Establishment of an adequate airway and close monitoring of vital signs.

The correct response is option D: Establishment of an adequate airway and close monitoring of vital signs.

Acute confusion may present as a psychiatric emergency that threatens permanent brain damage. Severe hypoglycemia, hypoxia, and hyperthermia are examples of critical conditions that may present as acute confusion. General therapy for the confused older individual, to be administered in parallel with specific therapy for the underlying cause of the acute confusion, begins with medical support. The initial treatment should include the establishment of an adequate airway to ensure that the patient is breathing. Vital signs and level of consciousness should be closely monitored (Inouye et al. 1999) (option D is correct).

Benzodiazepine use should be avoided, except in the case of withdrawal deliria (see Table 25–6, "Inpatient management of delirium") (option C is incorrect). Use of restraints should be kept to a minimum (option A is incorrect). Behavioral agitation generally can be managed by judicious use of antipsychotic medications, such as haloperidol (administered either intramuscularly or orally), olanzapine, or risperidone, in low dosages; yet if possible, medications should be avoided (option B is incorrect). **Chapter 43 (pp. 1214–1215); see also Chapter 25 ("Neurocognitive Disorders"), Table 25–6 (p. 690)**

43.3   What is the most common disorder contributing to memory loss?

A. Alzheimer's disease.
B. Parkinson's disease.
C. Alcohol use disorder.
D. Vascular disease.

The correct response is option A: Alzheimer's disease.

The prevalence of major neurocognitive disorder (NCD) due to Alzheimer's disease, the most common disorder contributing to memory loss, has been estimated to be 6%–8% in community-dwelling persons older than 65 years, and more than 30% in persons 85 years or older (Alzheimer's Association 2018). More than 50%

of persons with chronic memory loss will, at autopsy, exhibit the changes of Alzheimer's disease only (option A is correct).

Vascular NCD often is comorbid with Alzheimer's disease. In contrast to Alzheimer's NCD, however, vascular NCD is more common in males than in females (option D is incorrect).

Many patients with Parkinson's disease develop brain changes late in the course of the disease that are similar to changes found in Alzheimer's disease (option B is incorrect).

Approximately 5% of older persons experience memory loss as a result of chronic alcohol use (option C is incorrect). **Chapter 43 (p. 1216)**

43.4   A 73-year-old woman is brought to the physician by her children because she is becoming more forgetful. Until recently, she managed her finances independently and enjoyed cooking, but she has begun to receive overdue payment notices from her utility companies as well as from her landlord. She also is beginning to find it difficult to prepare balanced meals, having lost 4 kg in the past 5 months, and she recently left the water running in her bathtub, which flooded the apartment. When her children express their concerns, she becomes angry and resists their help. Lab tests reveal normal values for metabolic, hematological, and thyroid function. Which of the following would be the most appropriate next step in the diagnostic workup of this patient?

A. Genetic testing.
B. In-depth cognitive testing.
C. Mini-Mental State Examination.
D. Positron emission tomography.

The correct response is option C: Mini-Mental State Examination.

The nature and severity of memory loss should be assessed in conjunction with a chronological account of the onset of the older adult's problems and specific behavioral changes. Degree of the neurocognitive dysfunction should be assessed by both a thorough mental status examination and objective testing. The physical examination should include not only a thorough neurological examination but also a general physical workup to determine the health of the patient. Genetic testing, however, is not recommended (option A is incorrect).

The nature and degree of the neurocognitive dysfunction should be assessed by both a thorough mental status examination and objective testing. Standardized mental status examinations, such as the Mini-Mental State Examination (Folstein et al. 1975) and the Montreal Cognitive Assessment (Nasreddine et al. 2005), are available and provide a useful means of quantifying and documenting memory loss at the initial evaluation (option C is correct).

The in-office or hospital-based initial assessment of memory and neurocognitive functioning is followed by a more in-depth evaluation of cognition, with tests of specific functions such as executive functioning, language, memory, and spatial ability (tests of constructional praxis) (option B is incorrect).

Magnetic resonance imaging (MRI) or computed tomography scans are now routine in the initial evaluation of memory loss. Much interesting research is emerging to explore the association of memory loss and functional imaging (e.g., positron emission tomography and functional MRI), but the utility of these functional scans is limited to clinical scenarios in which there is a high index of suspicion for frontotemporal neurocognitive disorder (option D is incorrect). **Chapter 43 (pp. 1217–1218)**

43.5   Most pharmacological therapies for memory loss target the breakdown of a naturally occurring substance in the body. What is the name of this substance?

A. γ Secretase.
B. Acetylcholine.
C. *N*-methyl-D-aspartate (NMDA).
D. Estrogen.

The correct response is option B: Acetylcholine.

Most pharmacological therapies are based on the cholinergic hypotheses of memory and include primarily the acetylcholinesterase inhibitors donepezil, rivastigmine, and galantamine, which are available to physicians in office-based practice (option B is correct).

Treatment of Alzheimer's disease with selegiline, estrogen, prednisone, nonsteroidal anti-inflammatory drugs, statins, rosiglitazone, chelating agents, and the naturally occurring substances huperzine and Ginkgo biloba have not been shown to be successful in slowing cognitive deterioration in clinical trials (option D is incorrect).

Memantine, an NMDA receptor antagonist, has been approved by the FDA for the treatment of moderate to severe Alzheimer's disease (based on the theory that glutamatergic overstimulation may cause excitotoxic neuronal changes) (option C is incorrect).

Treatments addressing amyloid-related pathology—including inhibitors of γ secretase (the enzyme co-responsible with β secretase for abnormal cleavage of amyloid precursor protein)—have been successful in mouse models of Alzheimer's disease but have not yet been demonstrated to be effective and safe in humans with neurocognitive disorders (option A is incorrect). **Chapter 43 (p. 1218); see also Chapter 25 ("Neurocognitive Disorders"; pp. 701–702)**

43.6   A 65-year-old woman visits her primary care physician and complains of difficulty falling asleep, low energy during the day, difficulty concentrating, and low mood. On further questioning, the patient explains that every night after she gets into bed, she experiences leg discomfort for several hours before she can relax and fall asleep. Which of the following would be the most appropriate treatment for this patient?

A. Sertraline.
B. Polysomnography.

C. Quetiapine.

D. Ropinirole.

The correct response is option D: Ropinirole.

Nocturnal myoclonus, or restless legs syndrome (RLS), is a sensorimotor condition that can interfere with sleep and that also can be precipitated or worsened by commonly prescribed drugs, especially antidepressants (option A is incorrect). RLS may respond to medications such as dopamine agonists (e.g., ropinirole, pramipexole, rotigotine), anticonvulsants (e.g., gabapentin), or benzodiazepines (e.g., clonazepam) (option D is correct). RLS does not require polysomnography to diagnose (option B is incorrect). Although atypical antipsychotics such as quetiapine have been used for treatment of sleep problems, this practice is not recommended (option C is incorrect). **Chapter 43 (pp. 1221, 1223); see also Chapter 20 ("Sleep–Wake Disorders"; p. 549)**

43.7   Which of the following effects may occur when benzodiazepines are prescribed to older persons?

A. Reduced levels of fatigue.

B. Memory improvement.

C. Confusion.

D. Decreased risk of falls.

The correct response is option C: Confusion.

Benzodiazepines (e.g., alprazolam, oxazepam, lorazepam) are the key class of pharmacological agents used in the management of anxiety disorders. These drugs consistently have been shown to be efficacious in treatment of anxiety when compared with placebo, and they are relatively free of side effects. While they are generally well tolerated by persons of all ages, benzodiazepines present unique problems when prescribed to older persons. For example, their half-life may be increased dramatically in late life, with diazepam (2.5–5.0 mg) having a half-life nearing 4 days in persons in their 80s. This age-related increase in half-life means that repeated doses over an extended period can lead to a significant accumulation in fatty tissues, with subsequent disorientation, confusion, and slurred speech (option C is correct).

Older persons are also more susceptible to benzodiazepines' potential side effects, such as fatigue, drowsiness, motor dysfunction, falls, and memory impairment (options A, B, and D are incorrect). **Chapter 43 (p. 1225)**

43.8   Which of the following has been most closely linked to Alzheimer's disease?

A. Apolipoprotein E gene (ε2 allele).

B. Presenilin 1 gene.

C. Presenilin 2 gene.

D. Apolipoprotein E gene (ε4 allele).

The correct response is option D: Apolipoprotein E gene (ε4 allele).

Genetic risk factors for Alzheimer's disease have received much attention in recent years, especially the relationship between the disease and the ε4 allele of the apolipoprotein E gene (*APOE*) (Roses 1994). The ε4 allele has a direct correlation with brain amyloid plaque burden, and its presence is the strongest genetic risk factor for the development of late-onset Alzheimer's disease (Liu et al. 2013). Persons who carry at least one copy of the *APOE* ε4 allele are at increased risk of developing Alzheimer's disease (option D is correct). By contrast, the *APOE* ε2 allele appears to confer some degree of protection from this condition (option A is incorrect).

Much less common forms of Alzheimer's disease have been linked to chromosomes 14 and 1 (presenilin 1 and 2 genes) (options B and C are incorrect). **Chapter 43 (p. 1217); see also Chapter 5 ("Laboratory Testing and Neuroimaging Studies in Psychiatry"; p. 127)**

43.9 An 84-year-old man with mild vascular neurocognitive disorder comes to his physician's office for a routine checkup. During the appointment, the patient discloses that his neighbor has been stealing his mail and spying on him, and because of this, he has been having trouble sleeping. The patient asks for "sleeping pills." What is the most appropriate next step?

A. Hospitalize the patient.
B. Confront the patient's delusion.
C. Interview family members of the patient.
D. Prescribe zolpidem 5 mg qhs.

The correct response is option C: Interview family members of the patient.

In general, paranoid older patients do not adapt well to the hospital. Change from familiar surroundings and interactions with strange persons tend to exacerbate the suspiciousness (option A is incorrect).

It is rarely necessary for clinicians to confront patients regarding suspicions or delusional thinking; therefore, older patients' responses to questions can be supported emotionally (e.g., "I understand your concern"), and clinicians do not need to agree with or challenge statements made by patients that are known (or suspected) to be untrue (option B is incorrect).

Clinicians evaluating a suspicious older person should nonetheless remember that older adults are occasionally abused by family members and friends; therefore, a seemingly delusional description of persecutory behaviors may contain some truth. Because delusional thinking and agitation usually render the patient's history inaccurate, family members should be interviewed to review the patient's behavior, especially any change in behavior (option C is correct).

If the delusion does not create subjective stress and/or problems in management, regular evaluation of the patient and family without the use of medications is the preferred intervention (option D is incorrect). **Chapter 43 (pp. 1227–1228)**

43.10 A 74-year-old nursing home patient with dementia has been exhibiting many behavioral symptoms, such as frequently isolating in her room, becoming agitated
when showering, losing weight, and is uninterested in participating in group activities she once enjoyed such as karaoke and bingo. She has told nursing home
staff that she hears the voices of her children talking to her in her room when she
is alone. The staff members are worried that the patient may be depressed. What
is the best first step in the diagnostic workup?

A. Thyroid panel.
B. Psychological testing.
C. Magnetic resonance imaging (MRI).
D. Screening for HIV.

The correct response is option A: Thyroid panel.

The laboratory workup of the depressed older adult is presented in Table 43–1.
The thyroid panel—triiodothyronine (T_3), thyroxine (T_4), free thyroxine index,
and thyroid-stimulating hormone (TSH)—is essential in the diagnosis of the depressed older patient, given that subclinical hypothyroid disorders are often uncovered in the workup (option A is correct).

Tests such as the blood count and measurement of vitamin B_{12} and folate levels are useful in screening for medical illnesses that may present with depressive
symptoms. Psychological testing may be implemented to distinguish depression
from dementia but should not be performed in the midst of a severe depressive
episode (option B is incorrect).

Screening for HIV as part of the workup for depression in the older adult is
elective (option D is incorrect). MRI is also optional despite the association of sub-
cortical white matter hyperintensities with late-life depression (option C is incorrect). **Chapter 43 (pp. 1231–1232; Table 43–6 [p. 1232])**

TABLE 43–1. Laboratory workup of the depressed older adult

Routine

    Complete blood count (CBC)
    Urinalysis
    Triiodothyronine (T_3), thyroxine (T_4), free thyroxine index, thyroid-stimulating hormone
      (TSH)
    Venereal Disease Research Laboratory (VDRL) test
    Vitamin B_{12} and folate assays
    Chemistry screen (sodium, chlorine, potassium, blood urea nitrogen, calcium, glucose,
      creatine)
    Electrocardiogram

Elective

    Polysomnography
    Magnetic resonance imaging or computed tomography scan
    Thyroid-releasing hormone stimulation test
    Screening for HIV

43.11   A 74-year-old woman visits her primary care physician and complains of worsened insomnia and anxiety over the past several months. The physician has been prescribing alprazolam for both of these symptoms for over a year, and the patient is distressed and frustrated that her symptoms have worsened. She admits that she has been taking more alprazolam than prescribed to relieve her worsening symptoms. She also admits to stealing her daughter's lorazepam when she runs out of her own medication and is feeling tremulous, sweaty, or anxious. Which of the following would be the best initial step in treating this patient?

A. Referral to a 12-step program.
B. Confrontation regarding her substance use.
C. Referral to a psychiatrist.
D. Detoxification.

The correct response is option D: Detoxification.

The first step in treating the older adult with a substance use problem involves detoxification and withdrawal (option D is correct). Older adults should be withdrawn gradually.

Evidence-based studies have demonstrated that nonpharmacological treatment of both alcohol and substance use problems in later life is effective, although the studies have been sparse and small. The least-intensive approaches to therapy should be employed initially in the office if serious withdrawal symptoms are absent. A brief intervention (such as a 10- to 15-minute discussion with the treating physician) is the recommended initial treatment. If this is not successful, a variety of interventions may be employed. The Center for Substance Abuse Treatment (2005) recommended that any approach to treating substance use in older adults include the following components: 1) emphasis on age-specific treatment (e.g., mixed-age 12-step programs may not be appropriate for the elderly) (option A is incorrect); 2) use of supportive, nonconfrontational approaches that build self-esteem (in contrast to confrontational therapies often used with younger adults) (option B is incorrect); 3) focus on cognitive-behavioral approaches (as opposed to more nondirective therapies); 4) development of skills for improving social support; 5) recruitment of counselors who are trained and motivated to work with older adults; and 6) use of age-appropriate pace and content. Adherence to treatment is usually improved if the setting for treatment remains in the primary care office (option C is incorrect). **Chapter 43 (p. 1235)**

References

Alzheimer's Association: 2018 Alzheimer's Disease Facts and Figures. Alzheimer's & Dementia 14(3):367–429, 2018. Available at: https://www.alzheimersanddementia.com/article/S1552-5260(18)30041-4/fulltext. Accessed January 13, 2019.

Blazer DG, Yaffe K, Liverman CT (eds): Cognitive Aging: Progress in Understanding and Opportunities for Action. Washington, DC, National Academies Press, 2015

Center for Substance Abuse Treatment: Substance Abuse Relapse Prevention for Older Adults: A Group Treatment Approach. Rockville, MD, Substance Abuse and Mental Health Services Administration, U.S. Department of Health and Human Services, 2005

Folstein MF, Folstein SE, McHugh PR: "Mini-mental state." A practical method for grading the cognitive state of patients for the clinician. J Psychiatr Res 12(3):189–198, 1975 1202204

Inouye SK, Bogardus ST Jr, Charpentier PA, et al: A multicomponent intervention to prevent delirium in hospitalized older patients. N Engl J Med 340(9):669–676, 1999 10053175

Liu CC, Liu CC, Kanekiyo T, et al: Apolipoprotein E and Alzheimer disease: risk, mechanisms and therapy. Nat Rev Neurol 9(2):106–118, 2013 23296339

Nasreddine ZS, Phillips NA, Bédirian V, et al: The Montreal Cognitive Assessment, MoCA: a brief screening tool for mild cognitive impairment. J Am Geriatr Soc 53(4):695–699, 2005 15817019

Roses AD: Apolipoprotein E affects the rate of Alzheimer disease expression: beta-amyloid burden is a secondary consequence dependent on APOE genotype and duration of disease. J Neuropathol Exp Neurol 53(5):429–437, 1994 8083686

CHAPTER 44

Culturally Diverse Patients

44.1   Which of the following best captures the DSM-5 definition of *culture*?

A. Systems of knowledge, concepts, rules, and practices that remain static over time.
B. Systems of knowledge, concepts, rules, and practices with minimal impact on an individual's identity.
C. Systems of knowledge, concepts, rules, and practices that are learned and transmitted across generations.
D. Systems of knowledge, concepts, rules, and practices that are easily intuited by a seasoned clinician.

The correct response is option C: Systems of knowledge, concepts, rules, and practices that are learned and transmitted across generations.

In DSM-5, *culture* is defined as "systems of knowledge, concepts, rules, and practices that are learned and transmitted across generations. Culture includes language, religion and spirituality, family structures, life-cycle stages, ceremonial rituals, and customs, as well as moral and legal systems" (American Psychiatric Association 2013, p. 749) (option C is correct).

DSM-5 explains that "cultures are open, dynamic systems that undergo continuous change over time; in the contemporary world, most individuals and groups are exposed to multiple cultures, which they use to fashion their own identities and make sense of experience" (option A is incorrect).

These characterizations of culture illustrate central issues in cultural psychiatry that are relevant to the practice of all clinicians: 1) all individuals, as social beings, belong to at least one culture whose interpretations about the self, others, the world, and human predicaments (Who am I? Why are we here?) are debated in relationships and institutions across the lifespan (option B is incorrect); 2) individuals use their relationships and social groupings to fashion a unique sense of self (i.e., "identity") that informs their "psychology" (their understanding of thoughts, emotions, and behaviors); and 3) clinicians cannot make assumptions about anyone's cultural affiliation(s) lest they risk assigning stereotypes that can endanger therapeutic rapport (option D is incorrect). **Chapter 44 (p. 1241)**

44.2   You are conducting an evaluation for a new patient with a history of bipolar disorder. During the interview, the patient talks about a prior major depressive episode following the death of her grandmother, to whom she was very close. She later mentions that she still communicates with her deceased grandmother on occasion. Which of the following DSM-5 components would be most helpful in developing a case formulation for this patient?

A. The "Culture-Related Diagnostic Issues" subsection in the descriptive text for bipolar disorder.
B. The "Glossary of Cultural Concepts of Distress" in the DSM-5 Appendix.
C. The "Cultural Formulation Interview" in the "Cultural Formulation" chapter in DSM-5 Section III.
D. The "Cultural Issues" subsection of the DSM-5 Introduction.

The correct response is option C: The "Cultural Formulation Interview" in the "Cultural Formulation" chapter in DSM-5 Section III.

DSM-5 includes cultural considerations for clinicians in multiple sections:

1. Section I: the "Introduction" (pp. 14–15)
2. Section II: the descriptive text for each disorder
3. Section III: the "Cultural Formulation" chapter, including "Outline for Cultural Formulation," "Cultural Formulation Interview (CFI)," and "Cultural Concepts of Distress" (pp. 749–759)
4. Appendix: the "Glossary of Cultural Concepts of Distress" (pp. 833–837)

The Cultural Formulation Interview (CFI) is a standardized 16-item questionnaire that can be used at the beginning of every initial patient assessment. It includes instructions to clinicians that precede the questions and a guide to the interviewer on content designed for elicitation through each question (option C is correct).

For each DSM-5 disorder in Section II, the new subsection "Culture-Related Diagnostic Issues" provides data on explicitly cultural features of the disorder (e.g., cultural variations in disorder symptoms that did not warrant criteria revision), as well as culture-related information on development and course, risk and prognostic factors, interpretation of stressors, impairment, and severity (option A is incorrect).

The "Cultural Issues" subsection of the DSM-5 Introduction outlines how cultural factors influence the diagnostic and treatment process, such as in symptom presentations (e.g., alternative symptom variants), clinician assessments (e.g., diagnostic accuracy, evaluation of severity), and patients' responses (e.g., coping strategies, help-seeking choices, treatment adherence) (option D is incorrect).

The "Glossary of Cultural Concepts of Distress" in the DSM-5 Appendix includes nine examples of cultural concepts of distress from around the world that typify syndromes, idioms, and explanations and their interrelationships (option B is incorrect). **Chapter 44 (pp. 1249, 1251, 1252, 1258)**

44.3   Criteria for which of the following disorders were revised in DSM-5 to better ac-
        commodate cultural variation in psychiatric presentation?

A. Major depressive disorder.
B. Illness anxiety disorder.
C. Social anxiety disorder.
D. Bipolar disorder.

The correct response is option C: Social anxiety disorder.

Some disorder work groups used the DSM-5 revision process as an opportunity
to conduct systematic reviews of cultural factors that are relevant to each disorder. Most reviews elicited studies that did not meet the evidentiary standards
needed to propose changes to central DSM criteria on the basis of cultural variations. Nonetheless, data were robust enough at times to warrant proposed revisions. This was the case for social anxiety disorder, agoraphobia, specific phobia,
posttraumatic stress disorder, and dissociative identity disorder, among others
(Lewis-Fernández et al. 2010). For example, decades of cross-cultural research
have shown that the fear of negative evaluation by others (i.e., the hallmark of social anxiety disorder) can manifest as a fear that the individual will cause offense
to others, in addition to or instead of the fear that the person him- or herself will
feel embarrassed by engaging in social behavior (Choy et al. 2008). Labeled
"other-directed" or "allocentric," this type of fear is characteristic of local idioms
of distress in East Asia, described as *taijin kyofusho* in Japan and *taein kong po* in
Korea. The fear of offending others is also observed among individuals with social anxiety disorder in many cultural settings, including Australia and the
United States (Kim et al. 2008). Across cultures, the fear of offending others and
the fear of also suffering embarrassment can occur simultaneously, rather than being mutually exclusive, indicating that they are related presentations (Lewis-
Fernández et al. 2010). In acknowledgement of the strength of this evidence, the
Work Group on Anxiety, Obsessive-Compulsive Spectrum, Posttraumatic, and
Dissociative Disorders revised the social anxiety disorder criteria (option C is correct) to clarify this relationship and thereby reduce the potential for misdiagnosis
in settings where "other-directed" fear is the primary or initial presentation. The
revised social anxiety disorder Criterion B reads as follows: "The individual fears
that he or she will act in a way or show anxiety symptoms that will be negatively
evaluated (e.g., will be humiliating or embarrassing; will lead to rejection or of-
fend others)" (American Psychiatric Association 2013, p. 202).

The DSM-5 diagnostic criteria for a major depressive episode are essentially
unchanged from the DSM-IV (American Psychiatric Association 1994) criteria
(option A is incorrect).

Notably, DSM-5 departed from DSM-IV by eliminating the mixed episode as
a specific episode type and replacing it with the "with mixed features" specifier,
which can be applied to major depressive, hypomanic, or manic episodes (see Table 11–1, "Bipolar and related disorders: summary of major changes from DSM-
IV to DSM-5") (option D is incorrect).

Illness anxiety disorder is a new DSM-5 diagnosis characterized by a preoccupation with having or acquiring a serious illness (option B is incorrect). **Chapter 44 (p. 1250); see also Chapter 11 ("Bipolar and Related Disorders"; pp. 280, 281) and Chapter 17 ("Somatic Symptom and Related Disorders"; p. 481)**

44.4   A relatively new patient presents to your office for a follow-up visit. He reports that he had an *"ataque de nervios"* last week. You explore the experience with him in session, but you are still puzzled by the term. Which of the following DSM-5 components would be most helpful for learning more about this phenomenon?

A. The "Glossary of Culture-Bound Syndromes."
B. The "Outline for Cultural Formulation."
C. The "Glossary of Cultural Concepts of Distress."
D. The "Cultural Formulation Interview."

The correct response is option C: The "Glossary of Cultural Concepts of Distress."

The "Glossary of Cultural Concepts of Distress" in the DSM-5 Appendix includes nine examples of cultural concepts of distress from around the world that typify syndromes, idioms, and explanations and their interrelationships: *ataque de nervios*, *dhat* syndrome, *khyâl cap*, *kufungisisa*, *maladi moun*, *nervios*, *shenjing shuairuo*, *susto*, and *taijin kyofusho*. Only high-prevalence concepts with considerable research are included, and for each concept, the glossary lists related conditions across cultural contexts, including the scientific context that has produced DSM-5 (option C is correct).

The "Glossary of Culture-Bound Syndromes" appeared in DSM-IV/DSM-IV-TR (American Psychiatric Association 2000) but was revised in DSM-5 to produce two new sections: "Cultural Concepts of Distress" in the "Cultural Formulation" chapter in Section III of DSM-5, and a Glossary of these concepts in the DSM-5 Appendix (option A is incorrect).

Although options B and D would be helpful in understanding the patient's cultural context and values more broadly, these resources do not contain further information about the term in the question stem. The "Outline for Cultural Formulation" (OCF) is a framework for cultural assessment that can be used to evaluate patients within their life contexts by inquiring about sources of identity, the relationship of identity to the presenting problem, the effects of the illness on social relationships and daily functioning, and the extent to which the personal backgrounds of the patient and clinician affect the clinical interaction (option B is incorrect).

The "Cultural Formulation Interview" (CFI) is a standardized 16-item questionnaire that can be used at the beginning of every initial patient assessment and covers the same topical areas as the OCF. The CFI includes instructions to clinicians that precede the questions and a guide to the interviewer on content designed for elicitation through each question (option D is incorrect). **Chapter 44 (pp. 1247–1252, 1257, 1258)**

44.5   Which of the following best defines the term *cultural competence* in health care settings?

A. A highly encouraged but optional component of a physician's career.
B. A theoretically useful strategy for reducing health disparities.
C. A form of political correctness that emerged during the civil rights era to promote care of diverse societies.
D. The ability of an individual or organization to provide effective and equitable care that is responsive to diverse cultural beliefs, practices, preferred languages, and communication needs of the patient.

The correct response is option D: The ability of an individual or organization to provide effective and equitable care that is responsive to diverse cultural beliefs, practices, preferred languages, and communication needs of the patient.

In 2016, the National Academies of Sciences, Engineering, and Medicine defined *cultural competence* as "the ability of an organization or an individual within the health care delivery system to provide effective, equitable, understandable, and respectful quality care and services that are responsive to diverse cultural health beliefs and practices, preferred languages, health literacy, and other communication needs of the patient" (National Academies of Sciences, Engineering, and Medicine 2016, p. 12) (option D is correct).

Why should all clinicians consider cultural competence to be important? First, cultural competence has become an expected professional standard in the education of all medical professionals. At the undergraduate medical level, the Association of American Medical Colleges (2015) has identified clinician cultural competence as a critical mechanism for reducing chronic health disparities (option B is incorrect).

For academic medical institutions, the Accreditation Council for Graduate Medical Education's (2014) Clinical Learning Environment Review Program now requires residents, fellows, and faculty to be trained and engaged in health disparity reduction, cultural competence, and quality improvement initiatives. Cultural competence is not optional; it is expected at all levels of a physician's career (option A is incorrect).

A second reason why cultural competence should be considered important is that clinical evidence demonstrates that cultural competence is not merely a form of political correctness that emerged during the American civil rights movement (option C is incorrect) but also a framework for understanding culture's various manifestations in all aspects of patient care, such as patient perceptions of what is considered appropriate and inappropriate to discuss in mental health settings, clinician interpretations of patient experiences through professionalized systems of knowledge such as DSM-5, and patient and clinician interpretations of acceptable and unacceptable treatments (Lewis-Fernández et al. 2014). **Chapter 44 (pp. 1242–1243)**

44.6   In an effort to bridge the gap between formal theories of various psychotherapies and the cultural values of patients, mental health professionals have adapted interventions in multiple ways to increase their alignment and compatibility with patients' cultural perspectives and models. Which of the following cultural adaptations was shown in a peer-reviewed meta-analysis to have minimal benefit on treatment outcomes?

A. Matching race and ethnicity of provider and patient.
B. Substituting colloquial expressions for technical terms used in psychotherapy.
C. Making modifications that allow family members to participate in psychotherapy treatment.
D. Training therapists in local customs and metaphors to better facilitate communication with patients.

The correct response is option A: Matching race and ethnicity of provider and patient.

Research in cultural psychiatry has examined the extent to which patient–clinician cultural matching produces superior outcomes compared with unmatched dyads. Meta-analyses demonstrate significant variations in effect sizes when patients and clinicians are matched by race or ethnicity. A pooled analysis of 52 studies showed that patients exhibited strong preferences for therapists of their own race/ethnicity (Cohen's *d*, 0.63), and another analysis of 81 studies showed that patients perceived therapists of their own race/ethnicity more positively than therapists who were not of their race/ethnicity (Cohen's *d*, 0.32). However, a final analysis with 53 studies (Cabral and Smith 2011) showed almost no benefit in treatment outcomes resulting from patient–clinician racial/ethnic matching (Cohen's *d*, 0.09) (option A is correct).

Psychotherapy rests on assumptions that individuals can cognize and articulate aspects of themselves, which further rest on conceptions of personhood derived from Euro-American practice contexts that prioritize individualism and autonomy that are not shared in many sociocentric societies (Kirmayer 2007). To overcome these problems, clinicians and researchers have sought to align formal theories of various psychotherapies with patient cultural values. Culturally adapted psychotherapies may demonstrate greater efficacy than standard treatments because the adaptations are compatible with the patient's explanatory models of illness (Chowdhary et al. 2014). Cultural adaptations may include substitution of colloquial expressions for technical terms (e.g., "therapeutic exercise" instead of "homework" in cognitive therapy) (option B is incorrect); incorporation of local terms rather than biomedical categories to refer to illnesses; training of therapists in local customs and metaphors to facilitate communication (option D is incorrect); inclusion of local illness explanations, such as stressful circumstances and interpersonal difficulties, within treatment manuals; and modifications to psychotherapeutic techniques that allow relatives to participate (option C is incorrect) (Chowdhary et al. 2014). **Chapter 44 (pp. 1248–1249)**

References

Accreditation Council for Graduate Medical Education: Clinical Learning Environment Review (CLER) Pathways to Excellence. Chicago, IL, Accreditation Council for Graduate Medical Education, 2014. Available at: http://www.acgme.org/Portals/0/PDFs/CLER/CLER_Brochure.pdf. Accessed August 21, 2017.

American Psychiatric Association: Diagnostic and Statistical Manual of Mental Disorders, 4th Edition. Washington, DC, American Psychiatric Association, 1994

American Psychiatric Association: Diagnostic and Statistical Manual of Mental Disorders, 4th Edition, Text Revision. Washington, DC, American Psychiatric Association, 2000

American Psychiatric Association: Diagnostic and Statistical Manual of Mental Disorders, 5th Edition. Arlington, VA, American Psychiatric Association, 2013

Association of American Medical Colleges: Assessing Change: Evaluating Cultural Competence Education and Training. Washington, DC, Association of American Medical Colleges, 2015. Available at: https://www.aamc.org/download/427350/data/assessingchange.pdf. Accessed August 12, 2017.

Cabral RR, Smith TB: Racial/ethnic matching of clients and therapists in mental health services: a meta-analytic review of preferences, perceptions, and outcomes. J Couns Psychol 58(4):537–554, 2011 21875181

Chowdhary N, Jotheeswaran AT, Nadkarni A, et al: The methods and outcomes of cultural adaptations of psychological treatments for depressive disorders: a systematic review. Psychol Med 44(6):1131–1146, 2014 23866176

Choy Y, Schneier FR, Heimberg RG, et al: Features of the offensive subtype of Taijin-Kyofu-Sho in US and Korean patients with DSM-IV social anxiety disorder. Depress Anxiety 25(3):230–240, 2008 17340609

Kim J, Rapee RM, Ja Oh K, et al: Retrospective report of social withdrawal during adolescence and current maladjustment in young adulthood: cross-cultural comparisons between Australian and South Korean students. J Adolesc 31(5):543–563, 2008 18076980

Kirmayer LJ: Psychotherapy and the cultural concept of the person. Transcult Psychiatry 44(2):232–257, 2007 17576727

Lewis-Fernández R, Hinton DE, Laria AJ, et al: Culture and the anxiety disorders: recommendations for DSM-V. Depress Anxiety 27(2):212–229, 2010 20037918

Lewis-Fernández R, Aggarwal NK, Bäärnhielm S, et al: Culture and psychiatric evaluation: operationalizing cultural formulation for DSM-5. Psychiatry 77(2):130–154, 2014 24865197

National Academies of Sciences, Engineering, and Medicine: Integrating Health Literacy, Cultural Competence, and Language Access Services: Workshop Summary. Washington, DC, National Academies Press, 2016. Available at: https://www.nap.edu/catalog/23498/integrating-health-literacy-cultural-competence-and-language-access-services-workshop. Accessed September 15, 2018.